JOIN MY CLUB

The Ultimate Survivor Story
Volume I

The Chickens Come Home to Roost

JOIN MY CLUB

The Ultimate Survivor Story
Volume I

The Chickens Come Home to Roost

D Basil MulQueen

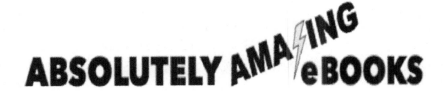

ABSOLUTELY AMAZING eBOOKS

Published by Whiz Bang LLC, 926 Truman Avenue, Key West, Florida 33040, USA

ISBN 978-1-955036-15-3

For information contact:
Publisher@AbsolutelyAmazingEbooks.com

This book is dedicated to the memories of Pat and George MulQueen, two more special people this world has never known.

"May the road rise up to meet you.
May the wind be always at your back.
May the sun shine warm upon your face;
the rains fall soft upon your fields and
until we meet again, may God hold you
in the palm of his hand."

JOIN MY CLUB

The Ultimate Survivor Story
Volume I

The Chickens Come Home to Roost

~ 1 ~

LIFE IS A CIRCUS

No wonder she took him to the circus that night. A little entertainment, a little diversion.

A momentary respite.

Maybe more than that?

Much more than that, he would find out later, as the familiar aromas of the concession stands and the sawdust and the animal scents greeted them at the front doors of the State Fair Coliseum.

The buzz was immediately apparent in the concourse as mothers and fathers scurried and chased after their runaway progeny while vendors on the go everywhere barked out their calls of "peanuts, popcorn, hot dogs."

Once inside the arena proper, the excitement continued to build as colorfully attired children throughout the grandstands hoisted gobs of pink and chiffon and pale blue cotton candy on white conical sticks high in the air like so many toy soldiers trying to protect and hang onto their childhood world of innocence and dreams.

All the while, the swirling, smoky, musky-scented air all about rose steadily to the rafters, continually bathing the crowd in what were intended to be future memories of all that was good about being a kid at the circus.

As they took to their seats in the lower bowl, the ringmaster entered center ring decked out in his shiny red tails and black satin tuxedo pants, his trademark black top hat and ebony and brass walking stick gleaming in the distance as he welcomed everybody to the Greatest Show On Earth with his resonant baritone drawl.

He first introduced the gracefully muscled creamy Hanneford horses, who galloped into the arena with their snow white manes waving in the foggy air as they circled center ring while their acrobatic riders somersaulted mid-air from one speeding bareback to another.

The poor chimps and the dear poor elephants were next up, kindly performing their forced labor routines flawlessly, as all the while the 10-foot-tall man on stilts with his garish mile-long turquoise pants and extra-long black and neon mustard yellow tuxedo-tailed jacket purposefully stumble-bummed his way around the arena perimeter.

Of course, the centuries-old universal circus constant kept the children cackling throughout – the chaotic cacophony of a cadre of candy-throwing clowns who pranced and danced and darted about the arena floor every which way, some riding helter-skelter on backfiring mini motor bikes, others piloting diminutive alarm-shrieking fire engines with constantly clanging strident brass bells, while others whizzed by on lit-up unicycles of varying height.

The superstars of the clown world made their entrance on foot, with the mandatory first in line being the one-and-only world-famous Emmett The Clown, who bopped around court side in his tiny black bowler and green blow-up shorts with red suspenders and bright yellow purple-polka-dotted shirt to go with his gaudy red-and-white painted face.

Bozo The Clown bounced into the arena behind him in his blue and white striped one-piece wizard suit highlighted by his enormous spoon shaped red shoes, pausing intermittently to do a deliberate skipped-step flop of the sole designed to throw a mini dust-bowl protest in the air, with his round white wrinkled cheeks and white-domed bald head accentuating his flaming red ring of scraggly wide hair that stuck out from the sides of his head like frozen stiff red mop heads twisted to a point.

Of course, it wouldn't be a Detroit Shrine Circus without the other home-grown favorite, Milky the Clown, who lurched herky-jerky around the coliseum like a human jack-in-the-box in his garishly blinding all-white garb.

At times some of the children looked confused, shy or scared and sat motionless, only stealing furtive glances at the wild spectacle of noise and color parading past them, in contrast to the many others who screamed and howled with hysterical laughter as they crowded the aisles and pushed and shoved their way to the coliseum end boards with outstretched arms and hands begging for more candy from their clown-faced entertainers.

Then it was time to get serious, as the infamous Clyde Beatty arrived center ring looking like Clark Gable with his finely tailored thin black-waxed mustache and tanned skin all done up in his trademark white-domed safari hat and khaki pants and starched white shirt, strutting cockily about the round steel cage snapping his long black whip, firing his blank pistol to taunt a cage full of very unhappy Lions and Tigers who growled and roared their displeasure with bursts of saw dust clouds filling the ring like bubbling froth from a medieval forest cauldron as they leaped to and fro through flaming rings.

Always a circus mainstay, the black-helmeted "human cannonball" was next, with his iridescent orange-and-red jumpsuit exploding with a tremendous bang from a 30-foot-long black steel cannon shaft across the arena at a mile-a-

3

minute, hitting the strategically placed net at the opposite end dead center.

All the while, the familiar aroma of roasted peanuts and popcorn and hot dogs continued to drench the arena with more balmy thoughts of how wonderful life is as an innocent little kid at the circus.

Until the moment of truth arrived, as the ringmaster entered center ring one more time, silver microphone erect once again, for the night's most important introduction.

His double-decker coal-black top hat genuflected forward this time as he asked for prayers and complete silence for the next performers.

The sold-out crowd froze in their seats as the lights were switched off and the arena plunged into darkness.

As the MC turned quickly from center ring to make his exit, you could barely see his swirling red-tailed coat slice through the dark thick air as a collective sigh of eerie tension spread across the building like a giant reverberating sound wave, leaving in its wake almost gasp-like sounds as if every single man, woman and child in the building inhaled and exhaled at the very same moment.

Goose bumps and prickly skin and sweat beads and nervous twitches popped out arena-wide as giant spotlights suddenly pierced the glaucous air from above and below and there they were high in the coliseum sky, three brilliantly costumed performers festooned in identical crimson pants and shimmering gold vests, perched precariously on a 3/8 inch steel cable three stories above the concrete coliseum floor, silhouetted in incandescent fluorescent white light.

There they were, the three of them with their customary long balance poles, the tightrope and all the rigging wires lit up in the blinding white light like a Marvel comic book Spider Man scene, a group of brightly costumed human spiders about to attempt traversing a gauzy sky-high web.

4

They slowly moved out onto the high wire in a pyramid formation, two on the bottom supporting one guy on top.

You could hear a feather helicopter to the ground as the aerialists continued to inch their way across the wire.

The three of them.

The young lad at the end of row three in section 106 poked his mother in the side and pointed in the air toward the men on the wire as they reached the opposite platform in front of them and began to descend a rope ladder.

"Mommy, why is that man crying?" he said.

"*Shhhh*, that's Karl Wallenda," the woman with the pixie and stone blue eyes said as she turned to the boy with raised index finger to her lips, before pointing back at the three aerialists who were now on the ground in front of them.

There were three on the wire this night – instead of the customary seven – because this was Thursday, Feb. 1, 1962 – less than 48 hours after Karl Wallenda's nephew and son-in-law law were killed, and his son paralyzed for life, after falling from this very same wire, in this very same building.

After Karl Wallenda's wife Helen had barged into his hospital room afterward and shouted at him, "How could you let this happen, how could you? Go in the other room and see what your crazy ideas have caused."

After his daughter Jenny, who had lost her husband in the fall, walked up to him in the same hospital the day before and in front of reporters called him a murderer, not once, but twice.

Only hours after, against his doctor's wishes, Karl Wallenda walked out of the same Hamtramck General Hospital his paralyzed son was still a patient at.

To return to the wire.

This night.

In this building.

On the very same wire of death.

5

With a cracked pelvis and a double hernia.

Why?

"We owe it to those who died to continue," the man known as The Great Wallenda told reporters on his way out of the hospital. "We can't let them die in vain. The show must go on."

So here he was, back on the very same wire once again, in the very same building that was filled with shrieks of terror and screams of horror less than 48 hours ago, the same building that now erupted in deafening applause as he made it to the other end and graciously bowed to the crowd after climbing down from the same dismount platform he and the troupe fell three feet short of two nights before.

The woman with the chestnut pixie at the end of row three in section 106 turned again and looked directly at the young boy with her, with almost a vague detached look of prescience emanating from those blue stone eyes, as if she already knew what the future held.

Now she turned away from the boy and looked straight ahead again, at the guy they called the Great Wallenda, the tears now twinkling lines of silver-blue light streaking down his ashen cheeks.

She continued to look straight ahead, with a blank, unfocused look on her face as her own eyes now also welled with water.

"Mommy, Mommy, what's the matter," the boy said as he tugged at his mother's sleeve.

She said nothing, as she continued to stare ahead, like she wasn't looking at anything in particular now, like she didn't hear him. Then she spoke, while she continued looking straight ahead, as if she wasn't just talking to the boy.

"See there, Denny, the show goes on," she said. "Don't forget it."

"What Mama?"

Again she didn't answer, as if she was now in a trance as she calmly rose to lead them out of the building.

The boy had no idea what she was talking about, why his mother brought him with her this night to witness Karl Wallenda's return to the wire, two days after tragedy struck in the city of Detroit.

He was in his eighth year of life now.
But he would always remember that night, as he was destined to find out what she meant, as the clock ticked on into the future and he found himself walking his own tightrope to death's doorstep and beyond.

~ 2 ~

LIFE IS A RIOT

"**H**ey Baby, what about a date? You don't have to be afraid of me, I've been with white girls."

That's what he said. A stocky, 150-pound kid, a 14-year-old African American kid. Fourteen going on 40.

A kid from Chicago with attitude, down visiting his uncle in Money, Mississippi. A curiosity road trip to the heart of the Mississippi Delta where his mother was born, to check out his roots.

And hang with his cousins, and some of the local kids. He showed them the picture in his wallet of his integrated school class from Chicago. He pointed specifically to one white girl in the pic he bragged was his girlfriend.

His cousins and some of the locals challenged him.

Hey dude, you're so bad, why don't you show us? There's a white girl works in that store over there, one of them said.

So he did.

And that's what he said after he walked in Bryant's Grocery and Meat Market.

"Hey Baby, what about a date? You don't have to be afraid of me, I've been with white girls."

After he asked "baby" out for a date, the 21-year old clerk at Bryant's grocery store ran scared out the front door toward her car that had a gun in the glove box. He followed her into the street and there he whistled at her – in front of the whole gang.

~ ~ ~

About a week later, at the end of August, 1955, a different 14-year-old African American teenager stood on a street corner in Louisville, Kentucky, holding the latest edition of Jet Magazine, a popular African American tabloid.

On the cover was a gruesome picture of the 14-year-old kid from Chicago in a coffin, after he was found mangled and disfigured in the Tallahatchie River in Mississippi. The caption identified the savagely murdered youth as a 14-year-old black kid from Chicago named Emmett Till.

When he read the accompanying article, the Louisville 14-year-old learned that Emmett Till had the same exact birthday and the same exact birth year as himself. It was a kinship that would stick with the Louisville teenager the rest of his life.

Outraged, the Kentucky 14-year-old recruited some of his buddies to help him destroy the local rail yard that night. One of the trains was derailed and the depot ransacked.

The experience sent the young Louisville teenager on a mission that would never be derailed.

In an interview years later, his mother put it this way: "My son was never the same after he saw those pictures."

The incident lit a fire inside him that would burn forever.

Never mind the time he saw his mother refused a drink at the diner one night, after she had worked on her hands and knees all day scrubbing rich white folks floors and toilets. Never mind a whole string of other heinous racist attacks he would witness along his journey to adulthood.

The one thing foremost on his mind was that picture of Emmett Till, the 14-year-old birth-sake African American kid with one eye gouged out, a bullet through his head, face bashed in and teeth knocked out.

For whistling at a white girl.

That picture helped make the Louisville kid a champion. A world famous champion.

The anger and the injustice became a thirst to conquer. The desire to be great. A craving to make a difference. A desire to become the greatest.

The 14-year-old Louisville kid with the same birthdate as Emmett Till was named Cassius Marcellus Clay Jr.

He had begun boxing in 1954 on the advice of a white police officer friend who recommended the sport after the young Clay said he was going to "put a whuppin' on" whoever stole his 60 dollar red Schwinn Varsity bicycle.

Now, after seeing those pictures, he was ready to take it to the next level.

The cop became his first trainer and oversaw Clay's quick rise through the Kentucky AAU golden gloves ranks. Soon he became an Olympic gold medalist in 1960 at the age of 18.

After a quick succession of impressive victories in the ring, the once thin and gangly Cassius Clay found himself in line for a shot at the heavy weight championship of the world.

This fight would be different.

Clay was now in the big leagues. He was going up against the undefeated and feared heavyweight champion of the world, Sonny Liston. A devastating puncher, Liston was an ex-con who hung out with mobsters and backed up his threats with a string of brutal knockouts.

But Clay – the world had never seen swag like this before. After that night on the street corner in Louisville, this man feared nothing.

The big fight was set for February 24, 1964 in Miami Beach, Florida. Las Vegas oddsmakers made the formidable Liston a 7-1 favorite.

The undeterred Clay now formally introduced himself to the world as the mother of all trash talkers.

"He's an ugly bear, he even smells like a bear," Clay taunted the Liston who terrified everybody else, inside and outside of the ring. "I'm gonna donate him to the zoo after I whup him," he said at the pre-fight weigh in.

Liston laughed in Clay's face. He said he was a punk who didn't belong in the ring with him. He said he was going to kill him.

When asked how he planned to avoid the deadly power of the vaunted Liston, purportedly the hardest puncher in boxing, Clay said, "I'm going to float like a butterfly and sting like a bee. His hands can't hit what he can't see."

The fight started out with Liston aggressively pursuing Clay across the ring. But Clay was quicker and used his speed to make Liston miss. By the sixth round he was completely dominating Liston, hitting him repeatedly and opening a cut above Liston's right eye, the first time the burley fighter had ever been cut.

The trash talking Clay backed his taunts up as Liston could not answer the bell for the seventh round and in one of sport's greatest upsets he was declared the winner by TKO. At 22, he was the youngest boxer to ever take the crown from a reigning champion. After the decision was announced, Clay dashed across the ring and climbed up on the ropes waving his arms and gloves at the crowd, shouting "I am the greatest! I shook up the world. I'm the prettiest thing that ever lived."

Almost immediately following the fight, Cassius Marcellus Clay Jr. disappeared. He who was, was no more – at least in the boxer's mind.

The newly crowned heavyweight champion of the world announced he was changing his name to Muhammed Ali and joining the Nation Of Islam. Asked why, he said Clay was a "slave name."

Few knew, but by now he was already heavily ingrained in the Nation's culture. In fact, while training for the Liston fight, he stayed at the house of a young black radical named Malcolm X. He had initially changed his name to Cassius X Clay, before switching to Muhammad Ali.

He proclaimed himself "King Of the World" and "The Greatest" through the national media but the white establishment refused to recognize anything about him – especially his new name.

But he was attracting a huge following in the black community.

That quickly earned him the earnest attention of the federal government.

FBI Director J. Edgar Hoover opened a file on the Nation of Islam convert and placed the new Muhammad Ali under immediate surveillance.

The wheels to silence the outspoken boxer spun into motion like an Indy car.

Back in 1960, when the man then named Clay had won the Olympic light-heavyweight gold medal, the selective service system classified him 1-Y, or to be drafted only in time of national emergency. He had supposedly failed the reading and writing portions of their exam, which would be consistent with his dismal performance in school, as he dropped out of high school early.

Now, in 1966, it was time for the government to change the rules of the game.

The Selective Service System arbitrarily decided to lower the standards such that all soldiers above the 15th percentile – which thus now included Ali – were reclassified A-1. This made Ali immediately eligible for the draft.

Though he wasn't book smart, Ali was plenty street smart and he knew what was coming. Sure enough, the government promptly called his number.

The man named the "Louisville Lip" by a sports columnist, would not hesitate to run his mouth on this one. The Vietnam war was raging, but Ali wasn't buying in.

"I ain't got nothing against those Viet Cong.." he said in an interview from the front yard of a house he had rented in Miami, Florida. "Why should they ask me to put on a uniform and go 10,000 miles from home and drop bombs and bullets on brown people in Viet Nam while so-called Negro people in Louisville are treated like dogs and denied simple human rights?"

"No, " Muhammed Ali continued, "I'm not going 10,000 miles from home to help murder and burn another poor nation simply to continue the domination of white slave masters of the darker people the world over."

He wasn't done making his point.

"I ain't got nothing against those Viet Cong," he repeated. "They don't call me niggah. My enemy is right here."

Thus opened the floodgates of national scorn and vilification.

In fact no establishment figure – except sportscaster Howard Cosell – would call him by his new name. Even the New York Times insisted on still calling him Clay.

The Times famous sports columnist Red Smith led the way, in one piece calling "Clay" an "unwashed punk" just like all the other anti-war demonstrators out there.

The guy considered the greatest sports writer of all time, the L.A. Times Jim Murray, also refused to call him anything but Cassius Clay. After he beat Liston and declared himself the greatest, Murray begged to differ. In comparing him to Detroit's Joe Louis, the "Brown Bomber," Murray wrote, "Cassius Clay couldn't carry Joe Louis' gloves."

While Ali couldn't do much about the vitriol, what he could control, that rectangle of white space inside the ropes, he did control.

His next opponent was another bad ass undefeated heavyweight named Ernie Terrell, who was the undefeated WBC champion and considered at the time as tough a challenge as Liston.

Terrell had a three inch reach advantage on Ali and, like Liston, he too brought tremendous power. And nobody liked to mock Ali more, with Terrell repeatedly calling him Clay in the pre-fight buildup.

Ali was not amused.

"I'm going to torture him," he promised. "A clean knockout is too good for him," Ali said the day before the fight, which was held on February 6, 1967.

True to his word, Ali toyed with Terrell, beating him mercilessly around the ring round after round. He staggered him so badly in the seventh everybody watching knew it was over, expecting Ali to end it right then and there.

But Ali laughed, and stepped back, hands at his side, as if true to his taunts he deliberately declined to knock out the already savagely beaten Terrell.

"What's my name, Uncle Tom, what's my name?" everybody ringside heard Ali scream at Terrell as he circled him, suddenly lurching back inside to land another vicious left jab, then an uppercut, then another overhand right to the head as he backed off again from the staggering and helpless Terrell.

"What's my name, is my name Clay, what's my name fool?" he again taunted Terrell mercilessly. "What's my name

15

now fool?" Amazingly, the fight went the full 15 rounds with Ali declared the unanimous winner.

After it was all over, a badly swollen and cut up Terrell claimed Ali thumbed him in the eye in an early round, and then rubbed the same eye into the ropes later in the same round, effectively making Terrell fight with only one eye.

When asked about Terrell's remarks, Ali responded with a smile and a hearty laugh and that was all.

Another well-known writer named Tex Maule famously called the fight "a wonderful demonstration of boxing skill and a barbarous display of cruelty."

Many still consider it Ali's best fight ever.

~ ~ ~

He had turned right on Northend Ave and was approaching the brown-and-red brick corner house on Kipling Avenue when he heard a lively discussion going on inside.

The marching orders were to wait 20 minutes in the back of the Our Lady of Fatima church and if no powder blue Ford station wagon appeared, then start walking. The red-and-gold clock on the kitchen wall read 10 minutes to four when he finally spun the gold knob open and walked in to 21471 Kipling Avenue in Oak Park, Michigan.

"I'm telling you, George, enough is enough. You have to quit. I mean to give your all and have those filthy gutter snipes try and kill you for it. The money just isn't worth it."

"It's not about the money Pat. "

"You have the Ford job and that is enough."

She referred to his job as a full time safety engineer for Ford Motor Co. He worked midnights so he could do what he loved most – teach special ed at Lyster School in Detroit during the day, and coach high school football in the afternoon.

"We will get by, we can economize, we're doing better with circulation with the papers, you can do something else. It's just not worth it, George."

Lyster was located in one of the worst parts of Detroit and his students, well, at least some of them, were the worst too. Many were emotionally disturbed, some were mentally disabled, others already had rap sheets.

On this particular day, a couple of burly teenagers were getting into it in his classroom and when he tried to break it up, one of the guys pulled out a stiletto and lunged at him.

"God damn it Pat, cut it out, can't you see I'm in pain?"

He wasn't hollering at her, but he nonetheless had the football coach part down pat, gruff and surly, as he sometimes was, such that when he spoke his voice carried and often came off as loud and scary even when he wasn't.

Peering from the safety of the kitchen around the corner into the living room, the kid could see his father's left arm was bandaged from his hand to his upper arm. The kid could see blood stains permeating the gauze in several spots. But it could have been much worse, if not for the wooden desk chair that landed across the top of the attacker's body – including his head, he heard his father explain to his mother.

Thank God for those MulQueen Irish genes.

Grandpa MulQueen was president of the AOH in Detroit in the 1930s and 1940s and he was also a golden gloves boxer. Not to say he was John L. Sullivan or Jack Dempsey, but he could fight, and outside of the ring, too.

He wasn't Ali, but he actually did have a fight as famous as any of Ali's fights, at least in the MulQueen lore, against a guy who would turn out to be as famous – or notorious – in southeast Michigan as Ali himself. And like a good Ali fight, this fight was also a knockout. More on that later.

At any rate, George MulQueen Jr. apparently inherited some of his father's skill. And he wasn't afraid to use it.

Although he earned bachelor's and master's degrees from the University of Detroit and worked midnights at Ford Motor Company as a safety engineer, teaching special ed to these disadvantaged kids and the football coaching after school were his life.

This was the path he chose – a life without much sleep – and he wasn't giving it up.

"I'm not quitting," he said to her. "I know there aren't many, but if I can save just one, it's worth it to me, Pat. So stop worrying, everything is okay. Let's not talk about it anymore."

He was back at his desk, sitting in the same desk chair that probably saved his life the very next day.

Bandages and all.

~ ~ ~

Despite the establishment's wishes, Ali's following grew and as opposition to the Viet Nam war grew, he found himself in popular demand as a speaker on college campuses. He willingly obliged.

The Black Power Alliance at Howard University asked Ali to speak on their campus on April 22, 1967.

"See, we have been brainwashed," the heavyweight champion of the world said to the attentive crowd of mostly black students. "Everything good and of authority was made white. We look at Jesus, we see a white with blond hair and blue eyes.

"Now, I'm sure if there's a heaven in the sky and when the colored folks die and go to heaven, where are the colored angels? They must be in the kitchen preparing the milk and honey.

"All the good cowboys ride white horses. Angel's food cake is white and devil's food cake is chocolate. Even Tarzan, the king of the jungle in black Africa, he's white."

He told the crowd the white establishment has concealed the truth from black people.

"Black dirt is the best dirt. Brown sugar causes fewer cavities, and the blacker the berry, the sweeter the juice."

Ironically, Ali was speaking on the steps of the Frederick Douglass Building, Howard University's most famous building named after the iconic abolitionist.

Six days later, per court order, Ali appeared before the Houston, Texas draft board. Three times that day, April 28, 1967, he refused protocol to step forward at the call of his name. He was arrested on the spot by the MP's and charged with a five-year felony, although the typical charge for the crime of refusing the draft board's order was only one year.

Later in the afternoon, the New York State Athletic Commission suspended his boxing license and stripped him of his title. The other state commissions quickly followed suit.

Almost four years would pass before he could fight again. That made the price of his stand, during the prime of his career, tens of millions of dollars.

~ ~ ~

Little more than three months later, two of Detroit's finest managed to return home safely from that same Viet Nam war that cost Ali his title.

That called for a celebration – Motor City style.

So the whole neighborhood made it happen.

More than 80 people gathered on July 22, 1967 in the offices of the United Community League for Civic Action at 9125 12th Street in Detroit to toast the returning vets. The group rocked and rolled in Motown fashion into the wee hours of the morning at the makeshift speakeasy when suddenly the party was over, in unfortunately what was at that time very Detroit Police-like fashion.

19

At precisely 3:45 a.m. on Sunday, July 23, a squadron of Detroit cops smashed the door in to bust the illegal after-hours drinking club they called, in the parlance of the day, a "Blind Pig."

The police officers swooped in like Green Beret commandos and arrested all 82 people inside.

While the Blues waited for transportation to arrive, a sizable crowd began to gather in the street surrounding the club and suddenly out of nowhere the speakeasy's doorman, Walter Scott III, threw a bottle at the cop nearest the door.

That would be Detroit's version of 'the shot heard round the world.'

The crowd ignited like napalm and from there the conflagration spread until it engulfed the city in what became the second deadliest race riot in the history of the United States (behind only the 1863 New York City draft riots during the US Civil War).

Things got so bad, the following afternoon, Martha Reeves, who was performing at the nearby Fox Theatre, canceled her concert mid-set and urged her audience to "go quietly" because of the trouble in the streets.

A little later in the day, after the Detroit Tigers finished their matinee ball game at Tiger Stadium, left fielder Willie Horton, who grew up blocks from the epicenter of the riot near 12th St and Clairmount Ave, got on top of a car, still in his Tigers' uniform, and urged the rioters to stop.

His pleas fell on deaf ears.

So too for legendary Detroit Congressman John Conyers, who, driven by an aide down 12th street on top of his car with a megaphone in hand, also urged rioters to go home. "We're with you, but please, this is not the way to do things. Please go back to your homes."

Conyers' car was pelted with rocks and bottles and he was lucky he escaped injury, or worse.

Decades of racism and job discrimination and housing discrimination and education discrimination and overall economic and social hell – exactly what Ali was talking about – had simmered for years in Detroit prior to the summer of 1967. But it was the years of mistreatment by the police – and systemic racist police brutality – that finally boiled over into what turned out to be five days of intense violence and destruction that left 43 dead, more than 1,189 injured, more than 7,200 arrested and more than 2,000 buildings burned to the ground or otherwise destroyed.

Detroit police were overwhelmed, and even with the help of the Michigan State Police and the Wayne County sheriff, the violence could not be contained. Only after the Michigan National Guard sent 8,000 guardsmen and 4,700 paratroopers from the 82nd Airborne Division and the 101st Airborne Division of the U. S. Army were deployed, was calm eventually restored.

One of the most infamous events of the Detroit riots was the Algiers Motel incident, where three black men were murdered by police in cold blood at the Woodward Ave. Manor House. Their confessions to the crime were covered up by authorities. Journalist and author John Hersey wrote a book about the incident called The Algiers Motel Incident.

Thank God for "The Lake" as the MulQueens always called it.

The MulQueen's Canadian summer home on Lake Erie allowed the family to stay out of the city and out of the crossfire, safely holed up over the Ambassador Bridge in southern Ontario while the carnage played out across the river. This four-bedroom colonial "cottage" on the Erie shores in Colchester that George and Pat MulQueen worked tirelessly to build was in front of the very same spot where the infamous Battle of Lake Erie was fought, one of the deciding battles of the War of 1812 against the British. An apt location, as George L. MulQueen Jr. was a Navy veteran who served as a medic in WWII aboard the USS Gosper. (George L. MulQueen Sr. was an air force pilot in WWI.)

The family stayed there out of harm's way for the rest of the summer – except one person.

He was getting dressed in the upstairs bedroom overlooking the shoreline when Pat MulQueen walked in on him.

"Where are you going, George?"

"Back to work honey."

"Oh my God, no, the city is still burning."

"I gotta get back to work, Dearie. I got a couple kids I hope I can keep out of jail. If they're not dead already."

"George, that's crazy. That can wait."

"Besides, I've got to check on the house."

The Oak Park house was three blocks from 8 Mile, the vast east-west road that defined the northern border of Detroit.

He grabbed his black valise and wallet off the dresser, walked downstairs and grabbed his keys off the fish hook key holder in the corner of the kitchen.

"See you in a few days, Dearie."

"Oh George, please be careful. Why don't you stay?'

"Can't, he said. "Too much to do."

As he turned and made his way toward the back door, he pointed to the painting she had done of the Battle of Lake Erie that hung on the dining room wall.

"Don't give up the ship honey. See you in a few days." The screen door slammed shut behind him.

He fired up his brand new blue metallic 1967 Firebird and "in a cloud of dust and a pile of crap" as he often joked when he took off with the kids in the car, he was off and gone just like that.

Straight into the belly of the beast.

~ 3 ~

LIFE IS WAR

A slightly built hunched-over oriental man of about 60 in yellow gingham shirt and pea-green cotton pants and woven loafers stood impassively in the dirt road, eyes downcast, head slightly bowed forward, casting a slight gray shadow in front of himself.

A fully decked out US soldier from the 1st Platoon Charlie Company casually walked up to the man, stopped for a frozen second in time and stared blankly ahead, seemingly not focusing on any particular place in space or time, or the man in front of him – as if in a trance.

Suddenly and without warning, he thrust his rifle bayonet in the man's chest as if he was casually spearing a fish.

The peasant villager lifted his hands as if in a pastoral embrace like he was reaching out to offer forgiveness to his camo-clad killer, as he gasped and gurgled and dropped slowly to his knees, his eyes still open as he slumped forward facedown as if kissing the ground in a final symbolic gesture, instantly and mortally wounded.

Just that simple, that's how it all started – the carnage that day.

And it went from there.

His appetite for killing now whet, the same US soldier just as suddenly whirled and pushed another villager into a

23

nearby well he was standing next to, then threw a hand grenade into the well. The explosive deafening force boomed smoke and ashes and singed body parts in the air like some kind of morbid confetti. The killing circus, on behalf of our country, upon the orders of the US Government and the president of the United States, was fully underway. You couldn't stop it now.

Now, it had a life of its own.

A short distance away in the Quang Ngai Province, about 20 people, mostly women and children, knelt solemnly around a temple with the slowly swirling smoke of burning incense escaping the golden chamber pots to fill the air with sweet white smoke amid the gentle hum of the peasants' chanting. The Vietnamese citizens gathered, mostly farmers and common laborers in the rice paddies, to pray and cry at the same time, as if they knew a horrible secret, about to be revealed to them.

The secret they would momentarily know is that it's all about circumstance – it could be all good, or depending where we are at in life, voluntarily or involuntarily, it could be pure evil. The most basic truth in life we all need to know, if never to understand, is that each and every one of us are fully capable of either.

And these circumstances weren't right – they were perfect – for the latter.

The Viet Cong in the area in recent weeks had ambushed and killed numerous members of Company C. Retribution was in the air, and there were reports the Viet Cong were hiding in the same area.

They were not.

But it didn't matter.

The praying and chanting was over in an instant as a group of US soldiers opened fire in unison with M-16 rifles on the peasant temple-goers, amazingly and instantly killing all of the unarmed villagers with shots to the head.

Meanwhile, in the nearby Xom Lang Hamlet, soldiers of the 1st Platoon rounded up a group of approximately 70 to 80 villagers, including women and children, marched them to an irrigation ditch east of the settlement, where they pushed them into the ditch and then methodically executed them with machine gun and rifle fire after repeated orders from Second Lieutenant William Calley, who personally led by example with his own rifle.

The women held up their hands in the air and said "No Viet Cong" as they attempted to shield their children just before they were executed. Some of the women had thrown themselves on top of their children and after the initial shooting, some of the children who were old enough to walk got up and Calley himself began to shoot the children.

The killing was out of control across the province.

Another group of up to 50 villagers was walked to the south of Xom Lang and killed on another dirt road paved red with their blood. Less than 100 yards away from this bloodbath, yet another grisly scene was taking place. As a group of about 15 South Vietnamese walked slowly down the same road another band of Charlie Company soldiers opened up with their M-16's while other US soldiers shot at the people with scatter shot and M-79 grenade launchers.

As if not to be outdone, members of the 2nd platoon killed up to 70 citizens as they swept through the northern half of the My Lai Hamlet. Meanwhile, only two miles away in the sub hamlet of My Hoi and the Co Luy Hamlet, an additional 150 villagers were slaughtered, again including significant numbers of women, children and the elderly. The US soldiers set fire to the hooches and huts and waited for the people to come out and they shot them as they exited their makeshift homes. Piles of bodies could be seen in every direction the eye could see.

By midmorning, members of Charlie Company had killed hundreds of civilians, raped or assaulted and mutilated an uncounted number of woman and young girls, killed all the livestock and burned to the ground every single building in the area.

The orders from their Captain were to destroy everything in the village that was "walking, talking, or growing."

So they did.

Despite the fact the American soldiers encountered no enemy fire, and found no weapons in My Lai.

When it was over that day on March 17, St. Patrick's Day, in the Vietnamese Province of Quang Ngai, where the massacre occurred, up to 70 percent of all villages were destroyed by air strikes and artillery bombardments, including napalm bombs.

The US Government had an optimistic take on the day's activity.

According to an official US Army news release, "128 Viet Cong and 22 civilians" were killed in a "fierce fire fight."

A post in Stars and Stripes Magazine stated: "'US Infantrymen killed 128 Communists in a bloody day-long battle."

General William Westmoreland, the US Vietnam commander, congratulated the unit for an "outstanding" job.

This "outstanding" work wasn't limited to My Lai.

In a confidential report to Westmoreland that was leaked, one American general described the Vietnamese countryside in totality as akin to "The Battlefields of Verdun." Civilian casualties alone were exceeding 50,000 per year.

The above actions of the US troops in those rice paddies of Vietnam described above were described thusly in public judicial testimony only as a result of great journalism.

Independent investigative journalist Seymour Hersh, after extensive interviews with Calley and many others from Company C and other military sources, first broke the Mỹ Lai story on November 12, 1969, on the Associated Press wire service. Soon, Time, Life and Newsweek magazines were all covering this incredible story. CBS televised an interview with Paul Meadlo, a soldier in Calley's unit during the massacre.

"It was just like the Nazi's, we had them all lined up in front of a ditch. I shot 20 to 25," Meadlo said. "I shot the first one. ... We all felt like we knew there was lots more killing to come."

The next day after the massacre, there was a loud explosion and the same soldier had his foot blown off.

Said Meadlo: "I felt this was my punishment for what I had done the day before. I told Calley his Judgement Day was coming too."

The Plain Dealer (Cleveland, Ohio) published explicit photographs of dead villagers killed at My Lai.

After a huge public outcry and a lengthy investigation, Calley and several others were charged with varying war crimes and the trials dragged on and on with a steady drumbeat of press coverage of the atrocities that saturated the airwaves everywhere, no place more so than Michigan, the home base of the University of Michigan and a hub of the national anti-war movement.

The tension that gripped the nation over this war exploded the following spring, when on May 4, 1970, the Ohio National Guard, called to the campus of Kent State University in Kent, Ohio, opened fire on a group of student protesters, killing four students and wounding nine others. Hundreds of students had gathered on the university commons in opposition to US President Richard Nixon's recent expansion of the Viet Nam War into Cambodia.

The fatal shootings, known as The Kent State Massacre, sparked massive outrage on campuses across the country, with ultimately more than 4-million students nationwide walking out of class in what became known as The School Strike of 1970.

~ ~ ~

In the midst of all the chaos, Barney pulled into an alley off of Fenkell and Livernois in south west Detroit and slammed on the brakes.

"Okay, guys, time to do your thing."

The two backseat passengers jumped out and ran up to a large blue-and-white truck with sliding aluminum doors on the sides. The truck, a Hamm's Beer truck, was parked in the alley behind Luvert's Liquor Store. They slid a louvered side door upward, grabbed three cases each out of the open vehicle, threw them in the trunk of Barney's blue 1965 Impala and they were outta there like Mexican bandits.

Three Schlitz, one Hamm's, one Stroh's and one Pabst Blue Ribbon. A little of everything.

Barney took a right hand turn on Livernois Ave and headed for Six Mile and a brown brick bungalow east of the University of Detroit where Mooney, another classmate that lived there, helped them sneak the contraband into the basement.

They were there, ostensibly, to make campaign signs for their buddy, the Shankster, who was running for high school class president. And they needed refreshments.

About eight hours later, at 3:40 a.m., she heard the noise.

"George what is that," a woman with stone blue eyes and short brown hair said as she shook her husband out of a deep slumber.

With the body of an offensive lineman, it was a tough fit.

And thus, the noise.

But he made it in. The side window. The frame bent a bit, and the window wouldn't close afterward if he could have tried. He hit the toilet with a loud bang as he rolled off the porcelain reservoir top and hit the cold tile floor.

After he had pried the side window open and descended into that dark basement he crawled around the corner to sleep it off by the side of the train table.

His father wanted to call the police. There was no response as he called downstairs to get out or get killed. But his mother had her priorities straight. And thank god or he probably would have had a cop's bullet through his head.

Being the editor of the local newspaper, she didn't want to be the lede story the next day on the front page of a competitor's paper. Any more than she wanted the local Oak Park Police to see her cluttered and filthy basement.

"No George, I think they were scared off, I don't think there's anybody down there right now, just go down and check for sure nobody is hiding down there," she insisted.

George Jr. and his son George III "Chip" MulQueen had just flipped on all the basement lights and rounded the corner by the train table when Chip shrieked, "No, Dad, no, it's Denny!" as his father froze with a raised baseball bat over his head.

George MulQueen and Chip MulQueen (he had a nine iron in hand) dragged Dennis MulQueen to his feet and ushered him up the stairs.

"I could smell vomit on him but not much else. I don't think it's booze Pat. I think he must be on goofballs," George MulQueen Jr. said.

29

"Oh My God George what are we going to do with him?"

"I think he needs a shrink. He's a total screw up."

Dennis MulQueen felt like he needed an undertaker less than four hours later as he simultaneously leaned on the rake and the aluminum fence post in the back yard as he puked his guts out over the chain link fence for the third time.

Boss's orders.

Clean up the yard.

At 7 a.m.

~ ~ ~

"Okay, Bokker Lee, how many cases do you want to give me?"

"I'll take one from you for starters. Then four more. Let's make it for five. Winner take all."

"Bokker you know I'm going to enjoy every last drop. My guy is going to kill your guy."

"Doon, you've got to get off the heroin. My guy Smokin' Joe is gonna shut the Lip's mouth for good."

"Oh, so you think so, eh Bock?"

Muhammed Ali was back in the game after he won a lawsuit in New York allowing him to fight again after an almost four-year layoff. After beating Jerry Quarry, he fought a mostly boring fight at the Garden in December against Oscar Bonavena.

Boring that is, until the 15th round when Ali exploded on Bonavena and won a dramatic technical knockout.

This set "The Louisville Lip" up for "The Fight of the Century."

"Okay, Bokker Lee, you're on. A case of what? It better not be the wine coolers we made Tremmer drink that almost killed him, okay? I'll put yours in the field and make you drink them a year later this time."

"Doon, you are not a nice man. So okay, you motha. I'm gonna make you pay up big time, ya hear me?"

~ ~ ~

"It's going well, Señor. We need just a little more time, and we'll be through."

His brown, twinkling eyes looked enlarged and spooky through the small owl lenses of his thin-rimmed black glasses. They were like mini Jack Benny's, but looked bigger on Mr. Pascuale's small, pointed, Poindexter-like head. He was not that much older than his students, this young Jesuit scholastic. He was from South America, Paraguay, or was it Uruguay, he couldn't remember.

He spoke very broken English and was demure and reticent.

He scrunched his eyebrows and shook his head back and forth in an uncertain way, as Dennis MulQueen shook his head up and down in a very certain way. Yes, it will be great, he promised, don't worry, he told his languid-looking language instructor.

"Two more weeks, Mr. Pascuale, okay," he said as he exited Pascuale's first floor classroom, turned right and bounded down the shiny red clay tile stairs towards the breezeway connecting the school proper with the gymnasium.

He pushed through the swinging doors that led to the gray tile walls of the gym and quickly descended another red tile stairway to the main hardwood floor. Dennis had arranged with Mr. Pasquale for he and Bokker Lee to do a "special project" the last semester in lieu of attending class. Their ninth-hour class now had a new location – the gym.

Bokker Lee just finished a layup en route to another ridiculous domination of the ordinary gym rats. Well, everybody was inferior to Bokker Lee on this court, he really was one hell of a player. His older brother Hondeau said he was the best all-around athlete in a family of great athletes. One intramural game Dennis watched him from the stands as Bokker Lee scored 62 points. In a single intramural basketball game. He counted what had to be an all-time record for an intramural league game.

"So what did he say?"

"Nuttin'. I told him we needed a couple more weeks for more research. A piece a' cake, Bocks. We're in the library right now, okay, doing research, if anybody asks."

"Gotcha, Big D. Good job. The library bar and grille, here we are."

They moved to the upstairs grandstands to watch the next game.

Dennis pulled out the sling shot his Grandmother Helferty bought him on her recent Arizona vacation. Just happened to have a sackful of BB's with him, too.

Mr. Leary, the gym teacher, he didn't think it was too funny. He never saw any of the actual shots hit several students, but when Dennis MulQueen nailed Mr. Leary in the ass with a beautiful mark, it was game over. The head gym teacher bent over and picked a spent BB up off the hardwood floor. He straightened up, instantly pirouetted on his black umpire-like gym shoes and looked up in the stands directly at MulQueen.

MulQueen tried to keep a straight face but the smirk must have given him away as Leary was in the grandstands in his face about 30 seconds later.

Barely enough time for MulQueen to slide his trusty sling down his back under his shirt and under his underwear.

"Get the hell out of my gym right now MulQueen." He was glowering red-hot pissed.

But he let MulQueen go, with no office visit. Or detention. Or a single demerit. Thank god Dennis MulQueen was a football player.

And Leary was the former AD. Ever seen one cop arrest another?

Very fortuitous. He needed to avoid another suspension. He already held the school record anyway. They told him one more thing – expulsion only.

About a week later, Leary followed him into the varsity locker room during lunch hour while the courts were full of kids playing intramural games.

The door slammed as Leary entered and MulQueen sauntered over to the drinking fountain in the corner.

"What the hell are you doing in here MulQueen?"

"Just getting a drink, Mr. Leary."

"I know what you're doing in here MulQueen. Do you want to graduate from this high school MulQueen?"

"I suggest you clean up your act or it's going be too late. It's not going to be a suspension when I catch you It's not going to be pretty MulQueen."

Several kids had recently reported money stolen out of their wallets, rifled from their pants hanging on coat hooks in the locker room while they were out competing on the gym floor.

~ ~ ~

He went to the sock hop that night with the best of intentions. Swear to god he was sober as a Baptist preacher as he walked to the bathroom about 9:30 p.m. that night. He let go of the spring-loaded door like he had done dozens of times before only this time it smacked the burly guy behind him square in the face.

He continued to the urinal but before he could even get set the guy behind him dressed in all black grabbed him by the shirt from behind and spun him around and cold cocked him with a vicious shot flush to the jaw.

Dennis MulQueen was lucky he didn't spit out any front teeth right then and there. But three front teeth were definitely loose now and eventually would turn black, die and have to be removed.

This guy was no punk. Dennis recognized him as a guy named Rick Uleson. He was a few years older, in his early 20s, but he already had a black belt in karate. He wasn't built like a typical Asian martial arts guy. He was a stocky dude with a brick shit house physique.

The force of the blow staggered Dennis, he flew back into the urinal and to make matters worse the back of his head slammed into the back tile wall. He was almost knocked out. By the time he gathered himself, Uleson was already out the door. At 6' 4", Dennis MulQueen peered above the crowd and could see the black-clad guy that assaulted him exit the main gym doors. He barged through the crowd after him.

He pursued his attacker outside where he had stopped with his back to the doors to brag to his buddies.

One good turn deserves another, MulQueen thought.

He sneaked up behind Uleson and pretty much copied his enemy's maneuver from a few minutes before. But with one big difference. MulQueen had a trick up his sleeve he had learned as a kid from one of the National Hockey League's most feared fighters.

As he came up behind Uleson, Dennis MulQueen reached over the guy's right shoulder and with his left hand firmly grabbed the front collar of the blue oxford dress shirt Uleson was wearing as he spun him around.

Now face-to-face, MulQueen fully extended his left arm while holding onto Uleson's collar and T-shirt at the same time he twisted his arm clockwise as tight as it would go and with a superior reach and three inch height advantage,

MulQueen hit the guy as hard as he could over and over again in lightning quick succession as he had him helplessly pinned in a stationary position.

An old hockey trick he learned from a good friend of his father's, a legendary Detroit Red Wing named Hec Kilrea, who gave Dennis MulQueen a boxing lesson one day when he was a kid visiting his Canada home in Belle River with his father.

Blood was now streaming from Uleson's nose and mouth, but being a black belt, Uleson had a few tricks of his own.

Before Dennis MulQueen could finish him off Uleson somehow managed to deliver a hard swinging leg kick with his left leg and the two of them tumbled to the ground in a bloody pile. At precisely that moment there was loud hollering as a different man in all-black appeared over the two combatants sprawled on the ground.

"Get off him now, let go of him MulQueen, break it up right now you two, the cops are on the way here. Cut it out right now both of you or you're both going to jail."

Dennis MulQueen looked up and standing over them was Fr. Richard Polakowski, S.J., the most unlikely of interveners. He was an amazing guy, a phenomenal English teacher, but a mild mannered intellectually superior man of great compassion and a human being with the softest of voices, to go with his much-less-than-athletic frame.

Thank God for small favors. Although Uleson's face was as bloodied by now as Dennis MulQueen's lip was fat and his teeth were loose, who knows what additional damage would have occurred had Fr. Polakowski not appeared like Raphael in the dark.

Barney was outside having a smoke and said he saw the whole thing. "Way to go, Mulky," he said after they got in his car to leave. "Let's find this punk. I wanna see you finish him off."

"Yeah me too Barney. Man I thought I broke my hand I hit him so hard."

"Yeah, I know, I saw it, he ain't no frat boy that guy. Good job, Mulky. You kicked his ass good. I was afraid you were going to kill him."

Dennis MulQueen was afraid his father would kill him before anybody else had the chance. He knew, like he was told, one more incident and it was out the front door for good.

He was afraid what Polo, as the students nicknamed him, might say to the assistant principal in charge of discipline. He was sure Polo would call the cops if he hadn't already if he saw him near the school again, so he hopped in the trunk of Barney's old Impala as Barney slammed the lid shut and circled the school parking lot several times looking for Uleson.

But they couldn't find the dirty SOB. Thankfully, nobody hit Barney's Chevy in the ass that night.

~ ~ ~

The March 8, 1971 Ali-Frazier fight was billed as "The Fight Of The Century" for good reason. The hype and buildup were ridiculous. It was so big even Frank Sinatra couldn't get a ringside seat. So he went to the fight as the Look Magazine photographer.

Ali was his usual nasty pre-fight self, calling Frazier a "gorilla" and an "Uncle Tom" and promised to destroy him.

"Joe Frazier is too dumb to be champ." Ali said. "Joe Frazier is too ugly to be champ. I'm gonna destroy him."

But Smokin' Joe was no dummy in the ring.

The fight lived up to the hype.

In his characteristic crouched fighting stance, the shorter Frazier bobbed and weaved and bulled his way inside, repeatedly getting underneath Ali's arms and constantly attacking him from within and while Ali was able to hit him on the way in Ali couldn't get full extension on Joe while Frazier was able to deliver terrific interior punishment to Ali with vicious body shot after body shot. And Smokin' Joe could bring it when it came to punching power, with devastating knockouts in most of his fights.

Frazier used that power to stagger Ali in one of the early rounds, but like only Ali could, he managed to dance out of it.

Through the first 10 rounds, the fight was scored mostly even. In the 11th, Frazier tagged Ali with another vicious left hook which wobbled him, but again Ali stagger-stepped his way backwards across the ring and Frazier thought perhaps Ali was clowning and trying to set him up for a counter-attack so he didn't pursue his advantage to take the injured fighter out.

In the 15th round, Frazier knocked Ali down with another vicious left hook. Referee Arthur Mercante said afterward it was as hard as he had ever seen a man hit.

But somehow Ali staggered back onto his feet – within three seconds.

He managed to finish the fight, but Ali lost by unanimous decision, the first loss of his career.

The "Fight of the Century" was indeed the biggest fight in history, broadcast to countries all across the world, with several hundred press credentials alone issued for the extravaganza.

Nobody knew it at the time but as the country was obsessed with the fight taking place at Madison Square Garden, a small group of radicals was obsessed with carrying out a burglary on a government office about 100 miles away.

Under cover of the fight hysteria, members of a group calling itself the Citizen's Committee to Investigate the FBI pried open a side window of the FBI Building in Media, Pennsylvania, and quickly made off with more than 1,000 pages of classified documents.

They immediately mailed these documents to newspapers and TV stations across the country.

As the secret FBI files became public, it was revealed that FBI Director J. Edgar Hoover had initiated a top secret spy program code named Cointelpro (counter intelligence program) that involved FBI agents secretly investigating and following and wiretapping a whole host of American citizens involved in the civil rights movement and the anti-war movement, including politicians, journalists and anti-war activists.

At the top of their list: "The Greatest" himself, Muhammad Ali.

The break-in revealed that the federal government was after Muhammad Ali beginning with his selective service case where by the feds changed his draft status. He was followed and surveilled relentlessly, including having his phones tapped and conversations recorded as his whereabouts and movements were scrutinized even to the point they accessed his elementary school records in Louisville, Kentucky.

Little Cassius Clay "loved art," his teachers reported in the classified government files.

The FBI records even contained a word-for-word transcript of Muhammad Ali's recent appearance on the Johnny Carson show.

~ ~ ~

He came straight home from school that Friday in late March and his mother greeted him in the kitchen with downcast eyes.

"Hey, Moms Mabley, what's wrong? You look tired."

"Not feeling too great, Denny. Grandma had a bad spell and she's in Providence Hospital right now."

"Oh shoot, Mom, that's terrible."

"She's in room 223. I know how close you are, Denny, and what it would mean for her to see you. All those summers you have stayed with her, she adores you, Denny. I'm going back to visit her in a couple hours. You want to go with me, Denny?"

"Aww, I love her too, Mom. I'd love to go see her with you."

About 20 minutes later, the phone rang, and it was Bokker Lee. Preoccupied with thoughts of his grandma, the Ferndale grandma he stayed with every summer, he almost forgot.

He and Bokker had still not squared up on their pre-fight bet and they had made plans to go out on the town this Friday night and get 'er done. He hung up and told his mother he would go see Grandma with her tomorrow. Bokker buzzed over a little after 7:00 p.m. and off and running they were.

They polished off all but four short of an entire case. This time it was Stroh's.

They hooted and hollered like drunken fools into the wee hours.

A little after 2 in the morning, Bokker Lee pulled his silver Barracuda up in front of 21471 Kipling Ave and dropped his buddy off.

Moms Mabley surprised him at the top of the landing this time. She was quiet but he could see tears were pooling in the corners of her eyes. Her face was pink and she looked drawn and spent in the few hours since he last saw her.

Before he could mount the top step to the kitchen, she wrapped her arms around him and whispered garbled words he couldn't make out.

"What Mom, what Mom. What happened?"

Silence.

"What Mom?"

"I went to the hospital after you left. We were talking a while and Grandma got up to go to the bathroom.

"I heard a loud thump come from the bathroom, I called out 'Mother' and ran in and Grandma was on the floor next to the sink."

His mother, his best friend from birth, was sobbing now.

"It was too late. It was too late Denny. She had a massive heart attack and keeled over dead on the spot. I looked at my watch, it was 8:32 p.m."

Just about the time he was finishing his first Stroh's of the night.

He felt his mother's tears dropping now with a light patter on his right shoulder, a diminutive barely audible sound that echoed in his mind like a 21-gun-salute.

~ 4 ~

RATHER BE LUCKY
THAN GOOD ANY DAY

"Come here, oh my God, come here and look at this George," said the tall slender brunette with blue stone eyes dressed in a white-and-black apron, gray blouse, dark navy slacks, and white tennis shoes.

She looked like she was straight out of an old '50s Spencer Tracy black and white movie, or maybe an old Father Knows Best episode.

Here she is, the all-American house wife, busy cleaning house.

She flipped the switch on the pink-and-white Hoover as she jabbed her long and pink big-knuckled fingers at small piles of white down on the floor in the corner near the picture-window sill.

The small frothy white piles looked like they could have been from a new born chick, a baby robin or a handful of gosling feathers blown hither and there by an invisible puff of wind.

She was anything but the house cleaner.

A striking brunette with a turned up pixie, tall for her time at 5'8", she was an accomplished journalist and an early glass ceiling breaker. In a totally male-dominated industry she started out as an editor of the Varsity News at the

University of Detroit, she later worked at the Wyandotte Tribune and the Detroit News and ultimately became the editor and publisher of her own newspaper company, owning and publishing seven weekly newspapers that included the Oak Park News, The Southfield Record, the Northwest Detroiter and the Northwest Record.

This woman could have run a country, in her sleep, let alone an upright vacuum cleaner.

Such was her acumen, the nuns at St Gregory Grade School in Detroit skipped her two grades in elementary school – she was always ahead of the curve, this gal. She was a woman who could have had anybody.

Must have been the cow eyes.

The girls often joked how he hypnotized them with those big brown eyes that danced, sparkled and entranced – or could stop a man dead in his tracks if there was danger or provocation. Or anger from something stupid one of his family members did.

Yes, she could have had anybody, but those eyes were all it took – they were the drive-through window to an inner passion and smoldering spark of life that gave him swagger, power and a charisma she found irresistible.

He was president of the church council, started and was president of his own credit union, The Our Lady of Fatima Credit Union, and after he left Lyster he ran the job upgrading program for Detroit Public Schools out of Chadsey High School in Detroit. Although he earned a master's degree from U of D in history and he was a safety engineer at Ford Motor Company, his true love was being an assistant football coach at Pershing High School in Detroit and later St. Mary's of Redford and Saint James High Schools.

Together George and Pat MulQueen were the center of attention in any room they entered. Meet the quintessential metro Detroit power couple.

He sauntered into the living room of their home at 21471 Kipling Ave in Oak Park, Michigan that day with those cow eyes bigger than ever.

"What is it Dearie? What in hell's half acres did you find?"

She was pointing at the downy pile on the floor.

"Oh My God," he said as he surveyed the scene. "What the heck is going on here?"

They looked at each other with simultaneously raised eyebrows. Their two young sons, 13 months apart, were both towheads.

But at the moment, the oldest was in his kindergarten class at Einstein Elementary. So they both knew where this came from.

He called his son's name, then again, in a louder tone – he knew how to be loud – heart-stopping loud when he was mad.

"Where are you, Son? Come here, Son."

Into the powder blue walled living room sauntered a four-year-old tow-haired boy in a light blue flannel shirt with dark blue pants, his head down, looking at the floor, a small bald spot in the middle of the back of his blonde head standing out like a flashlight in a cave.

This was vintage George and Pat McQueen in the living room of their Oak Park bungalow circa the fall of 1957.

Along with the kid destined to be the anti-hero of their lives – their son, the little kid sporting a self-inflicted bald spot in the middle of the top of his head, Dennis MulQueen.

~ ~ ~

That was then – this was now – almost 15 years later, those same cow eyes bouncing their magnetic spark off the rear view mirror directly into the now17-year-old's face in the back seat as they rolled down I-75, with the father

43

retelling the story of his son's infamous bad-hair day of long ago.

They were on the road again.

And it didn't really matter where they were going – it was always special being on the road again.

No matter if they were in the car, on a train, a bus, an airplane or a bicycle.

Just as long as they were going somewhere, it could be downtown, uptown or just down the street.

It's about purpose, being on the go, having a destination, it was always fun going places. This purposeful pattern was established way back in the beginning, with the holiday traditions.

Every December since the kids were little they would pile in the station wagon and drive from Oak Park to nearby Royal Oak, about a 15 minute ride, to the Royal Oak train station, where they would take the 8:05 downtown to visit the iconic J.L. Hudson's Department Store to shop at the children's shop and see Santa Claus, and catch a movie after lunch and then the 5:23 back to Royal Oak and home.

If the MulQueen love affair with the road didn't originate with the Christmas trips downtown, then it had to be their annual Thanksgiving pilgrimage over the border to their Canadian lakefront cottage, where they would gather with the family every year to celebrate the turkey holiday.

The minute they piled in the car to go to "The Lake," as Pat and George always called it, whether it was Thanksgiving, winter, spring or summer – it didn't matter when, but the minute they got in the car the switch was flipped and nobody was allowed to be anything but happy on the way to the lake again.

If it wasn't getting pumped up with courage at the cottage, taking the train to downtown Detroit to visit Hudson's, or flying somewhere locally in their uncle's plane, then it was the long distance car excursions that fueled their love of being on the road together.

One summer that was a journey to the "City of Brotherly Love" and the Liberty Bell and the Old Bookbinders with the huge ornate wood bar with the etched glass booths separating the fancy tables and chairs and the huge glass tanks filled with giant live lobsters.

In 1963 they piled into the '62 powder blue Ford station wagon for their first of many trips to New York City and all those winding steps to the top of the Statue of Liberty, before later ascending even higher to the observation platform atop the Empire State Building, feeling the building sway as the people like soldier ants in the streets 100 stories below made their way about.

Of course there had to be a mandatory stop for lunch at the world famous Automat where you loaded the stainless steel slit with quarters and like a Jetson's cartoon out popped your steaming hot roast beef and gravy sandwich, or whatever else you wanted.

Who could forget the 3:30 a.m. trek from their Edison Hotel room down to Times Square with the wall-to-wall people fascinating the MulQueen brothers as only the city that never sleeps could.

But nothing would compare to this trip – the trip-to-end-all trips.

Grandma Helferty was not in the ground one day when George MulQueen announced they were "hitting the bricks" the very next day – destination Paradise.

Paradise as in South Florida Paradise – George's present to Pat MulQueen to help salve the wounds of her mother's death. The anticipation continued to build as their getaway faux-wood-sided LTD wagon rambled down I-75 through Ohio, Kentucky, and Tennessee. They had just crossed the

Georgia state line when he was putting the wraps on Dennis' bad-hair day description of long ago.

"There are several small piles of hair, it almost reminded me of dog hair, only it was white and we didn't have a dog," he recalled from the front seat of the 1968 Ford wagon.

"I knew right then, you were a little off, Son," he said, his Hollywood smile and mesmerizing cow eyes now using the rear view mirror to light up the back seat like a halogen light you couldn't not stare at.

As he tilted his head back in a preamble to what was coming next, you could see the kid would have had to pull out a lot more hair than he did that day to match his father's well-established adult manhood bald spot.

"Why you would want to look like me, I'll never know," he said as then like clockwork his hearty trademark belly laugh shook the car again. "But alas, you may get your way someday, and I doubt you'll need any help."

"Just wait."

The car shook again.

You could hear Dennis MulQueen laughing from the back seat, his mother was laughing, his brothers and sisters laughed, everybody in the car was laughing now including their one remaining grandparent, Grandma MulQueen, who was making the journey with them.

Just like when he was mad you couldn't help but be terrified, when he was happy, everybody was happy. When he laughed, everybody laughed.

And that was never more the case than when they were on the road again, when the good old MulQueen vibes always spread smooth and easy like grammy's apple butter.

Until their on-the road-again bubble burst.

When several hours later, after everybody was sleeping, an ear-piercing screech and the smell of burning rubber filled the car with terror.

Time froze in slow motion frames as they came out of a curve and his father slammed on the brakes and everybody was thrown violently to the right as the car spun 90 degrees to the left and swerved across the asphalt before coming to rest – what seemed like an eternity later – half on the left shoulder, half on the median, only yards from where a semi moving so slowly in the right lane it looked like it was stalled in the middle of the road in front of them was so close they could reach out and touch it.

Not too far from the Tennessee-Georgia border I-75 was about to narrow to one lane because of construction and the speed limit dropped in a heartbeat from 70 to 35. There was no warning save one inappropriately placed sign. They were still far enough north the air was a bit foggy and the road visibility was tough. George MulQueen had to guess right or guess left, a split-second decision with life in the balance – everybody's.

He guessed the left and he guessed correctly, as a deafening, booming horn that sounded like the whistle of a freight train bore down on them from behind with earthquake-like force that rattled the doors and the windows of their station wagon as all 18 wheels of a second semi that was behind them with no chance to brake blurred by them like a giant UFO in the night.

Everybody was wide awake now.

"Wow, Dad, that was really close. Oh my God, how did you manage to pull that off?"

He inhaled slowly and deeply and straightened his arms against the steering wheel and from the back seat Dennis MulQueen saw the plastic steering wheel bend like putty in the hands of his father's firm grip.

"I'd rather be lucky than good any day," he said as he arched his eyebrows and slowly accelerated the lumbering Ford wagon back onto the highway.

Those cow eyes in the mirror were like saucers now. There was a reason he was president of just about any organization he was ever in. He could have been president of NASCAR too, or at least a member, the way he got the gang out of that jam.

"Hell," he said as he shrugged his shoulders nonchalantly and glanced in the mirror at his son in the back seat again. "I didn't even have to be lucky or good this time. I had my good luck charm with me awake in the backseat – you. Just like on Lake Erie, you always out fished all of us 10 to 1."

His father made him think, yeah, maybe you're right, Dad. I don't know about the good part, but you talk about a charmed existence – the MulQueen's really were a lucky bunch. As youngsters, the MulQueen kids never worried about anything. Both parents were workaholics, and none of the MulQueen kids ever wanted for anything. And nothing bad ever happened to them. Yet they were surrounded by bad things happening all the time to people they knew.

Maybe Thoreau was right, the vast majority of people lead lives of quiet desperation. But not the MulQueens. They lived nothing but large.

He would never forget that day his mother walked in the living room and told him to get ready to go for a ride.

"We're going to visit the Whites," she said as about 10 minutes later they pulled out of the driveway in the trusty 1962 Ford powder-blue wagon.

Mary Ann and Jim White were family friends of Grandma Helferty's and lived right down the street on the same block as his mother's childhood home at 1276 W. Marshall, in Ferndale, Mi.

Their son, fourteen-year-old Richard White, came down with bone cancer and had to have his right leg amputated above the knee, his mother explained in the car on the way there. She handed him a hardcover copy of "Treasure Island " by Robert Louis Stevenson, to give the poor kid. And a box of Sander's chocolates.

They strolled inside, he gave Richard the goods, they talked a little and then they left.

Six weeks later, Richard White was dead.

Ahh, to be out on the lake fishing again.

It was only the next year, Dennis was about thirteen now, when his mother's closest friend, Betty Barsdorf, died from lung cancer at age 39 (she was a smoker). He would always remember her forlorn kids crying at the funeral.

Same for the Shepherd kids. Dave was the mayor of Oak Park, he died of a heart attack. The MulQueen's friends the Cronks from the old neighborhood, same story. Their Dad died suddenly of a heart attack one day.

But nothing ever happened to the MulQueens.

Ahh, to be out on the lake fishing again.

They were now well into Georgia, when out of nowhere from the back seat he blurted out, "What's it like getting stabbed, Dad?"

"I mean, what were you thinking of, looking at that guy with a big knife lunging at your throat that day?"

"I wasn't thinking of anything, Son, except getting out of the way."

"Oh, come on, Dad, weren't you afraid of dying? Weren't you thinking about dying?"

"Hell no, Son, why would I think of that? I'm alive. Life is for the living. When you're alive, you think about living. Everything else is a distraction.

"There will be plenty of time to think about that stuff when the time comes."

49

'There is usually plenty of notice," he added, locking eyes again with his son in the rearview mirror.

"How's that, Dad?"

"Because, Son, the vast majority of people choose when and how they are going to die."

There was a pause.

"Don't worry, Son. you'll see what I mean."

There was another pause as his father's words had a chance to sink in.

"But what about the Franks, Dad?"

He wasn't talking about Anne Frank and WWII and Hitler.

He was in seventh grade when on November 13, 1965, the parents of an eighth grader he knew named Ken Frank, a friend of his older brother Chip, set off on a cruise from Miami to the Bahamas on the Yarmouth Castle cruise ship. Shortly after midnight that night, about 60 miles from the Nassau port, the ship caught fire and sank, taking 87 passengers down with it, including Ken Frank's mother and father.

"I don't think the Franks had much choice in the matter, Dad," he said.

"Yeah, I know, notice I said a majority. But they did buy the ticket, Son," he said as he tilted his head to the right and then back upright again as he broke out in a frown.

Then he changed the subject.

"Remember when your mother took you to the circus that day, Son?"

"Huh?"

"Not too far away over there we can capture some of that magic."

"What, Dad?"

"We could take that highway east and visit a monument to the man over there if we wanted. But it would take us out of our way and we don't have enough time on this trip."

His mother sat up in the passenger seat.

"What are you talking about George?"

'Over there Pat, Tallulah Falls, that's not too far over there in the eastern part of the state, not too far north east of Atlanta.

"Yep, that last road, we could take that for a while and we'd be right there."

That's where his father said Tallulah Falls State Park is located, where 65-year old Karl Wallenda had recently crossed the falls above the Tallulah Falls Gorge, and the river at the bottom, some 700 feet below, to complete a 1,200-foot sky walk that saw the ageless acrobat stop to do not one but two separate handstands in the middle.

At age 65.

To celebrate 50 years on the wire.

In tremendously unfavorable conditions, with the wind blowing and the wire swaying and nothing but air between him and the granite-floored valley 700 feet below.

~ ~ ~

When he awoke a couple of hours later, Dennis MulQueen realized they were now in the Sunshine State as they passed under a streetlight at the top of the exit ramp and he saw his first palm tree, although it wasn't a good look, silhouetted as it was in front of a street light in the midnight hour.

They turned right and pulled into the Howard Johnson's parking lot. 'No vacancies' the sign in the window said.

Rain started to pour from the tropical skies as they drove to three more filled-up motels before George MulQueen announced they had found their lodging for the night.

Right here, bed for the night, in the station wagon in the parking lot of the filled-up Ramada Inn. They cracked the windows, oblivious to the weather, the time of night or anything else.

As the Gods continued to empty the skies, they all slept exactly as they were – upright in the now fogged-up car, sitting in place, scrunched together like herring in a jar.

Ah, to be on the road again, the MulQueen way.

Not a care in the world, safe, happy, finally in the land of beauty and paradise.

Florida.

The surcease of all void.

The impossibility of any concern.

The beauty of serenity – scrunched up in a parking lot car.

Paradise.

The only thing Dennis MulQueen heard the rest of the night was his 76-year-old paternal grandmother, immediately to his left, trying to protect her turf.

"Git over, Denny, darn you," she said about once every hour it seemed like as she swatted him on the thigh, imploring him to quit crushing her with his big-man legs.

~ 5 ~

EVERYBODY LOVES A HERO

But for a matter of inches, it could have been him, and history much different.

But for the grace of God – who knows how destiny really works – in another place and time it could have been any of us.

But fate called this day for the man's childhood best friend, who only a second before stood nobly by his side manning a massive US Naval cannon.

The violent boom came at them from across the water, rattling his ribs like an airborne earthquake and just like that it was over and the buddy beside him no more.

The commodore stood stoically on deck as the blood ran beneath his feet and he wiped his friends brains and skull fragments off the front lapels of his blue navy jacket as casually as you would clean up after a food fight.

Without hesitation, the head of the US Navy Great Lakes Operations immediately stepped forward to personally man his fallen comrade's battle station.

He loaded the black powder and packed it ferociously with the long-handled tamper and fired a booming reply to his friend's death at the enemy ship in the distance.

But the captain's gallantry notwithstanding, by all appearances this battle was already over.

Another enemy cannon blast took the main mast down and the ship's gunnels were already blown apart with vast splintered holes like dark craters in a slowly sinking swiss cheese moon ship.

Indeed, the clock ticked rapidly toward zero hour as the ship continued to take on massive gallons of water and began to list.

His top aide ran up to the captain with a pleading, open-mouthed look on his face.

"Sir," he said, "we are almost out of ammunition and manpower. With all due respect sir I believe we are about to sink and it might be time to save who we can."

Codeword: surrender. Time to give up. Time to hoist the white flag. It's over.

The indignant captain said nothing, only a bitter scowl stamped across his sullen mien. As he whirled and walked away across the deck to make his own assessment, he nearly slipped and fell on the pools of blood that rendered the wooden planks as slippery as moss on a rock. As he mounted the steps to ascend the foredeck, the commodore had to step over human body parts splayed across the landing.

As he surveyed his stricken vessel, he realized he was down to 15 standing crew members.

But instead of calling for the white flag, he called for the boatswain to climb the mizzenmast and retrieve the blue and black flag, a gift from his dear friend and colleague, the recently killed-in-action captain that he had named his ship after: Captain Lawrence.

The commodore retraced his steps back to the aft stairwell leading down below to the ship's makeshift hospital that was formerly the galley – now pretty much a morgue – and called out for his 14-year-old brother who he had earlier sent below to assist the ship doctor with mostly amputations and mercy killings.

He turned and ordered his midshipmen to prepare the wooden lifeboat for launch.

With the folded flag in hand he barked out final instructions to the crew he was leaving behind and jumped in the wooden 12-oar, 18-foot vessel with a dozen of the remaining crew as it was slowly lowered by rope to the sea.

This would be no surrender.

There he stood, larger than life, decked out in full sartorial military splendor, in the blue and white navy uniform of his country, hand pointed in the air, index finger extended toward the enemy in the distance, exhorting those under his command to row the diminutive wooden dinghy with all they had from the burning sinking flagship of his fleet onward, despite near certain death and defeat, to the remaining 500-ton brig in the distance.

Cannonballs dropped in the water all around them like the sky was raining bowling balls.

Bullets seared the air, the whizz inches from human ears, as he insisted against all odds on one final attempt to defeat the most vaunted military force in the world – the undefeated, never-before beaten British Navy.

About 6 feet even, with long dark brown mutton chops, wavy brown hair and serious, never-to-be-doubted penetrating brown eyes, he stood dignified and majestic – and utterly defiant – in the wooden rowboat.

He looked as fearless and confident as his reputation, and if you believe in victory, and the fight to survive and conquer the odds he was facing, how else could you carry yourself, how else could you stare in the eye of the dragon and spit – if not for that magnificent swagger that defines any a true hero?

And hero he was, as he did reach the other ship and he climbed the rigging of the USS. Niagara and personally hoisted the flag that would define his legacy as he proceeded to attack the enemy and by miracle win the battle that ultimately won the War of 1812 for the United States of America.

As Dennis MulQueen purveyed the scene before his eyes it was like slipping on a comfortable old pair of Italian loafers. After all, he knew everything about this guy he could reach out and touch in front of him – save the glass wall that separated them.

How could he not know him? He was raised with him. The epitome of the MulQueen philosophy of life. Another reminder, lest he forget.

Who would have believed this guy would be the first person he came face to face with at their first tourist trap stop – the Miami Wax Museum.

Dennis MulQueen's jaw dropped in disbelief as he continued to stare at the amazingly realistic wax sculpture of Commodore Oliver Hazard Perry, the centerpiece of this realistic voice-activated recreation of the famous Battle of Lake Erie scene that was plastered all over the walls of Dennis MulQueen's boyhood summer home in Canada.

Of course the flag dominated everything. Slate Blue with grease black letters, "Don't give up the ship," it read.

Same as a photo on the bathroom wall in Canada. And a print on the dining room wall. And a painting on the living room wall, too.

The same exact scene comprised the Perry exhibit that was the very first, inside left upon entering the pink and white stucco building located on US-1 just south of downtown Miami.

If you love a good hero, this place was heaven.

No sooner had Dennis and his family walked past Perry and his men and rounded the corner they heard the familiar booming voice of another American icon.

"No, no, we are not satisfied, and we will not be satisfied until justice rolls down like water, and righteousness like a mighty stream.

"Let us not wallow in the valley of despair, I say to you today, my friend, for I have a dream today! "

There stood a very life-like wax figure of Martin Luther King Jr., who was assassinated on April 4,1968 in Memphis Tennessee. He was wearing his black bowler hat and long black wool coat, in a recreation of his famous 1963 "I Have a Dream" speech in Washington D.C. in front of the Lincoln Memorial. His actual voice filled the room, a breathtaking true-to-life recording of the historic speech King gave, replete with the gasping and "Oh Yes Lord, " "tell it like it is preacher," "tell it to us preacher," that put all listeners right there in the audience that day.

"I have a dream that one day... little black boys and black girls will be able to join hands with little white boys and white girls as sisters and brothers.

"I have a dream today! I have a dream that one day every valley shall be exalted... and the glory of the Lord shall be revealed and all flesh shall see it together. This is our hope and this is the faith..."

A young guy and his girlfriend had pushed the metal button to play the recording through a small silver speaker box mounted on an aluminum pole in front of the window. They stayed to hear it a second time as Dennis pushed the button again.

"With this faith," Dr. King continued, "we will be able to work together, to pray together, to struggle together, to go to jail together, to stand up for freedom together, knowing that we will be free one day.

"And this will be the day – this will be the day when all of God's children will be able to sing with new meaning: My country 'tis of thee, sweet land of liberty, of thee I sing. And so let freedom ring."

All of the MulQueens were stuck to the tile floor like Velcro as the climax of probably the greatest speech of all time played out before them.

"From every mountainside, let freedom ring. And when this happens, and when we allow freedom to ring, when we let it ring from every village and every hamlet, from every state and every city, we will be able to speed up that day when all of God's children, black men and white men, Jews and Gentiles, Protestants and Catholics, will be able to join hands and sing in the words of the old Negro spiritual:

Free at last! Free at last! Thank God Almighty, we are free at last!"

This exhibit alone made it worth the $2.00 price of admission.

But there was more.

A little further down, President John F. Kennedy sat upright on the open back ledge of his jet black Lincoln Continental limousine, a smile on his face, waving to the Dallas crowd.

Moments before Lee Harvey Oswald blew his brains out.

A push on another stainless steel button and another true-to-life recording resonated: the assassinated US President's famous "ask not what your country can do for you, but what you can do for your country" speech.

The very next window showcased a wax figure of his similarly murdered brother, US Sen. Bobby Kennedy, complete with his thin black tie and white shirt and black suit.

Lost in the moment was the fact that this was the same guy that as his brother's attorney general signed the warrants authorizing J. Edgar Hoover to spy on the guy two displays over – Martin Luther King Jr.

Wow Madame Tussaud, I guess you have to die violently to get on your stage, eh?

But Wait. Not true.

Over there – he would have no idea who this guy was, except he's standing next to a lunar rover on top of barren rocky ground – of course it's Neal Armstrong giving his "giant leap for mankind" speech after landing on the moon.

Dennis MulQueen had to push one final button – unfortunately.

The last big exhibit of the day in the far corner was entitled "Ponce DeLeon's conquest of Florida" and featured the Spanish explorer and his overlords standing over fallen-down, bloodied, shot-up and stabbed Native American corpses littering the ground.

In contrast to Perry and Kennedy, all-American heroes who looked like they were going to open their mouths and start walking they were so realistic, the fallen natives looked like over-inflated blow-up dolls, like clownish comic-book caricatures, nothing remotely resembling actual human beings.

But why not? Why would tourist trap revisionist history be different from mainstream revisionist history? Do we need more varnished history to explain how Key West got its original name, Cayo Hueso?

All told, the MulQueens were at the Wax Museum little more than an hour before heading back down US-1 toward the Tamiami Trail and the real reason to come to South Florida.

~ ~ ~

If you don't believe in God, test yourself – visit here. Because, if he's alive, he has to have a condo in South Florida.

If you've never been in person, it's hard to describe it in words, so surreal is the depth of her pure tropical beauty.

At least that was the case, as seen for the first time, through the eyes of a teenager raised in the concrete jungle of Detroit, Michigan.

For Dennis MulQueen, it all starts with the palm trees.

He had never seen one before. But here, they bombard you. Up and down the streets, in the middle of neighborhoods, downtown, uptown and in the middle of nowhere.

If it's hard not to be hypnotized by brilliant classical music, then the palms are the conductor's wand waving the South Florida tropical orchestra to full attention.

Amazing how many different kinds, and all unique.

The somnolescent and soothing foxtails, the first ones he noticed on the sides of the turnpike as they looked for a hotel that first Florida night, sway proudly upright in the gently moving tropical air like giant emerald feather dusters of the sky.

The centennial palms he first spotted at the local shopping center sported round clusters of leaves that looked like Chinese fans waving in the breeze to come on in and spend some more of those tourist dollars.

The Christmas tree palms with their skinny jean trunks were everywhere adorned with bright gobs of small red ornamental berries that hung like holiday baskets in the air. The signature coconut palms in the neighborhoods and parks displayed their round green and brown milk-filled loot waiting to drop like thirst-sating souvenirs from the sky.

But the royal palms, he found, are the rulers of this tropical kingdom, some more than 60 feet tall and 15 feet wide at the top with smooth gray bark as thick as a Roman colonnade, standing in ramrod-straight formation like obedient six-story toy soldiers with giant spherical green-plumed hats on top saluting the emperor in the sky.

Not to be left out, smaller, carefully pruned robellinis dotted the landscape along with the sylvester palms and their cousins the powerful-looking canary date palms with their massive girth and carefully sculpted thick pineapple bark.

Complementing this all-green palm tree tapestry is a spectacularly colorful array of flowering regular-leaved trees, some with clusters of amarillo blooms like tulips, some with neon cardinal red flowers like crimson sparklers lighting up the air, while still other deciduous-looking trees show off with purple clusters of flowers dangling high in the air like Easter egg baskets from the gods.

But of course it wouldn't be South Florida without the tropical fruit trees, with their neon fruits begging to be indulged of their succulent bounty, the fig trees and the banana trees and the lemon trees and the lime trees, and of course the omnipresent orangest of the green orange trees, begging to be picked of their juicy sweet harvest from orchards lining the highways and suburban backyards everywhere.

Notwithstanding all these resplendent tropical arboreal specimens, what takes the natural beauty of South Florida to the ultimate level are the jaw-dropping tropical gardens whose cornucopia of brilliant color tantalizes the optic nerves everywhere their breath-taking opulence is found, in the mall parking lots, the middle of the road way medians, surrounding the subdivision entryway signs or in just about anybody's yard in the neat neighborhoods with clean streets and manicured lawns framed in by row after row of salt water taffy stucco houses.

Bright fuchsia and purple and salmon-colored Bougainvilleas and shrubs with radiant dangling tulip blossoms, and orange and blue and yellow and white birds of paradise and simply stunning orchids of every gorgeous shade in the rainbow flash their Crayola-crayon colors in the sun like it was Christmas and New Years and the Fourth of July all at once, over and over and over everywhere you look, every single day of the year.

Paradise.

The surcease of all void.

Utter tropical magnificence visible from every street corner.

There is just no end to the panoramic beauty that surrounds every man woman and child that cares to look.

And why shouldn't every day be like Christmas, New Years and the Fourth of July? Indeed, all you have to do in South Florida is open your eyes.

If New York City is the city that never sleeps, South Florida is a world where beauty never quits.

After taking it all in for the first full day of sightseeing in the Florida heat they weren't accustomed to, it was early to bed at a relative's house for a good night's sleep.

But the excitement of their first tropical vacation saw them early to rise the next morning and back out the door heading straight south.

Not long down the way on SW 8th St, the Tamiami Trail as it is called, not too far past a town named Sweetwater, famous for its 24-hour liquor sales, the advertisements for the air boat tours started popping up and soon a congregation of thatched-roof huts off to the left could not escape attention.

A ticky-tacky 6'x 3' yellow and brown shoddy, hand-painted sign advertised "live alligator wrestling."

Beneath the squiggly, faded, hand-painted words sat a silhouetted native in another cartoon-caricature-like pose with a comical alligator sketched out in front of him, mouth agape.

Ponce De Leon we just saw your ghost again.

The 50-spot or so parking lot was nearly full.

The MulQueens though cruised right by without as much as a single lost mile-per-hour as they moved closer to that aforementioned real reason to come to South Florida.

They were about to enter one of the last remaining virgin frontiers in North America.

Little more than an hour drive from Miami proper was a visitor center with a gift shop and marked trails stretching more than a half mile into the authentic world-renowned "River of Grass."

They parked and disembarked from their station wagon en masse and proceeded down a winding asphalt trail into the pristine heart of the Florida jungle, if you will.

When the Jesuits talk about finding God's presence in the world, they could have been thinking about this place. Dennis MulQueen was entirely breathless now in the midst of this purest of natural beauty settings that stretched out for what seemed like forever. He had never known a world like this existed, which, despite an annual onslaught of tourists like himself and his family, appeared mostly undisturbed and pristine, save the occasional plastic bag or tin foil gum wrapper.

Great Blue Herons with their huge four foot stature and pointed tan beaks stood motionless like sentries in the water under the sizzling spring sun, snow white egrets with their cockatoo feathered heads perched on both sides of the trail in the distance with their long black legs and snowy white facades calling for immortalization in picture.

The black-and-white kites with their arrow pointed wings sliced the air overhead like an angry army of natural drones while the red-winged blackbirds sang their piercing spring mating calls over and over from perches in the tree canopy, while turtles of all varieties without a care in the world basked on partially submerged logs.

The long gray outlines of fish he could not identify lie still in perpetual trance beneath the surface, as did, ubiquitous in all directions, the main attraction, the primordial kings of the everglade domain, the alligators.

Over all of this natural panacea stood guard the magnificent mangroves in interlocking formation like a protective security fence circling the water with their tentacled branches reaching far and wide as if to keep the outside world at bay.

Further off in the visible distance, the silhouettes of the long-ago abandoned ancient Indian mounds stood out ominously above the horizon as a sorrowful reminder of what was once a complete natural balance, permanently sabotaged, as only humans could do, by the white man's perpetual conquest of other humans and the natural world, the barren mounds testimony to this relentless slaughter to obscurity of the indigenous population here and everywhere, reminiscent of the US Calvary at Wounded Knee or the Sherman tanks through Atlanta.

Nary a survivor.

Without a word, Dennis MulQueen valiantly sneaked off the main path about 10 yards into the thicket to get a close-up shot of about a 12 footer basking in the shallow water at the edge of the surrounding marsh.

He wasn't more than two feet from those primordial jaws when he heard her.

"Get back, get back right now Denny, oh my God what are you doing," his mother called out. "It's spring, there are babies around here you could be dinner getting that close, these are very powerful wild animals."

She was right. They look slow, they move slowly, he didn't know a gator can actually run a human down in a heartbeat, at 35 miles-per-hour no less, if he wanted to. He had no choice now but to put his white Polaroid swinger away and clamber back up onto the pathway, his two-minute Clyde Beatty moment over.

The timing was eerie as not another minute later, amid the loud croaking noises of the gators' mating calls and the cheery bird songs, a shrill scream from ahead, just around a bend in the path, pierced the sultry warm air.

A sobbing young girl of about 12 appeared, her mother's arms wrapped around her to no avail as she scurried to keep up with her inconsolable daughter. The reason for her tears was revealed later when the MulQueen's returned to the gift shop .

Her dog had wandered too close, and in the snap of two fingers the poor animal was lunch for a hungry gator.

~ ~ ~

He wasn't Ali, to be sure, but nonetheless there he was in a boxing ring, a gruff looking guy with a beard wearing black Everlast gloves in fighting pose, legs bent one in front of the other at an angle, arms raised at a 45 degree angle to his body, with gloved fists clenched, looking every bit as fierce as Ali, with similarly searing beady eyes and a cold-hearted scowl.

There he was larger than life on the wall, the centerpiece of a giant 5'x4' oil-on-canvas portrait with gold gilt wood frame.

He looked like a powerful dude, too, this guy whose works were among the inspirational trove resting in that black wrought-iron book stand in the Canada lake-house living room underneath the Perry portraits.

Dennis MulQueen was more than familiar with this guy, because he had to read not only "The Old Man And The Sea" but also "A Farewell to Arms" in English class at U of D High in Detroit.

And here he was reliving it all, right here at the source, looking at Ernest Hemingway's portrait on the wall at the one and only Sloppy Joe's on Key West, Florida, Hemingway's favorite old bar haunt on Duval Street.

"That must have been a heck of a fight there," George MulQueen said, gesturing toward the massive 10-foot blue marlin mounted on the far wall.

For the guy famous for defining courage as "grace under pressure," it didn't end up all that well. But as obsessed with war and death as he was, what a perfect spot to hang out and create, or re-live, so many of the iconic war and death scenes that permeated his writing.

For the history of Key West where he wrote Farewell to Arms in the 1930s is steeped in war, going back to the beginning. The island was first owned by the Spanish, who named it *Cayo Hueso* – translated as Bone Island, for the piles of bones covering its coral rock surface from the Native American tribe the Calusa. Ponce De Leon, the first non-native settler, allegedly "discovered" these skeletal bones when he arrived in the 1500s.

Later, in 1763, Key West was taken over and owned by the British, then Spain took it back again until Florida became part of the United States in 1821.

During the Civil War, while the state of Florida as a whole was part of the confederacy, the island itself was controlled by the North.

Even though Union troops were stationed here, most of the locals flew confederate flags.

As proof of that history, after leaving Sloppy Joe's to tour the rest of the island, the MulQueens quickly came upon Fort Zachary Taylor at the furthest southwest end, and later the two Fort Martellos on the south side, two Civil War garrisons still standing.

Moreover, Fort Jefferson, another military installation of this era located on the nearby islands named the Dry Tortugas, is only a short boat ride from Key West proper.

The US Military first came to the island in the 19th century to protect against Blackbeard and other marauding pirates who regularly attacked and plundered commercial vessels who travelled the nearby Straits of Florida for international commerce.

Things had come a long way since then as the MulQueens stopped by the main port to get a better look at the huge Naval ships and a US Coast Guard cutter docked there. As they exited the car to look, US Navy planes on their training missions screeched by overhead as they spun their milky webs high in the azure tropical sky.

The Conch Republic, as they like to call themselves, is not as independent as they think. Back in the car, the MulQueen entourage passed several blocks of what looked like giant gray Lego block buildings by the sea, but were actually barracks housing hundreds of seamen.

One of the main thoroughfares was named Truman Avenue after US President Harry Truman, the guy who dropped the atomic bombs on Japan to end WWII.

During his presidency, Truman visited Key West 126 times, for varying lengths of time.

A high security complex where Truman always stayed, soon came to be known as the Truman Little White House.

He was only one of numerous US presidents to visit Key West over the years going back to Ulysses Grant and including John F. Kennedy at the time of the Cuban missile crisis.

President Dwight D. Eisenhower had a presence here too, as he also spent time at the Little White House, his longest stay being when he came to recuperate from a heart attack he suffered during his presidency.

He too is honored with his own thoroughfare, Eisenhower Drive.

Ironic Eisenhower's name would be attached to Key West because the island's dominating military presence contrasts with the great fears Eisenhower had about the "Military Industrial Complex," a term he coined in his last national address to the American people while president.

One of the great US generals, Eisenhower warned of the explosive growth of the US defense industry following WW II.

In his farewell speech to the nation on Jan. 17, 1961, Eisenhower presciently warned the U.S responsibility to "enhance liberty, dignity and integrity among people and among nations" faced a grave threat from a military industrial complex run amok.

"Until the latest of our world conflicts, the United States had no armaments industry. But now...we have been compelled to create a permanent armaments industry of vast proportions. ...," Eisenhower stated.

"Three and a half million men and women are directly engaged in the defense establishment. We annually spend on military security more than the net income of all Unites States corporations. This immense military establishment has become the very structure of our society."

Therein lies the danger, Eisenhower warned.

"We must guard against the acquisition of unwarranted influence, whether sought or unsought, by the military industrial complex," he said.

"The potential for the disastrous rise of misplaced power exists and will persist."

Eisenhower also had a caveat for the intellectual profiteers that run the American higher education system and its technology labs.

He warned that the universities and their research arms are so intertwined with and dependent on the military industrial complex and government contracts that there is danger "our public policy could itself become the captive of the scientific/technological elite."

Ironic that Key West, which had such a special place in his heart, with its dominant military presence, was home to writers like Hemingway (Farewell to Arms), John Dos Passos (USA Trilogy), and John Hersey (Hiroshima) who made their reputations writing about war – the horrors of war.

More irony as the MulQueens drove by the Key Wester hotel on South Roosevelt Blvd near the airport where peacenik John Lennon stayed when he was on the island, and also passed by the gates to Bahama Village, which Muhammed Ali, who refused to fight in the Viet Nam War, paid to have constructed when he visited the island.

Before departing Key West, there had to be one final stop: the personal residence of the man himself.

They toured 907 Whitehead St, the house Hemingway called home from 1931 until December of 1939, like it was the Louvre or the Smithsonian, poring over every artifact. In his writing cottage behind the stately main house, his Royal typewriter was still there on the upright desk in the corner where he famously wrote standing up, the descendants of his legendary six-toed cats still prowling the grounds.

Hemingway might be the most famous, but actually Dos Passos was first – he came to Key West in the 1920s, and Hemingway followed him after he told his good friend about the tropical paradise when they were together in Paris as part of the famed "Lost Generation" of expatriate American writers who lived there in the 1920s and 1930s.

Once established by Dos Passos and Hemingway, the Key West literary tradition took off and over time the list of literary giants that at one time or another called the Conch Republic home would grow to include Tennessee Williams, Ralph Ellison, Robert Frost, Wallace Stevens, Elizabeth Bishop, John Ciardi, Tom McGuane, Judy Blume, Carson McCullers, Gore Vidal, Terrance McNally, James Kirkwood, Shel Silverstein, Ann Beattie, William Wright, Annie Dillard, James Gleick, John Malcolm Brinnin, Edmund White, Richard Wilbur, Allison Lurie, and James Merrill to name a few. Not to mention all the great musicians and painters and sculptors that would also call the place home. And one particularly famous musician, who is also a pretty good writer. Many people don't know Key West's own Jimmy Buffett is one of only seven authors to have a number one bestseller on the *New York Times* fiction and nonfiction lists.

What a great place this would be to live and write someday, Dennis MulQueen thought.

~ ~ ~

Moms Mabley never met a tourist attraction she didn't like. So the next day started off with a visit to the Monkey Jungle, "where the people are caged and the monkey's run free," before heading to the Miami Serpentarium ,where the main show consisted of watching a famous herpetologist named William Hass milk the venom of numerous poisonous snakes with the highlight coming as he removed the front side of a tall wooden box and out popped a giant King Cobra, only about 10 feet of grass and a single thin line of white rope suspended in the air between the spectators and the deadly reptile.

Keeping the daredevil theme alive, the last stop before heading back up north came at the Miami Parrot Jungle, where the highlight was the McCaw circus where the

MulQueens, seated in a mini-auditorium, got to see a group of very colorful parrot Wallendas ride tiny little blue bicycles across a tight rope strung between two platforms up in the air above the ground.

~ 6 ~

THE CHICKENS ARE GOING
TO COME HOME TO ROOST

On March 1, 1971, a bomb exploded in the men's room at the United States Capitol. The Weather Underground Organization, a leading group of anti-war, anti-government activists with ties to Michigan, claimed responsibility.

At the end of the month, on March 29, 1971, U..S. Army Lieutenant William Calley was found guilty in US Courts of the premeditated murder of 22 Vietnamese citizens, a scar on US military history forever known as the My Lai Massacre.

But the Vietnam war continued to rage despite Calley's conviction and escalating public dissent across the country.

By the third week of April after the MulQueens had returned from Paradise to the real world of Michigan, chaos was erupting everywhere, across college campuses, major city streets and the nation's capital.

On April 24th, 1971, more than 500,000 demonstrators converged on Washington D.C. demanding an immediate end to the war started to 'stop communism.'

On the same day, 150,000 protesters marched in downtown San Francisco.

Barely a week later, on May 1, 35,000 protesters gathered in West Potomac Park in Washington, D.C. and attempted to disrupt the government with a series of marches and sit-ins throughout the Capital. In response to what was called the May Day Protests, the government deployed 10,000 military troops in the area, including helicopters and 4,000 troops from the US 82nd Airborne Division, in addition to 5,100 D.C. Metropolitan Police, 2,000 National Guard troops and President Richard Nixon's own internal security force.

Pitting the vast government military and law enforcement machine against the people, 12,614 citizens were arrested between May 1 and May 4, making it the largest mass arrest in US history.

The local Detroit newspapers and TV and radio stations – as well at the national media – continued to saturate the airwaves with news of the protests and more details of the war and its atrocities. At local cafes and restaurants, local sporting and musical events, and on college campuses – particularly the University of Michigan – the war dominated the conversation. There were not enough jails, there were not enough soldiers, there were not enough cops to arrest the millions of protesters nationwide demanding an end to this war.

In the meantime, while all this chaos in the world continued to escalate, Dennis MulQueen's personal Vietnam continued to escalate at the red brick bungalow on Kipling Avenue in Oak Park, Michigan.

He had received 10 letters and numerous phone calls and scholarship offers from colleges trying to recruit him to play football for them.

One of the suitors was the Air Force Academy, which was where his father wanted him to go. But he wanted to go to U-Mass, that was his number one choice.

His mother wanted him to go to the military school also, but he told her there was no way, with what was happening in Viet Nam, that he was going to join any branch of the US military. Now they were both upset with him, now he wasn't talking to either of them.

For months he sent in no paperwork, no responses, anywhere.

Finally, after much maternal prodding, he sent a few apps out late in the year.

Timing is everything, he learned the hard way.

He had already missed several school's deadlines, and since it was very late in the year others were now requesting his latest grades.

To the tune of a 1.5 on his latest report card.

Not good.

His Mother handed him four letters after their return from Florida.

Worse than not good.

Four more lost opportunities.

Because he didn't qualify for admission with a 1.5 GPA.

Anywhere.

~ ~ ~

What sounded like a runaway truck crashing into the side of the house shook the walls and rattled the windows of the three-room edifice on the corner of Kipling and Northend.

That's one hell of a slammed door, he thought as he was in his room, lying in bed reading a little Doc Savage. Amazingly, no broken glass sounds.

What the hell is going on now, that was the question he asked himself.

He heard shouting, and what must have been a chair slamming into the kitchen table.

He heard moaning, heaving, groaning. Something else slammed, something else about it being over. The end. He couldn't make out too many words, but it sounded like somebody died.

Then he made out the name Pasquale. Then Comer.

There was more incoherent mumbling.

Then, the volume elevated and the words came through raspy but clear.

"He's done. He isn't going to make it."

"What do you mean he's not going to make it, George?"

"He's done Pat. Comer told me. He hasn't been to class in three months. He's not going to make it."

"He's not going to graduate."

Then muffled sounds, like the moaning of a wounded animal caught in a snare.

About 10 seconds later the door to the back side bedroom swung wildly open, the brass door knob crashing through the drywall on the far wall behind it.

His father stagger-stepped into his bed room bent over like he was carrying a very heavy weight on his shoulders. He faced his son, perpendicular to the bed, who was lying down in the bottom bunk.

Their eyes met and the guy that was president of everything was hunched over withered and wan like a beaten man, everything red, his bald head red, his face red, his hair disheveled, his eyes bloodshot red. His cheeks were shiny red.

Dennis MulQueen stared at his father with a winced look like he was indeed looking into the eyes of a very powerful wounded animal.

Then he saw the tracks. Lines of molten white fire running down his crimson red cheeks.

The guy he never saw cry before was standing over him, sobbing, his breath coming in gasps and heaves.

"You are done, you are not going to graduate." His voice was gravelly, almost a hoarse whisper now, the exact opposite of his normally booming baritone.

"You never went to class, you never showed up, you don't give a fuck, you are flunking three classes, why, why, why would you do this? What the fuck is wrong with you?"

Spit was flying out of his mouth as he struggled to get the words out.

"I'll tell you one thing you're going to find out, the chickens are going to come home to roost someday."

His father had been out somewhere, he could smell it on his breath. The next thing he knew, he smacked him, several times.

"Call the police, he's going to kill me," his son screamed.

George MulQueen was a good fighter in his day, he won boxing tournaments when he was in the Navy, but these were not a boxer's punches.

His son barely felt a thing.

These were feeble kid-glove shots, like an angry child lashing out at another child.

He laid there, motionless, in the fetal position in the bottom bunk with his arms around his head.

After all was said and done, there was no physical harm, zero physical damage to think about. That's not anything either would have to live with.

What he would carry with him forward from that day was the look in his father's eyes, the sound of his voice that day. The disappointment.

And the tracks of those white-hot lines, they would stay with him too, long on into the future, until that day many years forward when memories of those tears were replaced, that day when he found out, under way worse circumstances, what those cotton candy jabs and those white hot streaks that day really meant.

That day in the future when he figured out what those first tears were all about, on that horrible day in the future when he learned of his father crying for only the second time ever, in the afternoon, in the evening, and all night long.

Those would be the tears that he would never forget.

~ ~ ~

This was one of those carefully crafted work spaces you would expect to see on the top floor of the General Motors Building, or the back corner of a Wall Street investment bank – the hardwood wainscoting, the floor-to-ceiling multi-paneled glass windows, the solid polished wood desk against the far wall.

Not the type of office you would expect to find occupied by the vice principal at a local high school.

But this was no ordinary school. This was the University of Detroit Jesuit High School, the top-rated college prep school in the state of Michigan. And probably the entire Mid West, if they ever did a survey. This place was hands down superior in the way that counts – in regards to intellectual achievement. The class of 1971 had 45 national merit semi-finalists, with the next closest other local school being in the single digits. The place graduated literally over the years thousands of attorneys, medical doctors, engineers and business and civic leaders.

Maybe that's it – the office had to match the school – and the occupant.

Because this was the type of guy you would expect in a place like this, in a role like this. Like George and Pat MulQueen, this guy was a University of Detroit grad, and a starting lineman on the Titans' football team, which back in the day was a darn good team.

Tall and handsome, with a ramrod-straight back, he always sported neatly pressed dark slacks and a white shirt with short sleeves and meticulously shined see-your-face-in-the-mirror black wing-tip dress shoes. Jack-Benny-like black horn-rimmed glasses finished off the look.

You always knew he was coming before you spotted him in the hallway. Just follow the Old Spice trail and you could find him in the middle of a stadium.

He was the head basketball coach and the offensive line coach for the football team, and Dennis MulQueen knew him well – not because he played football and he was his history teacher but mainly because of his main job, Vice Principal in charge of student discipline.

His name was Dan Comer, and it was only apropos this tough hard-nosed Irishman had this job.

He was a hell of a guy, if he liked you – and you knew how to stay out of trouble.

But Dennis MulQueen? Trouble was his middle name. Trouble stalked this guy like a starving dog.

He was next in line, and he damn well knew it as he crossed the threshold to Mr. Comer's inner sanctum that day in late April of 1971. Dennis knew of a half guys from his class that Mr. Comer had already booted out the door. He would do whatever it took to protect the school.

"MulQueen, what the hell you think you've been doing around here? What on God's earth are you thinking, Son? I mean you haven't been to Spanish class all semester. And you haven't been to your film class and you haven't turned in your English paper either. MulQueen you are flunking three classes and you're not going to graduate like this. Do you understand me?"

"Sorry, Mr. Comer."

"Now, don't sorry me. What the hell is going on here? Why haven't you been to Mr. Pascuale's class?"

He said he made an offer to Mr. Pascuale to write a special term paper and spend the class time in the school library. It was going to be so spectacular that he needed an assistant to make it all happen. Enter Bokker Lee, his partner on the special project.

"MulQueen I wasn't born yesterday, and neither was Pascuale. And that's sure as heck not the story I get from him."

MulQueen kept at it.

"Mr. Pasquale has lots of trouble with English and he said yes. We must have just had a big misunderstanding."

"Don't even try and bullshit me MulQueen. Yeah it's big all right."

He leaned back in his wooden swivel chair and looked out the window, and then back at Dennis MulQueen.

"Now listen to me MulQueen. By all rights I should boot you right out the front door this very moment. You have been in how many fights, you show up late to class, late to your final exams, you skip classes, you've been suspended how many times now? You've had more jugs and more suspensions than anyone I know of in the history of this school. By far. And now this bullshit."

He paused and leaned forward in his wooden desk chair towards MulQueen.

"But you know what MulQueen? I don't know why I'm doing this. I talked to Harteau about you. I talked to your teachers. And I also talked to your parents. But I also coached you MulQueen and I know you have heart because I never saw you back down from anybody. But it's time you faced up to this and right now. Listen MulQueen, I know you're not a bad guy. So quit acting like it. I'm going to give you one last chance. Because in spite of all the evidence, I believe it's the right thing to do. So you know what MulQueen? I talked to Luttner about your English class. You can make up the paper there, but what about the film? You have to turn a film in to pass Kopeck's class."

"I will turn one in."

"Well you only have two weeks MulQueen. If you want to make an attempt at getting out of here with a diploma, I suggest you get your act together immediately and start with Pascuale. Turn this great big special project in that you and Harteau have been working on all semester in the library gym and maybe you'll get lucky and he will give you a passing grade also."

"By the way, when I talked to your father he's not too happy with you. He is very disappointed. And that goes for your mother also. They spent a lot of money over here. Is there anything else going on I should know about? Anything going on at home to explain why you are acting this stupidly? Because I had you in class and I know you're not stupid, MulQueen."

"No, nothing that I can think of."

"You're lying, MulQueen, but all right, we'll leave it at that. Whatever is bothering you, whatever you are worrying about, forget about it, okay. Forget about it, forget about the whole world, and just concentrate on the job at hand, okay? Let's get it together MulQueen, and right now. The party's over, you understand?"

"Yes, Mr. Comer."

"Come back in at the end of the day Friday and I want an update."

"Thank you, Mr. Comer."

~ ~ ~

The Jesuit scholastic looked up with his thin swarthy face and oversized dishwater-grey glasses lurching back and forth like he was a human bobble head.

No offense, but this guy was like a cartoon caricature, a funny pages kind of a guy.

That's the primary reason for this conundrum, Dennis MulQueen tried to rationalize to himself. He couldn't help it. Some people beg to be taken advantage of and he just couldn't help it. What do they call that? Sophistry?

Mr. Pascuale moved that bobble head of his slightly to the right as he inhaled and then back down again as he exhaled. His lips and cheeks shuddered slightly on the exhale like he was spitting raspberries.

But he wouldn't look at his student eye-to-eye and he stated not a word as Dennis MulQueen attempted his best groveling imitation ever.

"We are almost done, señor. We just need a little more time to make this thing really great. It will be on your desk by the middle of next week, I promise. I'll be back Mr. Pascuale. We are working really hard on this Mr. Pascuale and I'll report in every day from now on. Okay?"

He said nothing as MulQueen left and headed straight to the library. The real library this time, not the library gym. He pulled a book from the shelves entitled "Dias De Espana," with a worn green jacket cover of colorful adobe buildings on a hill side.

He proceeded to write – make that cowrite (along with the author of the book) – the best 35-page plagiarized term paper ever.

He said a prayer it works, as he left the library and headed back over to the gym.

Because if it doesn't work, he was afraid it wouldn't be kid gloves the next time.

~ ~ ~

The following week, three more rejection letters came in the mail. Time to take a walk.

South on Kipling. East on 8 mile. A five minute walk.

When he walked in the front door, there she was. Dolly Parton bellied up to the bar.

Or at least her twin. At least from his vantage point off to the side.

She had that bleached blond puffed-up coif with a row of black roots visible from underneath, a pushed-up inflated chest overflowing a smooth white satin blouse, to go with a tight gray skirt replete with the black fishnets.

Side views can be misleading.

Once he strutted in the 8-mile dive bar about three blocks down from Kipling and mounted the barstool next to her, she turned toward him and smiled and the perspective changed like somebody flipped the channel. The cake makeup topped off by grease-paint thick cherry-red lipstick took over the scene.

With the kerosene-like perfume and yellow smoke-stained teeth in his face now, Dolly was now low-end hillbilly.

When she opened her mouth to speak, he knew what they meant by kissing your sister – or more like being cornered in the living room alcove at Christmas as stinky old drunken Aunt Mabel rams her tongue down your throat.

"So what brings you here young man?"

"Oh just out for a stroll looking for a drink."

"Well hey kid let me buy you a drink. You don't look like you're old enough to buy ur own cocktail. What cha havin' there, good lookin'?"

"A martini please."

She barked out the order.

"And another highball for me too, please"

She started smiling and scooched her chair right up next to him, they were practically touching.

"Now tell me about yourself. Where you from kid. What cha' doin'? You're such a handsome young man."

She looked herself over in the mirror behind the bar and then back at Dennis MulQueen. Before he could even answer, she reached behind her back and appeared to fumble with the zipper. "Please can you zip me up and fasten the clasp on the back of my dress.?"

He looked at her. Oh my god woman, he said to himself, you want me to undress you right here at the bar?

Her blouse was open about two inches in the back. No problem closing the zipper, but fastening the clasp, that was another matter. That's when he saw movement behind him in the bar mirror. He saw a man in a black cowboy hat with a greased black mustache approaching them.

It was too late.

"Hey fuckhead, you ready to die today?"

"Pardon me?"

He noticed the guy had a black leather jacket on, a black T, and black boots to go with his black pants. A Jack Palance look alike. Only this was no movie.

He reached into his right pocket and pulled out a cobalt-colored Saturday night special and pointed it at Dennis MulQueen. Right in the bar, in front of everybody.

"Get your fucking hands off my woman before I blow your fucking head off."

The heavy set bartender in a white shirt and black bolo string tie looked down and pretended he was washing a glass in the sink.

"Oh I apologize sir, she just asked me to fasten the back of her dress I meant nothing by it honest to god sir I'm sorry."

His heart felt like a football in his chest, to go with the softball in his throat.

"Harry, no. Put that thing away, it's over Harry, this isn't Viet Nam any more. Remember you said you didn't want to do any more killing."

She looked at Dennis MulQueen, then back at Harry, then she called for another highball for Harry. The bartender retrieved a Jim Beam bottle from behind him and started talking to Harry about something Dennis MulQueen couldn't make out as he fixed another drink.

She motioned underneath the bar with her thumb toward the door.

Dennis MulQueen was already one foot out the door. In fact, he ran to the door so fast when he opened it he hit himself in the leg with it.

Only two blocks east was Bare Assets.

It's got to be better over here, he thought.

The flashing red sign said peep shows. A sign in the window to the right of the door said massage.

He turned the scratched up gold knob and walked inside.

There were books and magazines lining the back wall, and a glass covered counter on the right that contained every conceivable sex toy on earth. A red sign with a gold silhouette of a woman with an arrow pointing straight ahead caught his eye.

Then she caught his eye.

"Welcome sir," said a middle aged woman in a black pantsuit with a white blouse as she stepped into the room and bowed towards the 17-year-old high school student.

She looked like she could have been the server at the local jack in the box. Or a hostess at Bob Evans. She was apparently the MC here.

"Come follow me. You have your choice of the best of the best this evening young man. Only the best for you sir."

They walked straight ahead down that narrow corridor ahead until they came to the first door on the right, which was wide open.

A big-breasted woman with a black negligee and dark black hair sitting on a black vinyl chair against the back wall smiled and motioned with her right index finger to come on in.

When she stood up he could see through the gauzy see-through nylon fabric that she was wearing a turquoise g string with a matching bikini top that barely concealed her blow-up doll boobs.

She had uneven teeth but at least they were white. She dipped her chin down and in as she stood up and preened and pirouetted on her gold sequined pencil pumps as she leaned over toward the wall and thrust her rear in the air at him.

He kept walking to the next door, where he was greeted by a shapely thin and tall brunette with smaller boobs and bright red lipstick. There was a ditsy-looking red head in the third room. Oh My God. They have it all here he thought as he turned and pointed to the middle room.

He walked in and she closed the door behind him.

"Nice to meet you, my name is Marjorie. Please undress and sit on the table and get ready for the time of your life."

The back wall behind the table bed was lined with shelves of every kind of oil and cream – and incense – you could imagine.

It smelled like – well, exactly what you would expect a perfumed-up room at a place like this would smell like.

He sat on the edge of the table that was covered with a very thin white pad.

"Let me help you," she said as she walked over and reached out to unbutton his shirt. He turned his shoulders to the side and inhaled deeply.

She was on the second button when he brushed her hand to the side and stood up.

"Excuse me I'm sorry. I just remembered. I left my wallet in the car. I'll be right back."

"Oh. okay. No problem. I'll be here."

When he exited the front door he sprinted across all four lanes of 8 Mile Road like he was still running from the guy with the gun. He turned left and didn't stop until he was back on Kipling.

Instead of crossing back over to the other side where his parent's house was, he turned right on Northend and kept on walking. Straight down North End Avenue, it was about maybe 40 minutes until he got to Pearson Street in Ferndale. He knocked on the door. His best buddy Bokker Lee let him in.

The next morning, he heard Bokker's father downstairs in the living room.

"I hope I'm not feeding whoever those tugboats belong to," he said pointing to the 13 EEE black wing tips resting on the bottom stair.

Dennis MulQueen had officially run away from home. He stayed there over two weeks, until Bokker's mother insisted he call his parents and let them know where he was. She drove him back to Kipling the next day

~ 7 ~

A KNIFE TO THE THROAT

"**D**ennis MulQueen," the guy in the maroon robes up on the stage called out.

Before his name had a chance to reverberate off the soundproofed white walls of the stately Ford Auditorium in Detroit, Michigan, everybody inside – students, parents, teachers and even Mr. Comer – broke protocol and stood up and shook the rafters with a thunderous standing ovation, even though the principal's introductory instructions were no clapping for any individual, please, only collective applause at the end.

He couldn't believe it.

Nobody could believe it.

He made it. They let him walk.

Fr. Polakowski walked up to him in the lobby afterward.

"I've never seen that before, Dennis. Congratulations."

He said it again, as if in amazement. He could never recall an instance of a student getting that kind of ovation.

"I guess it takes a special record of achievement, to get recognized like that," Fr. Polakowski said with a wide smile creasing his face.

"Yeah, I guess one isn't the loneliest number, huh father?"

They looked at each other and smiled. He knew, the smirk gave it away. Dennis MulQueen didn't need to elaborate on that one.

"You're the only one in more ways than one, Dennis," he said.

One as in 1.0. His GPA for the last semester. That had also probably never happened before either. Talk about records you don't want to set.

But it was the truth. He was the only student to ever graduate with a perfect 1.0 on his final card marking, at least that Fr. Polakowski said he ever knew of.

But he made it. That's all that counts, right?

~ ~ ~

Several weeks later, in mid-June, the *New York Times* and the *Washington Post* alternated publication of the Pentagon Papers, with soon about 15 other papers jumping in with coverage of their own.

The Defense Department study, leaked to the press by Daniel Ellsberg, showed that a series of four U.S Presidents beginning with Harry Truman and on through Presidents Eisenhower, Kennedy and Johnson, systematically lied to the American public and Congress about US involvement in the war in Viet Nam, and US government actions and intentions regarding the war, such as the government's secret bombing of Laos and Cambodia and the coast of North Vietnam, all of which was hidden from Congress and the media.

Daniel Ellsberg, who released these classified documents, was immediately charged with conspiracy, espionage and theft of government property. During the Watergate scandal, it was revealed that officials in the Nixon administration had mounted a systematic campaign to smear and discredit Ellsberg and the charges were eventually dropped. Nixon's solicitor general said the Pentagon papers were an example of "massive over-classification" of government documents with "no trace of a threat to National Security." The big question for the public was if this is truly a democracy why is the United States government allowed to "classify" whatever documents it chooses so they can hide from the people the truth of what the government is doing at home and abroad?

In the meantime, despite graduating, Dennis MulQueen's personal Viet Nam continued with the final rejection letters all in now and no athletic scholarship, no college opportunity of any kind, and no job prospect of any kind on the horizon. He was in his bed room sitting on his bed re-reading the letter from U Mass when the door swung open and once again there he was in his face.

"Please get off your ass and get out there and get a job, will you please do something?"

Later that night after his father left for his Ford Motor Co. job, Dennis MulQueen joined his mother in the living room.

"He hates me."

"No, he doesn't. He just wants you to succeed. Come down to the newspaper tomorrow. I'll give you a job. You can write some stories. You can start out with Government Day on Thursday."

He gladly walked into her office the next afternoon, with her black metal and brown Formica top desk in the middle of the room barely visible with the papers and boxes and baskets of paper and notes and glue and notebooks and pens and pencils – a journalistic version of a haystack.

"A messy desk is the sign of a genius," a sign on the wall read.

This was the glass ceiling breaker's final career stop, this corner office in the Northwest Metro Newspaper building behind the shopping center and next to a pool hall at 9 Mile

Road and Coolidge Highway, the heart of downtown Oak Park, Michigan. After stints at the *Detroit News*, the *Wyandotte Tribune*, her present gig as Editor and Publisher – make that owner – of Northwest Metro Newspapers saw her producing seven weeklies including the *Northwest Record* and the *Northwest Detroiter* as well as papers in Oak Park, Southfield, Berkley, Huntington Woods and Pleasant Ridge.

She had pictures hanging on the wall of some of the people she had met and interviewed and written about over the years, including an autographed picture she got from US Sen. Ted Kennedy, a picture of his older brother John F. Kennedy from when he was in Oak Park campaigning for president in the fall of 1960, US Sen. Phil Hart, Michigan Gov. George Romney, State Representatives Joe Forbes of Oak Park, Detroit Mayors Jerome Cavanagh and Roman Gribbs, and numerous celebrities she had interviewed over the years for feature articles including Elizabeth Taylor, Charlton Heston, and Rock Hudson.

Her son wasn't going to be interviewing anybody comparable to those folks. His first assignment was to quote the Oak Park City Manager and a few other low-level municipal grunts from various departments about Oak Park's "Government Day."

He handed his 12-paragraph work of art to her a couple days later, the highlight of which was the inner workings of the Oak Park jail, with its thick green metal door and hardwood bed – sans any mattress and nary a blanket in site.

She pursed her lips as she perused his first story ever, which in a hot instant went from 12 paragraphs to nothing.

He was sitting in her office in the black vinyl swivel chair across from her desk when, after about a 30-second read, she balled it up and tossed it in the corner wastebasket.

"I can't believe my son wrote this. You can do so much better than this. Please do it over. You might want to start by describing the police department, and the work they do, what kind of people end up behind that green door and for what reasons, and after you create some interest then describe what the other city departments do so people have an idea how government actually functions and affects their lives – and in the process inform the reader how not to end up behind that green door."

"Yeah, okay."

He turned sideways with his head down so she couldn't see his face, as he quickly exited her office.

Clearly he wasn't cut out for journalism, or a writing career of any kind.

But he managed to fake his way through the piece in a re-do, but nonetheless it was time for a job transfer. He told her he didn't really like writing and she offered him a job in the circulation department, in the newly-created position of delivery manager. She phrased it as a necessary undertaking for the good of the company.

This is where we need you now, plenty of time to learn about the writing business later, she said.

~ ~ ~

"Step it up, will you please. Come on now, Goddamn it. How fucking lazy are you? Can't you work a little bit?

"Jesus Christ, move a little will you for God's sake? At this rate we'll be here a month just to get this one block done."

The spit was flying from Dennis MulQueen's face and his skin was red if not purple, as he screamed and berated the African American Kelly Services employee in front of him, one of dozens the company hired each week to deliver the newspapers door-to-door throughout the cities they covered.

He certainly heard Dennis MulQueen. And he apparently felt the sting of his words, too.

The newly installed delivery manager for Northwest Metro Newspapers flinched but otherwise had no time to react or utter a single word as the guy spun like lightning and grabbed him by the shirt collar and pinned him against the side of the white circulation department truck. Dennis MulQueen's heart and spinal cord seared a white-hot rope of terror up and down his internal viscera as he felt the silver blade press against his throat a mere angstrom from death.

"Listen to me, honky-tonk motherfucker, I don't know who the fuck you think u're talkin' to, but I 'm gonna slit your fucking throat and cut your fucking head off and roll it down the street like a bowling ball, you understand me, if you ever ever talk to me like that ever again. You understand me, you fucking honky-tonk racist punk?"

"A yeah, sorry," he managed in a low guttural voice.

"I just, ahh, you see, I'm not racist. I didn't mean it like that, these are my mother's newspapers and I'm just trying to, you know, do a good job for her. Sorry."

His chest felt like it was about to explode. His knees quivered.

"Yeah, motherfucker, that's what they all say when they put a bullet in your back for jaywalkin'. Well, listen motherfucker, it don't happen like that with me. You see, I'm not out here to take your fuckin' shit, I wouldn't be out here for no minimum wage suck-ass job like this takin' ur honky fuckin' shit if I had anywhere else to go. Got that, fat fuckin' white prick?"

Dennis MulQueen could see the whites of his eyes, and the thin red lines, filled with blood, about to burst with the fury of what he surely saw as just another white man slave master ripping him open with another racist rant, probably just like so many others.

"I ought to kill you, honky motherfucker."

"I'm sorry. I didn't mean it like that. I swear. I'm really sorry."

The temp worker from Kelly's twisted Dennis MulQueen's shirt just a little tighter for emphasis to make sure he could feel the veins swell in his neck. Then he instantly let go and slowly backed up, as he flipped the long silver blade back into the black handle of the switch blade he held in his right hand. Without saying another word, he turned and reached into the truck and grabbed another bale of papers. He brought the knife out again and slit the twine like it was butter, put the knife back in his right front pants pocket and stuffed a sheaf of papers into the orange-and-black canvas newspaper bag hanging from his shoulders. He walked up the sidewalk of the next house like nothing had happened.

About ten feet away from the door, he turned his head around and looked the boss in the eyes again.

Dennis MulQueen called out another weak, "Sorry, man."

They continued the same slow, steady pace of delivering that day's newspaper, up and down the streets of Oak Park, 8 hours in a row, a short half-hour lunch break the only interruption. His new job put him in charge of these crews making sure the papers got delivered.

At the end of the day they did all get delivered, with time to spare, and minus any further verbal entreaties from the new delivery manager. As he turned to get in the truck for the drive back to the office, he felt two sharp taps from behind on his right shoulder.

"Sorry about all that today, man. It's just there's only so much a man can take. Like I said, I wouldn't be out here if things was lookin' up for me, okay, man? But somebody needs to teach you, man. If you're gonna stay alive. Understand, man, you got to learn how to treat people if u're gonna make it, you understand, man? I get it now your

93

intentions are good and you are young and you don't want to let your Mama down. I didn't know it's your newspapers, but that ain't the way to do it. Cuz what you put out, you get back, man. It's called Karma. I know that much."

Dennis shook his head and apologized again, said thank you, and extended his hand toward the man he had insulted that morning.

They   shook   hands   and   embraced.

~ 8 ~

LIFE IS A FOOTBALL FIELD

With his left hand he turned the dial counter clockwise on the antique Arthur Godfrey-era square wooden box transistor radio on top of the adjacent bookshelf as he picked up the receiver with his right hand and dialed the number with his index finger as the cigar smoke swirled about him. When the phone began to ring, he leaned back in his wooden swivel office chair and propped his feet up on the old weather-beaten desk in Room 106 at Chadsey High School in Detroit, Michigan.

"Hi Dan. This is George MulQueen. Mike Rhoades told me to call you. Said you are interested but you might want to see him first."

"Oh, okay. Yeah, George. I talked to Mike again. He said he worked him out and he vouched for him. I don't need a workout, he sent me the films. I looked at the film from the Divine Child game, that guy was all-league and your kid totally dominated him. I think he pancaked the guy six or seven times I counted and the guy didn't have a tackle all game.

"And I talked to Frank Buford. He vouched for him too. Frank said they clocked him in the 40 under 5. He said he was 4.9 and he's benching 250 and he's tougher than hell. Frank said he is in the same mold as Pietrzak or Bob

Johnson, the guys before him over there at his position. Pietrzak is starting for us this year and he's going to be All-American and he's headed for the NFL. Frank thinks your kid has the same potential. We're happy to have him, George, if that's the case."

"I know you'll be happy with him, Dan. He had 10 other schools that wanted him. But the academics, Dan, that's why he's still available. The school was supposed to send you copies of his SAT's and his transcripts. Mike said you could help with the academic part?"

"Yeah, we already got all that, George. I talked to the admissions director, they are on board, as long as he's got the diploma, that's all he needs. I told him he had a car accident, that's why his marks are so bad at the end, but his SAT's are actually quite high, George. They couldn't figure out those marks with scores like that until I told them about the accident. As long as he's got the diploma, they know he can pass up here with the rug weaving and bicycling classes I'm going to set him up with. We just need a copy of his diploma, George. Get it in as soon as possible and we'll go from there."

"Okay, we'll get that to you right away. And thanks, Dan. You'll be very pleased, Dan. The kid's tougher than cat shit. I'm gonna tell ya, he doesn't back down from anybody, or anything. He brings the goods, Dan."

"I hope so, George. I've built a program here that's designed for the next level. I should have ten or eleven guys off the current team get drafted, more than State or U of M or Notre Dame."

"What about the money, Dan?"

"I'm giving him a full ride for this year, George. But I'm only going to guarantee the first year, okay? If he shows he's got what we think he has and he continues to develop then I'll get you the next three years, okay, George? It'll all be in the paperwork. You should get everything in a couple days. Have him sign everything and get it back to us as soon as possible, okay? He better be a hard worker, George."

"No problem there, Dan."

"Just tell him to show up ready to bring it; we start next week with three-a-days. I want him on the field by then so he doesn't fall behind.

"Okay, Dan. Thanks. I'll get everything taken care of right away. Talk to you soon."

~ ~ ~

"I'm gonna rip 'ur fuckin' head off, honky, but first I'm gonna stomp ur balls in the ground and then I'm gonna tear your fucking head off. You understand me, you fucking piece of shit, I am going to kill you. Today is the day you die. I hate you, motherfucker, you understand?"

Dennis MulQueen had just taken his stance across from this guy, he couldn't help but feel the fear singe up and down his spine, like he was looking down the barrel of a cannon.

He knew who this guy was. Everybody knew who this guy was.

He wasn't the most terrifying physical specimen – height-wise. Not much more than 6 feet tall, if that.

But he was as wide as he was tall. His legs were like tree trunks. His arms looked like they belonged to Thor. And he moved like greased lightning. And he exploded off the line like a cannon. He was fierce, he was nasty, he hit with explosive power, and he was dirty in vicious ways.

He was the meanest SOB on the planet.

Lots of guys have impressive physical skills.

But this guy had attitude.

The eyes were a dead giveaway.

They looked like you would imagine Satan's. The whites were almost dirty white, like an old faded cue-ball, from a lot of work or wear and tear, and you could see the little red capillaries bulging as if about to burst, like that Kelly guy with the knife, from extreme internal pressure.

Yeah, about ready to pop and explode. He pawed the ground with his right foot, then his left, setting himself in the turf like an enraged bull about to charge. We are talking about bull power here, the power of a bull about to explode from the pain of having his balls strapped tight against his ass.

Dennis MulQueen's first big-time scrimmage. He hoped it wouldn't be his last. Talk about baptism by fire.

The battle fields of Viet Nam – you didn't know when or how it was coming there. At least you could try and hide in the bush or a ditch. Here, there was no place to hide. And you knew what was coming and how. Everybody heard the stories of this guy putting people in the hospital.

Dennis MulQueen wondered if the man across from him also saw those Emmett Till pictures.

A few plays later, there was no wondering.

There was nothing, except the trainer helping him back on his feet. Concussion number one.

But heck, nobody keeps track of those things.

Welcome to the big time, Dennis MulQueen.

He didn't know he was playing against a future Pro Bowl caliber NFL player, a guy who would lead the Detroit Lions in sacks one year even though he missed four games due to injury. On an outstanding NFL defensive line with Al "Bubba" Baker and Doug English (nicknamed the "Silver Rush").

His name was Dave Pureifory, and he didn't care who he was lined up against.

Welcome to the big time, Dennis.

Coach Boisture indeed built himself a big-time program at Eastern Michigan University.

Actually, it was more than big time; it turned out the Hurons did end up with more players on that team drafted into the NFL than Michigan or Notre Dame. No less than 10 players on that team would go on to play in the NFL. If he wasn't going up against Pureifory, who started out with the Packers before he starred with the Lions on the Silver Rush, then he had the fun opportunity of going up against a guy named John Banaszak, who ended up winning three Super Bowls as the starting defensive end on the famed "Steel Curtain" defense of the 1970s. Most remember Mean Joe Greene or L.C. Greenwood from that famous defensive line, but playing alongside those guys it was Banaszak who was named the defensive MVP of Super Bowl XIII with 6 tackles, two sacks, and a fumble recovery when the Steelers defeated the Dallas Cowboys in a game many still consider the greatest Super Bowl ever.

So Dennis MulQueen considered it a treat when he got to face off against Bob Boone, another All-American who was drafted by the Minnesota Vikings. Occasionally – and luckily, only occasionally – he got to go head-to-head with middle linebacker Will Foster, who played in the NFL for the Philadelphia Eagles.

As a freshman, he was mostly fodder for these guys. But give him credit. He brought all he had, every play. He could actually block Bob Boone, who was the same year as he was. He could block Banaszak, a sophomore, some of the time. But Pureifory – a senior – he couldn't stop him. But he stood up to him, and played against him – every single day in drills and scrimmages. If anybody was going to make a man out of him, it was Pureifory.

~ ~ ~

A couple weeks later, with the headaches, on top of everything else, he was having trouble sleeping. He took the elevator downstairs to the main Pittman Hall lounge and flipped on the TV hanging from the wall in the corner.

"We're asking for world peace, okay?" said John Lennon, wearing a green shirt with sergeant epaulettes and stars on the sides as wife Yoko and Dick Cavett looked on along with a national TV audience.

"You've been accused of being the dragon lady who broke up the Beatles" Cavett said to Yoko.

"Well, if she did," John interrupted, "then she gets the credit for a lot of the nice music that Paul and Ringo and George and myself have made since then."

It was Lennon - Ono film night on Cavett as the two musicians debuted several of the 12 avant-garde movies they made together, including "Fly," which is nothing more, nothing less, than a fly crawling all over a woman's body, presumably Yoko, beginning with the foot and the leg, and of course the woman's bottom as close ups of the fly show him waving his arms and antenna in the air like a conductor's wand.

Lennon and Yoko chain-smoked the entire time as another short played, this one titled "Erection," which was a slow motion time-capsulated view of an industrial building going up from day one of construction to finish.

The main draw was the film entitled "Imagine," which opened with an outside shot of a magnificent large building with stately Romanesque white columns roof-to-ground as John and Yoko walk into the building, with high ceilings and a very dark almost black interior, with only thin lines of floor to ceiling light rays visible through the wall of windows lining the back.

John walks to a white baby grand piano off to the side of the room and beings to play as Yoko opens the blinds to let the light in.

Yoko's sparkle headband and white flowery dress contrasted with Lennon's black shirt and black neckerchief and black shoes neatly set off by his snow white pants as the former Beatle sang his classic paean to hope for a world of peace without countries, religion or war.

As "Imagine" plays, Yoko opens more white shutters as John continues to sit at the white piano and sing.

After a nice ovation for this performance from the studio audience, Lennon said he would like to come back in the near future and perform live for Cavett and his audience.

"A while ago, you said you wanted to be forgotten," Cavett said. "Now you're talking about going out and performing again."

"Well, I can still be forgotten when I'm dead. I don't really care what happens when I'm dead," Lennon said.

Cavett wanted to talk about drugs and music. He asked about "Lucy in the Sky with Diamonds" being about drugs.

"Mel Tormé said it is about LSD, that's the initials of the song's title, right? Well, my son came home from school one day with a drawing he showed me with a strange looking woman flying around in it.

"I said it is beautiful, what is it? He said its 'Lucy in the Sky with Diamonds.' I immediately wrote a song about it. It wasn't about drugs a'tall."

"They said 'Eleanor Rigby' was about heroin because I wrote a song about Mr. Kite and Henry The Horse. I actually got the idea for most of the lyrics from an old circus poster for an old fashioned circus in the 1800s.

"'Happiness is a Warm Gun,' it was banned. They said it was about shooting up drugs. Well, I saw the front of a gun magazine. It said happiness is a warm gun; they were advertising guns. I thought it was crazy so I wrote a song about it."

Cavett asked him if he knew Janis Joplin or Jimmy Hendrix.

"She sent me a happy birthday tape just before she died. Singing happy birthday to me in the studio. I got it in the mail the day after she died."

"What do you think about the drug overdosing in and outside of the profession?" Cavett asked.

"The basic thing you have to ask is why do people take drugs from alcohol up to hard drugs, that question has to be resolved first before you can ask what can we do for the poor drug addict.

"Why do we have to have these accessories for normal living, that means there is something wrong with society that makes it so pressurized we can't live in it without guarding ourselves against it.

"If people are allowed to be a bit more free to express themselves they wouldn't have to be protected from getting hurt. People take drugs and drink so they don't feel what's going on around them. Freedom for everybody is our goal."

Maybe I should try some of that, Dennis MulQueen thought. Maybe I'll be able to sleep a little better. Or at least the headaches won't be quite as bad.

~ ~ ~

The next weekend, during warmups, he took his usual place on the field with the first unit. The line coach came up to him and informed him he wasn't starting this game. Because he was late for practice the day before after staying out late with a teammate.

As he walked off the field, he saw his father in the first row in the stands with Coach Rhoades next to him. He got in the game later and played the whole second half, but the damage was done.

He apologized to his father after the game. "That's all right, Son. Coach Rhoades said you looked good out there, you fired out with intensity."

It was the only game he didn't start all year.

~ 9 ~

IMAGINE

"Is he really going to be there, Aurelius? Are you kidding?"

"That's what they say, D? And if so, we should be able to touch him. We'll be real close. We'll only be a few rows away. Are you up for it, man?"

"Ah, yeah, I think I can fit it into my schedule."

His friend told him to be at his house by about 6 so they could grab a pizza and some drinks ahead of time.

By the time they got there, and walked inside, a steady drone of white noise permeated the fog already in place that made barely discernible a bowl of gray space off in the distance that was surrounded by towers of black boxes inside of two-story aluminum-bar scaffolding.

As they sat down in their seats, through the gauzy haze of sweet pungent smoke that was everywhere they could see a guy in black pants and matching dark shirt stroll up to the microphone all herky-jerky like a Ray Bradbury character lit up by strobe lights.

They were indeed within spitting distance, just a few rows back.

"Make no mistake about it. This country is in as bad a shape today as Nazi Germany was at the rise of Nazism," he said.

103

Through the overhead projector they could see the man was wearing a Roman collar.

Some kind of priest.

"Who is this guy?"

"Says here, D, on the program he is some guy named Father Groppie. That's all I know."

You could see his thick Jack Benny-like glasses through the sweet, white smoke. People were smoking joints and cigarettes and pipes everywhere. A guy to the left was smoking a cigar.

"What allowed Nazism to spread is good people who were quiet and said nothing," the guy on stage with the white collar said.

'Today, in this country, Richard Nixon is killing as many Indochinese as Hitler killed Jews. In this country, we can no longer sit back and say 'Look what happened there.' What happened there is happening here and now."

Crisler Arena in Ann Arbor, Michigan, was packed wall-to-wall on Friday, December 10, 1971, for this event, the "Free John Rally" aimed at trying to get the local political activist John Sinclair out of jail.

"Kick out the jams, motherfuckers."

That was his anthem – the kind of music John Sinclair liked. The kind of music he helped create – and manage.

Sinclair followed Malcolm X and heard him speak in person. He emulated Eldridge Cleaver and Huey Newton, creators of the Black Panther Party, so much so that he created the White Panther Party and incorporated the former group's manifesto as his own.

He was close associates with Abby Hoffman and Jerry Rubin, Ed Sanders and the Yippies, and by association became one of the anti-war movement's top figures.

This same guy, John Sinclair, was the main guy behind the late '60s "rock and roll revolution" whose credo was "total assault on the culture by any means necessary, including through rock and roll, dope, and fucking in the streets."

In that effort, Sinclair managed Iggy Pop and the Stooges, Billy C and the Sunshine Band, as well as MC-5, whose song "Kick Out The Jams" became a rallying cry across metro Detroit and the Midwest. It was along with the MC-5 band and Pun Plamondon that Sinclair created the White Panther Party, making it the first and only band in history to form a political party.

A combination of all of this led Sinclair to form the Detroit Artists' Workshop, which morphed into Trans Love Energies, which formed a commune and at one point controlled a several-blocks-long stretch of homes in Detroit, with the group bringing free films, music, painting and literature to anyone in the community who wanted to participate.

But it was Sinclair's first-ever use of the bands to disseminate radical political statements to a national audience through rock and roll that the government found particularly alarming.

Yeah, kick out the jams all right, all the way to Jackson State Prison.

Sinclair was arrested for giving two marijuana cigarettes to an undercover police woman, his third marijuana offense. He was given the maximum 10 year sentence. The Free John Campaign was formed to try and get him released, which this event at Crisler Arena was the culmination of.

The air inside was dishwater cloudy by now with the pungent aroma of weed mixed with the nicotinic fumes of the tobacco addicts. The sweet acid smell of alcohol offered meek competition for the tainted air space.

A tall thin man with a wide afro followed the priest onto the stage

"The only solution to the problem is a people's revolution," he said.

Dennis MulQueen's friend Aurelius leaned towards him and said, "You know this guy, don't you?"

"No, who is it?"

"It's Bobby Seales. He's a bad ass from the Black Panthers."

"Oh, that guy. Of course. Of Chicago Seven fame."

With all of the ambient white noise, it was a safe bet many were not listening, but the guy on stage kept talking.

"Brothers and sisters, it's one thing to talk about doing something," Seales said. "It's another to get down to the nitty gritty and do it. The universe belongs to the people. We are the people. Power to the people."

Aurelius interrupted. "Here, D. Try this, it might improve your memory. I'm betting you'll like it even if it doesn't make you smarter than you already are."

There was a reason he nicknamed his friend with the curly black hair, Dr. Aurelius. He actually was enrolled in the pharmacy program at Michigan State. They must have taught him something in those classes. He could have been Victor Frankenstein with his knowledge of what affected the brain.

It was a dark brick, small, about half the size of a square of bazooka bubble gum. "What the hell is it, Doc?" It had a very distinct smell; it was sticky to the touch.

"It's brain food, D. Gobble gobble. Vitamins. Then Bobby Seale will make more sense to you. Go ahead."

'What, just eat it?"

"Yeah, just eat it, D. It's candy. It's better this way, and it lasts a lot longer."

Ah, Black Lebanese. Straight outta the Humble Pie song. Thirty days in a hole all right. How about thirty days on the moon.

"But here's to no more than that, okay," he said as he popped a square into the back of his throat.

But there was more. Doc had all the hors 'd oeuvres appropriate for the occasion.

Out came the flask, the dead worm floating in the bottom of the golden waters perhaps a reminder of the further brain damage they were about to enjoy.

Suddenly, it all made sense.

"Oh my God, Doc."

He looked out at the stage and the black top hat caught his eye.

"Now you're from Detroit, don't tell me you don't know who this guy is."

"Yes, that's the Master Cylinder." They both broke out laughing.

"The Master Cylinder is inside your head, D."

They both cracked up again as the arena sprung to life with the big energy of big time, old time rock and roll – as only a local – and national by now – icon could do it.

"Oh Carol, don't let him steal your heart away.

I'm gonna learn to dance if it takes me all night and day."

This was a revved-up version of "Oh Carol" that filled the arena as only Michigan's Bob Seger could do it, with his top hat, brown blazer and white sneakers surging the arena to life with his raspy high energy voice doing what he does better than anybody – 100 proof old time rock and roll.

"Can't get much better than this guy," D said to Doc.

"You got it, D."

Certainly can't get much better than the combination of Bob Seger and Chuck Berry (who wrote and first performed the song) – as well as Teegarden and Van Winkle, who took the stage with Seger for this set.

By now the smell of marijuana was so sweet and heavy it hung in the air like molasses.

The timing was perfect for Seger to take over and really get the place rockin'. The Ramblin' Gamblin' Man is local, an Ann Arbor guy no less (Down on Main Street) who had already earned his stripes with his own protest songs (Two Plus Two).

So no way he could not be here this night.

But they came from all over to take the stage for this historic occasion in Ann Arbor, Michigan.

After a short hiatus following Seger ,a thin gangly guy who looked distinctly out of place strode up on the stage with an ambling gait.

"Who the hell is that, Doc?"

"You got me on this one, D. I have no idea."

"What do you think, I'm clairvoyant? I know it's not Iggy."

"Hahaha."

He sang – and he talked.

"It's always good to have rallies like this," he said.

"I hope the people here are ready to direct their energies to getting rid of Richard Nixon. Because what he's been doing the last four years in office, sowing the seeds of fascism, step by step, beefing up the police, ordering different raids, working with the media, step by step he's been taking over the country, with more and more wiretapping, getting more and more supreme court justices, If he gets four more years there's not going to be any America left as you know it now."

"So here's a song," he said as he started singing.

"Here's to the land, you've torn the heart out of, Richard Nixon, Find another country to be part of."

They overheard a guy in the row ahead of them identify this guy as the folksinger Phil Ochs.

Another local but nationally well-known radical, Rennie Davis, was up next.

"We need John," Davis said. "Because the whole time John Sinclair has been in prison because of his opposition to the government, that government had dropped two and a half times Hiroshima in bombs per week every week since July 1969 when John Sinclair was imprisoned. We need John to sweep this warmaker Nixon into the sea."

As Sinclair's wife Leni came on stage and gave a short spiel, Doc lit another joint and their smoke billowed and mixed with that of the other 14,998 in the arena. The stage hands now scurried about in front of them like little gremlins, as another act was getting ready to continue the radical extravaganza.

A black man appeared front and center stage dressed in red velvet vest with gold shirt – the same colors Karl Wallenda wore that night in Detroit all those years ago when he reappeared at the coliseum right after losing family members. This guy could have been a Wallenda, only better, given the courage and inspiration he continuously gave the world.

If only he could see.

A woman in long shiny dress walked with him, her arms locked in his, guiding him to a piano and bench at the front center of the stage.

Everybody knew who this Motown superstar was. And Oh My God did he steal the show.

"For once in my life,
I have someone who needs me,
Someone I've needed so long..."

Dennis and Aurelius looked at each other and simultaneously said in unison: "Wow."

The Motown legend Stevie Wonder continued his stunning performance.

"For once in my life I won't let sorrow hurt me,
Not like it's hurt me before.
For once I have someone I know won't desert me,
I'm not alone anymore.
For once I can say,
This is mine you can't take it.
As long as I know I have love I can make it.
For onnnncceee in my life,
I have someone who needs me."

Talk about incredible. That's all that could be said.

It was beyond unbelievable to see this blind man gyrate and move his head back and forth as he took every man woman and child in that arena in the palm of his hand on a journey to the center of the universe where for those beautiful few minutes only peace and love dwelled.

D leaned over and bumped Aurelius on the arm.

"Look, Doc, over there, he's right there, I think that's him."

"You're hallucinating, D. That's a roadie."

He was low to the ground, sitting cross-legged it looked like, taking it all in. Right in front of Dennis MulQueen and Doc Aurelius. The guy was wearing a black leather jacket, with it looked like a pink t shirt. He had round gold-rimmed glasses on.

He just sat there, at the back of the stage, feet away from them, swaying to the sounds of the Motown soul God Stevie Wonder.

They could almost reach out and touch him. As the Wonder Man continued his show, the atmosphere in the arena was suddenly more magical than imaginable. Not just the "roadie" on the back of the stage, but as D looked around

110

people everywhere were swaying in unison, holding hands, lighting their lighters.

In between numbers Stevie Wonder got up with the help of another band member who held his left arm and walked him to the front of the stage, about three feet from the edge.

"This song goes out to all the undercover agents who might be out in the audience ... somebody's watching you," Stevie Wonder said.

"Before coming here today, I had a lot of things on my mind," he continued. "A lot of things you don't have to see to understand ... We're in a time in the world today where a man can get life in prison for stealing 50 cents. And another man kills four human beings – and is set free. A time in which a man can get 12 years in prison for possession of marijuana. And another who can kill four students at Kent state and come out free. What kind a shit is that?"

The crowd roared in response.

Then the one and only Motown legend broke into a stirring version of "Heaven Help Us All."

"You know, I know, and everybody knows," he sang, *"we neeeeeddddddd loooooooooooovvveeee.*

"We need you Lord.

"We need you Lord. You know. And everybody knows."

Just like that he turned and walked off the back of the stage in front of Dennis and Aurelius as Jerry Rubin walked up to the microphone. Dennis MulQueen was so stoned at this point he couldn't really focus on what he said. But this guy was the main reason the tikkies for this show set a record by selling out in three minutes. This radical Yippie leader had reportedly coaxed the night's superstar attraction into coming from New York to Ann Arbor.

What seemed like a terminal wait was now about to come to an end – but not for almost what seemed like another hour or more of exhortations from security and promoters imploring those in attendance to back off of the stage and to remain calm.

There was real fear of the swelling anticipation leading to crowding and pushing to get just a little bit closer. A steady buzz of anticipation was now being undercut by fears of some kind of dangerous stampede. Finally, after one last exhortation to the crowd to remain calm and stay back from the stage, suddenly there he was, he came right past Dennis and Aurelius wearing a black leather jacket and pink T shirt.

"I told you that was him, Doc."

He was the reason 15,000 tickets for the Free John Rally sold out in three minutes, the fastest sell-out of any show in Michigan pop music history.

"Oh My God, there he is, Doc. I can't believe it."

Now he understood the teeny boppers screaming on *Ed Sullivan* all those years before. He walked right by them and the goose bumps popped out everywhere. Dennis looked at his watch. It was 3:03 a.m.

He walked to the center of the stage carrying his guitar, a regular looking acoustic. His presence filled Crisler Arena with awe. It was one of those forever moments, as he strode to the center microphone.

"We came here not only to help John and to spotlight what's going on, but also to show and to say to all of you that apathy isn't it, and we can do something," John Lennon told the audience.

"Okay, so flower power didn't work, so what? We start again."

He wasted no time as he flew into the first number.

"Attica State, Attica State
We're all mates with Attica State ..."
Attica state Attica State,
we're all mates with Attica State.

The music wasn't stellar, the sound system was poor by modern standards, but it didn't matter.

It was about history. It was about the moment. It was about being part of it.

The band appeared to be a hodgepodge group, slightly out of sync, looked like David Peele was there, Jerry Rubin was onstage with Lennon. Sure enough, John Lennon was wearing a magenta T-shirt with a bright green cannabis leaf on the front. Yoko Ono, immediately to his right, wore an identical shirt.

The second song, "The Luck of the Irish," was about another cause dear to the Irish Lennon's heart.

"If you had the luck of the Irish,
You'd be sorry and wish you were dead," he sang.

With little fanfare they launched into the next number with Yoko singing "Sisters Oh Sisters."

Then it was time for the main cause d'célèbre.

"This is a little number I wrote for John," Lennon said.

With Yoko standing to his right playing a bongo, he launched into "Won't You Care for John Sinclair?"

"In the stir for breathing air," Lennon sang,

"It ain't fair, John Sinclair ..."

When this number was over, he turned quickly and walked past Dennis and Aurelius and was gone.

The Ann Arbor performance was Lennon's first since the Beatles broke up the previous year. Lennon was only on stage for about 15 minutes, playing just these four songs, in the middle of the night with poor acoustics at that, but the impact spoke for itself.

On Monday, December 13th, 1971, three days after the Ann Arbor concert, the man and his organization – the

White Panthers he headed that the FBI in 1970 referred to as one of "potentially the largest and most dangerous of revolutionary organizations in the United States" – was freed from his Jackson, Michigan, prison cell.

The Michigan Supreme Court overturned his conviction and Sinclair was released after serving two years of his 10-year sentence.

Later that day, the phone rang in Sinclair's Ann Arbor residence. (He and Lani and the gang had relocated from Detroit after the arrests and constant harassment from Detroit officials.)

"What happened, man?" John Lennon asked.

"I don't know, they just told me to go," John Sinclair said.

"Beautiful ..."

Lennon then handed the phone to his wife Yoko.

"We are so glad you gave us hope. I mean you became history, right? You gave us all incentive. You see, the people in New York and all over were very ... We can start all over again, right?"

"It's beautiful," John Sinclair said.

"It's never too late to start," Yoko said. "Sorry the music wasn't so hot; it was the message."

John Lennon interjected, "The music is the message, right? What happens next?"

There was a pause.

"We can't believe it happened," John Lennon reiterated.

Yoko quickly added: "We hope you are the first one. The start of many. It's good to have lots of people ... the number really counts."

Sinclair's wife Lani took the phone to thank the Lennons. She asked John what record he was working on

Lennon replied, "I've been recording David Peel right now. I'm producing it for him. You know it's a record. The Pope smokes dope."

He laughed before getting back on point.

"Nobody can believe it. I was calling all over the world. It is incredible. Apathy is no good, right? We're so happy for both of you. It's just beautiful. We'll say bye-bye now. Love to both of you."

He hung up the phone and that was that.

John Lennon would never be in Michigan again.

~ ~ ~

Little more than six weeks after Lennon unveiled his "Luck of the Irish" song in Ann Arbor, Michigan, highlighting the Troubles and centuries of British occupation of Ireland, the mood was upbeat as thousands of civil rights marchers set off from the Bishops Field in Derry, Northern Ireland, just before 3 o'clock in the afternoon.

The sun was shining on this day, January 30, 1972, and the air was crisp and the atmosphere was more akin to a kid at the circus rather than a somber march against centuries of oppression culminating in the recently instituted internment without trial policies of the Brits.

The march had been banned by the Stormont government, but there was no sense of fear as the marchers, singing and chanting, wound their way down from Creggan through the Brandywell and finally the Bogside. It was common knowledge that the IRA had withdrawn from the Bogside.

As the march reached the army barricade at William Street, the great bulk of protesters followed the platform party on a lorry. A minor confrontation occurred at this barricade, but by the standards of Derry in 1972 it was low key, and as 4 p.m. approached it looked like things had petered out.

But at approximately 4:07 pm., out of nowhere, the order was given for the 1st Battalion of the Parachute Regiment to begin an "arrest" operation. Then it all started. Exactly three minutes later, soldiers of the Support Company began firing.

"Hugh Gilmore was running beside me," said Geraldine Richmond in a public testimony given to a local historian. "He was going away from the soldiers and he had no weapon. The soldiers jumped out of the Saracens and started shooting. Some were standing or kneeling as they shot; they were not lying down or taking cover. There were a lot of people running to get away.

"Just as Mr. Gilmore and I reached the main section of Rossville Flats, he said, 'I'm hit, I'm hit.' I said, 'Try and keep running.'

"He started to stumble. I got my two hands under his arm at the shoulder and supported him till we got round the corner of the building. I was looking round as we ran.

"There was continuous firing all the time. People kept falling. A lot of them were diving for cover, but I think at least one of them was shot by the wall of the flats along Rossville Street.

"We got round the corner and against the end wall of the building near a telephone box. I put Mr. Gilmore down and opened his shirt. I saw a bullet wound in the lower part of the stomach, a small entry wound and a big exit wound. I knew it must be a fatal wound and in fact he died in a few minutes.

"There were about half-a-dozen people beside the telephone box taking cover. A man took me from Mr. Gilmore's body along towards the box. At this time we could hear the cries of wounded at the other end of the shops (the center block of Rossville flats).

"There was firing down Rossville Street and also between the two buildings from the waste ground in front of Chamberlain Street. This kept us pinned where we were.

"A man was shouting out that he did not want to die. We wanted to go to him but could not because of the gunfire. Mr. Barney McGuigan said, "I'm not going to let him die by himself. If I take my white hankie, they'll not shoot me".

"We tried to dissuade him, but he took out his handkerchief and moved out from the wall a few paces waving it in front of him. We shouted to him to come back because the shooting did not stop.

"Then he was hit, just about four paces out from the wall. He fell and he was dead as he hit the ground. He was hit in the back of the head.

"I could not remember much after this. I was taken to hospital and treated for shock."

Meanwhile, others crowded into the Glenfada Park on Rossville street to try and find shelter from the carnage. They were unaware that four British soldiers were approaching. When these soldiers came into view, the crowd attempted to escape. Joe Friel, Daniel Gillespie, P. O'Donnell and Joe Mahon were wounded.

Jim Wray, wounded and unable to move, lay just yards from his grandparents' home. A British soldier murdered him in cold blood as he lay wounded and defenseless.

Gerard Donaghy, Gerard McKinney, and William McKinney were also murdered as they sought to escape the rampage.

Malachy Coy, who was also at the march, said, "I saw a youth wearing a dark blue suit panic and start running. One of the soldiers shot him in the stomach before he had even made a step. The soldier had shot him from almost point blank range. On seeing this, I panicked and ran towards the opening on my righthand side. I heard more shooting but I kept running until I was well away from the gunfire danger."

When all was said and done, British soldiers shot 26 unarmed civilians on January 31, 1972, during the protest march against "Internment Without Trial".

Fourteen died. While most of the victims of what would be forever remembered as "Bloody Sunday," were shot while fleeing from the soldiers and some were shot while trying to help the wounded, two protesters were also injured when they were run down by Army vehicles.

All eyewitnesses (apart from the soldiers), including marchers, local residents, and British and Irish journalists present, maintained that soldiers fired into an unarmed crowd, or were aiming at fleeing people and those tending the wounded, whereas the soldiers themselves were not fired upon.

No British soldier was wounded by gunfire or reported any injuries, nor were any bullets or nail bombs recovered to back up government claims they were firing in self-defense.

Lieutenant Colonel Derek Wilford, who was directly in charge of 1 Para, the soldiers who went into the Bogside, was awarded the Order of the British Empire by the Queen, while other soldiers were equally decorated with honors for their part on the day.

Two government inquiries cleared all officers and soldiers of the British Military of all wrongdoing. Not a single British official, or soldier associated with Bloody Sunday was ever charged with a crime or held accountable in any way.

One paratrooper who gave evidence at a subsequent tribunal testified they were told by an officer to expect a gunfight and, "We want some kills."

They got their way, and these "kills" immediately sparked protests all across Ireland. In Dublin, the capital of the independent part of Ireland, outraged Irish citizens lit the British Embassy aflame on February 2nd. Tension and strife that dated to the 1920 Ireland Act, which severed off the six most north western counties in Ireland and annexed them to Great Britain as Northern Ireland, continued to boil.

The IRA revenge would come a few months later when the Republican terrorists exploded 20 bombs simultaneously in Belfast, killing dozens of British military personnel and a number of civilians.

In response, Britain instituted a new court system composed of trial without jury for terrorism suspects, and conviction rates topped over 90 percent.

Former Beatle Paul McCartney, who like his bandmate Lennon is also of Irish descent, recorded the first song in response to Bloody Sunday, only two days after the incident.

The single, entitled "Give Ireland Back to the Irish" was immediately banned from the airwaves by the British Broadcasting Company (BBC).

The very next week, his former Beatles colleague John Lennon, appeared outside the British Airways offices in New York City along with approximately 5,000 others to protest the massacre of the 14 unarmed civil rights marchers in Derry on Bloody Sunday a week before.

Lennon spoke out in behalf of the victims and families of Bloody Sunday. It was bright and cold outside as the crowd gathered to hear John and Yoko sing their new song, "The Luck of the Irish," to the demonstrators.

"My name is Lennon, and you can guess the rest," he told the cheering crowd which consisted of a majority of Irish-Americans.

Two days after the protest, Lennon and Yoko invited Irish American political activists to their home to explore ways they could help the civil rights movement in Northern Ireland.

Later in the year, Lennon's album "Some Time In New York City" was released, which featured a new song devoted to the tragedy simply entitled "Bloody Sunday," as well as the song he sang at the Ann Arbor Free John Rally, "The Luck of the Irish."

Lennon donated the proceeds from "Some Time in New York City," released in June 1972, to the Northern Ireland civil rights movement. Lennon was disappointed by negative reaction from disc jockeys to "Luck of the Irish," which he'd hoped to release as a single.

But his one-time partner, now rival, McCartney's "Give Ireland Back to the Irish," zoomed up the US Billboard charts.

~ 10 ~

LIFE IS NOT FOOTBALL

The Big House.

Tom Harmon played here. Gerald Ford played here. Brian Griese played here. Tom Brady played here.

And Dennis MulQueen.

By the time this game was over, he might have wished it was Gerald Ford or anybody else he was going head-to-head with instead of Jim Pietrzak (All-American and future New York Giants/New Orleans Saints 13-year NFL veteran) or Bill Dulac (All-American co-captain of the team, the LA Rams and New England Patriots.)

Nonetheless, it would be his finest moment on the grid iron. And Coach MulQueen and Coach Rhoades were in the stands watching.

They had switched him to defense and his first play of the spring green-and-white game at the U of M stadium, he split the two blocks and assisted on his first tackle of the contest.

Maybe it was self-defense – he knew if he didn't split the tackle they would split him in half, or maybe just bury him underneath the U of M artificial turf.

No matter if it was self-preservation or ego or trying to please the coaches, or his father, he came up with spin moves and bull rushes and submarine charges he never knew he had in him.

He gave it his all, and he had to.

Piertrzak and Dulac were superior physical specimens, heavier and stronger and maybe a tad faster too. But they weren't any tougher, and MulQueen had good technique and guile and he used his leverage – thanks to Coach Rhoades tutoring him off the field – to play as effectively as he ever had.

He played smart. He had to. He anticipated the count, he paid close attention to Pieterzak's stance, the look in his eyes. He knew ahead of time if it was going to be a pass or a run or a double team just by the way he lined up and got in his stance. He went after it with everything he had. With carefree abandon, he attacked, attacked, and attacked some more with carefree abandon. He fired out on every play like it was his last.

On one play he made a spin move to the inside, the next play he faked inside and spun to the outside. On third and two, when Pietrzack and Dulac telegraphed the double team, he knew the ball was coming his way so he tunnel bombed and contained the line of scrimmage allowing the linebacker behind him to make the play.

One play high, the next play low. On a slant inside, he broke through for a tackle behind the line of scrimmage. The next play he fake bullrushed him inside, then lightning head-slap spinned the other way (he could thank Purefoiry for teaching him this move) and in an instant outsmarted his guy again for another opportunity to disrupt the play.

"Way to hit out there, Pietrzack and MulQueen," he heard the offensive coordinator Nick Coso yell out after one goal line stand. To be included in that conversation, how sweet it is.

You couldn't help but hear the thunder out there that day on the field, if you were anywhere in the stadium. It was almost like he took his shoulder pads off and slammed them against a metal wall, that's what it sounded like, every play a thunderous clap of power and force as the sounds of helmet meeting helmet and shoulder pad meeting shoulder pad filled the stadium.

What a beautiful thing. He even had the look going that day.

Yeah, a dog can smell fear on a man, but he can also smell no fear. Dennis MulQueen had no fear out there, and it showed.

But it wasn't all pretty. A couple times he broke free of his guy but another All-American on the team, running back Mike Strickland (future Minnesota Viking) made him look like a fence post planted in the middle of the field.

"Stay broken down real low on that, MulQueen," the defensive coach Woody Widenhofer (future Pittsburgh Steelers defensive coordinator and architect of the Steel Curtain defense) came over and told him. "And keep your eyes on his belt buckle. And time your lunge like an uncoiled spring and make sure you run right through the guy," he said as he patted MulQueen on the backside.

All in all, it was his best day on the gridiron.

He knew so when Head Coach Boisture, (future head coach of the Detroit Wheels), the guy who gave him this big opportunity, smiled and nodded when he came over to the sidelines afterward.

"I see your body's not like a pear anymore, MulQueen. Keep it up and you'll have a future here."

When this guy talked, you listened. The fact there were 10 guys on the field that day with Dennis MulQueen who went on to play in the NFL speaks for itself. The team was undefeated in the 1971 regular season and finished the year ranked No. 3 in the country in the NCAA College Division. The only loss came in the nationally televised Pioneer Bowl against a Louisiana Tech team quarterbacked by a guy named Terry Bradshaw, who of course Banaszak and Widenhofer would hook up with in the near future to win all those Super Bowls for the Steelers.

The payoff for all that glory playing on that field of dreams that day came for Dennis MulQueen the following morning when he woke up and it took him 10 minutes to get out of bed. He couldn't raise his arms to drink a cup of coffee. His shoulders hurt so bad he thought he had broken his collar bone. To go along with one hell of a headache. Ahh, what a beautiful thing.

~ ~ ~

He looked like a frat boy, clean-cut, handsome, tall, nice features, sandy blonde hair and blue eyes with a blue Oxford button-down to go with tan slacks and blue blazer. But he pranced the stage like an evangelical minister at a pray-a-thon.

Dennis MulQueen wondered if he could be right. That there is something beyond us that we aren't aware of, a mysterious force out there that will rescue us and make it all better if we can somehow just tap in.

He doubted it.

He was an agnostic and he didn't go to church or pretty much believe in any kind of spiritual mumbo jumbo.

The guy must have sensed something wasn't right. He stopped right in front of Dennis MulQueen and stared him down like they were having their own little private seance. Despite the packed auditorium surrounding him.

"My Dad was a horrible alcoholic," the speaker said. "He abandoned me and my brothers and my mother when I was 13 months old. I never ever saw him or met him or heard from him ever again. My mother couldn't take care of us by herself. She put me in an orphanage and I ended up bouncing around foster homes most of my childhood."

Dennis had no idea as he watched this guy bounce around the stage at Mercy High School that he was witnessing the evolution of the soon-to-be very rich and very famous Wayne W. Dyer, the guy that would go on to be acknowledged as the all-time guru of inspirational speakers.

It was obvious he was in take-off mode already, although at this point he was only the high school guidance counselor at the all-girls Mercy Catholic High School in Farmington Hills, Michigan.

This guy knew how to connect with people.

Like landing the toy fishing rod magnet smack on the back of the floating magnetic plastic bathtub fish, first try, this guy knew how to reel people in, emotionally.

"This man, my father, the man that I never heard from again, the father I would never know who walked out on me and my two brothers and my mother, this man who was a con man and a thief, and an alcoholic. He turned out to be my greatest teacher.

"He turned out to be my biggest gift. Without interference from parents or teachers in the orphanage, I learned self-reliance, that there is only one thing that we need to rely on, and that is within, within each of us there is a divine force passed down to us from our source, and by just turning ourselves over to this power within you can do anything in life you want to."

This, he explained, was the true path to self-actualization, the state of happiness and peace achieved by all successful people as outlined by Abraham Maslow, who was one of his main mentors along with Albert Ellis and his rational Emotive Behavior Therapy.

This was Dyer's schtick, you can make any great result happen, you can overcome any negative circumstance, and will yourself to become a fully self-actualized successful happy person as long as you imagine that positive result coming to you ahead of time before it actually happens, and resolve to stay out of the self-defeating negative thinking zone, the realm of your "erroneous zones."

Sprinkled in the mix were a little Carl Jung, a little Lao-Tse, and a little Emerson. Along with a healthy dose of William Blake and his *Auguries of Innocence*.

"To see a World in a Grain of Sand,
And a Heaven in a Wild Flower,
Hold Infinity in the Palm of Your Hand,
and Eternity in an Hour ...
A Robin Red Breast in a cage
Puts all heaven in a rage ...
The wanton boy that Kills the Fly
Shall feel the spider's enmity ..."

But none of his teachers, he said, was a bigger favorite than the guy he discovered one day while sitting out a high school suspension for refusing an assignment.

"If one advances confidently in the direction of his dreams, and endeavors to live the life he has imagined, he will meet with a success unexpected in common hours," Dyer read as he picked up a copy of Henry David Thoreau's *On Walden Pond* that just happened to be sitting on a shelf in the principal's office next to the wooden bench he was anchored to that day for his punishment.

He particularly liked the essay Thoreau included in the back of Walden Pond entitled "On Civil Disobedience."

~ ~ ~

The voice had a wail to it, the sounds of desperation and grief, a cross between primal and childlike, ethereal and soft and even soothing at times, but overall, mostly vulnerable and hurt. This was the voice that filled Louis Scaboni's lower level that day. Dennis and Scaboni had gone to the Dyer show together along with another buddy named TJ, and

Phase Two of Dennis' awakening that summer took place back in the basement of Scaboni's Royal Oak house playing records.

The wail of grief in the first song Dennis MulQueen played for his friend was John Lennon and the title of the song was "Mother," off of his first solo album since breaking up with the Beatles.

It was all about him having his mother but his mother never having him. And another verse devoted to his father leaving him, while he never left his father.

In the last stanza of the song he calls for his parents to return as the tune ends with repeated wails over and over and over again, at least a couple minute's worth of wails. Lennon's voice was piercing the air at the end, almost like primal screams, probably related to his recent primal scream therapy in California with the controversial psychotherapist Arthur Janov.

"You know who he's talking about, don't you," Dennis said to his friend.

"Alf they called him. That was his father, Alfred, who ran out on him when he was four years old. And his mother Julia, who gave him up to his Aunt Mimi, who raised him."

Scaboni, who would later go on to become a pre-eminent psychiatrist himself, was already on his way. He said Lennon's wailing confirmed what he already knew. That most of the screwed-up people in the world can trace their problems directly to pathological parent-child interactions growing up that spill over into adulthood anxiety and depression and dysfunction.

This is it in a nutshell, according to Scaboni. "Everyone feels an obligation to fulfill at least a portion of their parent's dreams for them," Scaboni said. "And when that doesn't happen, which is frequently the case, major negative consequences can develop for everybody involved."

~ ~ ~

George MulQueen Jr. was at the iconic Walsh's Tavern in Detroit that day it all got started, along with a boisterous crowd of Lion's fans talking about the key play that had just happened at near-by Briggs' Stadium.

A blitzing San Francisco 49er's linebacker crushed legendary Detroit Lion's quarterback Bobby Layne like a door mouse with a hit that would have been lights out for anybody.

But not this guy. There he was, calling the next play after stumbling back to the huddle.

"Okay, guys, you all just block now this time and ole Bobby, I'm gonna git the ball to one a y'all downfield, okay, guys? Good ole Bobby'll git cha' the damn ball and we gonna win this dang thing, okay, guys?" he told his teammates in his familiarly unflappable Texas twang.

Sure enough, the very next play the great Bobby Layne dropped back once again, this time deftly pirouetting to his right to barely avoid another brutal hit, and floated a perfect strike down the far left sideline to the willing embrace of another NFL soldier, the great tight end Leon Hart.

The galloping giant tucked the slightly wobbly leather air bladder into his soft sticky hands and romped into the end zone with alacrity, giving the Detroit Lions the winning margin over the YA Tittle-led Niners on this fateful day in the Motor City.

The expertly executed score provided a victory that would propel the Lions to another NFL Championship that year.

But it wasn't all Lion's talk at Walsh's pub that day.

George MulQueen was busy reminding the most famous bartender in town who owned the joint, Billy Walsh, that his grandfather, Jack MulQueen, whose had emigrated from Askeaton, County Limerick to this Detroit neighborhood called Corktown in the latter half of the 1800s, was born in this very building, in an upstairs bedroom, the old fashioned way – the midwife way.

"Yeah, yeah, I know what's comin', Mulky. I didn't forget, Mulky. I know I promised ya the front doors of the building your grand pappy was born in, I promised 'em to ya, you'll get 'em soon enough. But no rush, okay, you don't get 'em until I'm dead but not a moment too soon, okay?"

"Never too soon to celebrate a life well-lived, Walshy," George MulQueen said as he hoisted his Guinness overhead with two hands like a chalice at a Catholic church mass.

Then a switch flipped and he jumped off the bar stool and hustled over to a pay phone in the corner and stubbed a nickel into the stainless steel slot at the top and dialed his home number. Pat MulQueen didn't answer. She wasn't home, it would turn out.

He recognized his mother-in-law's voice. She was home babysitting.

"Hello Margaret, it's George. Sorry I forgot to call at half time – "

She cut him off like a bandsaw as he was forced to hold the phone several inches from his ear to prevent tympanic damage.

"Where are you now, George. He was born an hour ago. I'm going to kill you, George. I can't believe you went to the Lions' game while your wife has had a baby."

George MulQueen dropped the receiver like a hot tamale and raced out of those promised doors and down Michigan Avenue to the Old Providence Hospital to greet his wife and new son – Dennis MulQueen.

The date was October 11, 1953, and for those that knew George MulQueen, it was no surprise he would squeeze in the most important Lions' football game of the season on the day his son was born.

~ ~ ~

Exactly 19 years to the day later, October 11, 1972, Dennis MulQueen knew it wasn't going to be a pleasant birthday. Especially when his father's favorite sport – and thousands and thousands of dollars – were involved.

It started with the car ride from his dormitory to the top restaurant in Ypsilanti, Michigan, a joint named Haabs. His parents had driven up from Oak Park to be with him on this day.

Despite the fact he had told his mother, who had told his father.

The concussions and headaches and other constant aches and pains had become not worth it. He wasn't enjoying it. So he gave up his football scholarship and walked out on the opportunity that had rescued him by getting him into college.

His father didn't call him a quitter that day – but his words conveyed the message loud and clear.

"Jesus Christ, look at those sideburns," he said as he turned in the car and looked at his son. "When you grow those goddamned sideburns out like that, you look like a goddamned hippie. The long-ass hair, its bullshit. Why don't you just cut it all off for Christ's sake, and clean up a little and quit looking like a goddamned freak."

The haircut – or lack thereof – certainly didn't help. The shaggy mane he now sported fell almost to his shoulders. And those sideburns – no greaser could top his mutton chops.

Completing this transformation, Dennis MulQueen now smoked cigarettes (and other things he knew the old man would kill him for if he knew) and wore bell bottom "hippie pants," as his father called them, and was a bigger rock and roll fan than ever.

No, he never called him a quitter. But his words stung nonetheless.

"Goddamned hippie."

"Freak."

And even though he didn't say it, that other unsaid Q word nonetheless bounced around inside his skull that day and thereafter like a croquet ball.

"Now what the hell is gonna happen? Now what are you gonna do?"

After an interminable silence that seemed like a lightyear, as they pulled in the parking lot he looked at his son and answered his own question.

"No problem. You'll just have to get a goddamned job now and support yourself," he said as he banged the steering wheel with both hands.

"Lots of jobs."

They slowly exited his 1970 navy blue Olds 98 and headed for the front door of the restaurant for this "happy birthday" celebration.

Dennis made sure he sat at the opposite end of the table from his father.

~ ~ ~

"I'll be a good boy, I'll promise you anything,
just get me out of this hell," the former Beatle
sang
   into the bright lights.
"Cold Turkey's, got me, on the run."

He was again dressed in his green military jacket with angled sergeant insignia on the sleeves, blue-tinted gold round glasses.

He was playing with the Elephant's Memory Band, at Madison Square Garden. His friend, ABC's Geraldo Rivera, got him to do a benefit concert there on December 15, 1972, for the Wildwood Home for Retarded Children.

There he was again, up on stage again, Lennon being Lennon, anteing up the way he wanted to, raising money for a school as a platform to again get his bigger message out to the world at large.

Stevie Wonder also performed at this benefit, singing a first-time-ever version of "Superstition," which wasn't scheduled for public release until months later.

But JW was able to turn the tables on the guy he sat on the back of the stage to watch that night in Ann Arbor – "This guy, he's my Beatles," Lennon said of the Wonder Man – the guy who had in fact stolen the show in Ann Arbor the previous year. This night though was JW's gig all the way. The audience was going crazy as he sang one of his best numbers ever, about "Instant Karma" going to get you.

It was a dynamite performance that also included "Come Together," which Lennon customized with the inserted phrase "stop the war" coming out of nowhere in the middle of the tune.

It was vintage Lennon from start to finish, which of course also included a performance of "Imagine." Yoko chipped in with "Sisters O Sisters" and "Woman is the Nigger of the World," before Lennon closed it out with a rousing rendition of "Power to the People."

Yoko also included some of her patented scream verses, once again reminiscent of Arthur Janov and his primal scream therapy, which John had recently completed a course of in California during his "Lost Weekend."

But Yoko could have been the original primal screamer this night.

Yeah, he thought. Maybe I should try some of that too. Just have to go home for that.

Yeah, JW, he said to himself, I'll do anything too, just get me out of this hell.

~ ~ ~

The following April, George MulQueen was in that same wooden swivel chair in Room 106 at Chadsey High School for a different kind of phone call.

"The Rouge? Yeah, that would be great, Ray. He'll be out the end of next week. Which plant would be the worst do you think?"

"The foundry, George. It's like Auschwitz in there."

There was a pause.

"But we don't have anything there right now. I can get him on the line in the Stamping Plant though. That's a pretty close second. He'd get a pretty good workout in there."

"Okay, Ray. Make it the worst job in the place, okay, Ray? He already dropped football, he's hanging out with a bunch of dope heads and hippies with hair as wide as the door, I'm afraid he's going to drop out altogether, I want him to know what it would be like out there with no college education."

"Gotcha, George. Will do. Tell him to report there the following Monday at 8 a.m. sharp. Tell him to skip the employment office line, that'll be a mile long. Just have him go around all that to the guard box out front at the main gate and the guy there will have his name and take him inside to fill out the paperwork and get started right away."

George MulQueen was on the phone with his good friend Ray Maly, who was a top executive at Ford Motor Co. in charge of personnel with his office in the Glass House one floor down and right below the Deuce's office.

"Let me know how it goes," he said. "And, George, it'll turn out just fine. Remember the painting on the wall. A victory will be gained if it is God's will. If not, there's always martinis."

They both had a good laugh on that one.

"Thanks, Ray. I'll relay the message. Really appreciate everything. And speaking of martinis, Pat wanted to know, what are you guys doing on the weekend? We'd love to have you guys over to the lake again."

"Thanks, George. That would be great. I'll tell Rita. I don't think we have anything planned."

"Terrific. I'll have Pat call Rita to firm things up."

"What do you want us to bring?"

"Oh, just the usual, Ray. Just bring yourselves. We'll have steaks and drinks and everything. Supposed to be a beautiful weekend."

"Always is with you guys, George. All right. We'll at least bring the dessert. Gotta run now. See you guys in no time. Can't wait. Thanks for having us. Bye now."

"Bye, Ray. Thanks again for everything."

~ 11 ~

QUITE A SHOCK

Battleship gray coveralls.

How apropos.

The uniform of choice, because there was no choice.

Everybody wore them, because everybody had to be there – and you had to wear them to be there, or you'd have no clothes left anyway.

No, this wasn't a southern Civil War battlefield; this was a different kind of battlefield. This was Detroit, Michigan, the summer of 1973.

Just like any battlefield, he was there because there was no choice.

And no sooner had he manned his station, he wished he did have a choice – to leave before he got killed or maimed, which is actually what happened in three separate incidents in a two-week span proximate to his start at Detroit's big bad Rouge Complex down on the Rouge River in Dearborn, Michigan.

He was on the fender line, the truck fender line, at the end of it. Thank God he was at the end of it, it's doubtful he could have made it anywhere else.

But he wasn't sure he could make it there either, especially Day One.

He had to take a truck fender – these were transport truck fenders, the big daddy semi fenders, so they were thick and huge, about five feet long, and curved dramatically more so than an ordinary car fender, and weighing probably ten times as much due to their thickness and girth, unwieldy to say the least – and he had to grab the fender off the line behind him (before it crashed to the floor, he was at the official end of the line) bend over rapidly with this albatross in hand and stoop almost to the floor and twist and turn the damned thing to get it underneath a hard plastic anti-spark and smoke shield, maneuvering the damned thing while awkwardly extended like this up and over onto the silver die whereby little indentations on the inside of the fender lined up perfectly with the spots on the die so everything matched up properly. And set it down exactly there, not a millimeter off one side or the other – or it wouldn't seat properly.

Complicated, huh?

Then he had to turn around 360 degrees behind him and push two buttons simultaneously as the 100 ton press lowered itself to spot weld the fender in numerous places for one final step in the process. Then he had to remove the completed fender and stack it properly on top of piles of other feeders in a large metal bin off to the side.

So, he thanked God he was last on the line, because when he fell way behind, which was immediately every day, he could cheat and stack the untreated fenders bunching up at the end of the conveyor belt on the floor next to his press and catch up later while the rest of the line shut down for break or lunch. And at the end of the day when everybody else got to go home.

About midway through his first morning on the job, he caught a guy out of the corner of his eye walking toward him wearing an immaculately pressed blue jacket with the white-

and-blue Ford oval patch on the upper right, the standard identifying feature of all the line bosses.

He was a lean and tall scraggly-haired guy with a large hooked nose and gray aviator spectacles and he moved with one of those halting, rollicking, off-kilter, herky-jerky gaits that combined with his swarthy almost-jaundiced-looking skin gave him a Stephen-King-character look.

Turns out it was Andy, the foreman on his line.

He was wearing darkened boots that looked like they had been treated with Neets foot oil a thousand times over to contrast with his tan khakis.

Dennis MulQueen flinched when he saw him, certain he was about to get reamed out as not even halfway through his first day on the job he had already stacked more fenders on the floor than he had processed through his "Green Monster," the affectionate moniker he had already bestowed on his machine.

But he walked right past Dennis MulQueen to the next press over.

This battle station, immediately to MulQueen's right, was operated by a taciturn, sullen-looking guy who stared unmoved and silent earlier in the morning when Dennis said "Hi" and extended an introductory handshake offer that went unreciprocated. Best leave a man in thought alone, he said to himself as he turned and walked back to his own unit.

Now Andy walked up behind this guy one press over, who was the only worker in the plant Dennis ever saw that day or thereafter not wearing the standard-issue gray coveralls – something about being allergic to the material, the scuttlebutt was.

This day he was dressed in a plain pea-green T-shirt (no writing) with beige-ish slacks that looked like the modern-day Car Hart workpants with the thick wide beltloops and that awful nondescript mustard yellow hue that was supposed to look like tan. The T was a couple sizes small which made the guy's ripped-out physique pop like GI Joe.

When Dennis MulQueen looked over there he realized the reason his unpressed floor fender pile wasn't deeper – his line mate was about as efficient as he was, judging by his advanced floor pile that was even deeper than Dennis'.

The noise in the place was so loud everybody was issued ear plugs on hiring day. But even though his were not a snug fit, they still made audibility even more implausible.

So what Andy precisely said to the guy will remain forever unknown, but Dennis didn't need to hear what he said to know it could not have been 'Hi, nice to see you today'.

That became crystal clear as Andy leaned in on the guy's space as he spoke and got up on his tiptoes and now he was inches from the guy's face as he was obviously berating him for either the piled up fenders or his flouting of the dress code, Dennis surmised. While he couldn't decipher the words, despite the factory racket the volume came through loud and clear as he was now yelling at the guy.

Then he knew it wasn't a dress code violation as he pointed to the pile on the floor and the rest of the conversation was history.

Out of nowhere, without uttering one word, the guy in the mustard pants and pea-green shirt who was built like a brick shithouse, even though he was four or five inches shorter than Andy, whirled like Smokin' Joe Frazier coming out of his crouch and hit Andy right smack in the middle of his face so hard he flew in the air like a rag doll.

It was like one of those slow-motion, car-wreck moments as big huge sweat drops flew from Andy's head right at the moment of impact, back-lighted by the fluorescent factory lights as at that same moment they flew all over the place and one bounced on the floor not two feet from where

Dennis MulQueen stood, and he realized they were not sweat beads at all.

They were Andy's chiclets. One that landed about three feet away had to be one of his front teeth; it looked like a horse tooth it was so big.

And there five feet away lay Andy, the geeky foreman, out cold as the blood ran from the corners of his mouth and his nose, mixing with the greenish-black greasy puddles of oil and water that littered his resting place on the grimy factory floor.

I wonder if he is dead, Dennis MulQueen said to himself as his line mate calmly turned and began walking east toward the plant's main doors, as casually as if he was walking a dog in the park.

Nobody was about to stop him.

Andy still wasn't moving as Dennis turned to go get help. He called out for the foreman the next line over and it wasn't two minutes later several guys in white coats arrived with a stretcher and black bags as they surrounded Andy and after listening with a stethoscope to his chest they lifted him onto the white sheets and off they wheeled him in the direction of the plant infirmary, probably to wait for an ambulance to the local hospital.

But you can't stop progress.

Not 10 minutes later, they brought a sub over and the truck fender line hummed back to life like nothing had happened.

Lunch break, a couple of hours later, couldn't have come soon enough.

"Sure hope he doesn't come back in here with an Uzi and kill all of us," said Larry, a grassy-haired Rouge veteran of almost three decades, as the two of them walked together toward the cafeteria.

The former linemate's name was Ralph, according to Larry, and he was one mean dude. It was common knowledge he had already killed three people in his neighborhood, Larry said, but everybody was too afraid to call the cops on him for fear they would be next.

Very believable, after the scene he had just witnessed.

"But probably not till tomorrow. Somebody told Gerry the foreman on the Mustang line, and the guards caught him at the gate before he ever got outta here," Larry said. "The police came and took him away in the paddy wagon."

Later in the afternoon on break, Dennis learned the damage. He was sitting on a stool near his press cleaning his safety glasses with a tissue when from behind he caught wind of the strong smell of booze, the sweet acrid garlic fumes penetrating through the smoky haze of the hi-los and the presses and he knew who it was.

He turned around and sure enough it was Larry again, the dangling Pall Mall hanging from his thin lips bobbing up and down like the needle on a Geiger counter.

"Just lost his teeth and busted his jaw in eight places but he's alive," Larry said.

"But hey, pal, losing teeth ain't nothin." He pointed with his right hand in the air to the right. "See that press over there, just last week they had to scrape Ron off the floor over there."

"Come on, man, cut it out," Dennis said.

"No, I'm not kidding. He put his fender in crooked, nobody knows if it was on purpose or not, he wasn't the fixer on his line, but the freakin' die bolts busted loose and, man, that's a 400-ton press and whatever that die weighs it came on him instantly and they literally had to scrape him off the floor with yard tools."

He wasn't done.

"And see that press over there?" He pointed to the left this time.

"A guy lost both his arms in that one. That's the danger of taping your buttons down. You can go like hell that way and meet quota for the guys to get out early but once in a while a guy pays the price.

"Welcome to the Rouge, man."

~ ~ ~

His buddy wanted to know what it was like.

"It's like being in a war zone, Bokker, that's what it's like."

"That bad, eh?"

He told him about Tuesday, how when he walked in there were four guys next to his locker, and the guy in the middle had a needle in his arm.

Shooting up in the locker room in front of him.

"I was smart enough to keep on walking like my locker was in Nebraska. Like I saw nothing. I know what happens to witnesses."

He told him about the two guys that got killed by their machines. And the foreman who almost got killed by the guy working right next to him on the line.

"Boy, the old man got you a hell of a job, didn't he?"

"Yeah, but the money's incredible." Andy was eavesdropping and couldn't resist. Not that Andy. A different Andy. He was the owner of the joint, and he doubled as the bartender. If Ralph had attacked this Andy, it might have been a permanent result.

"Now this is a real war zone here, buddy," Andy said. "That ain't shit you're talking about. This is real Detroit here. But I know how to make peace."

He reached into his back pocket and pulled out a silver plated, shiny flat hand gun that glistened in the dark bar lights like straight outta James Bond.

141

"Okay. I see," Dennis said.

"Yeah, man. Anybody fucks with me, I blow their fucking head off. That simple."

As if on cue, a loud buzzer went off and Dennis hoped he wouldn't have to give testimony.

Andy whirled to get a look-see. There was a two-way silver mirrored window in the front door that magnified an image of whoever was on the other side. He reached down below the bar counter and pushed a button that buzzed the guy in.

The door swung open and in walked Rick Uleson

Now Dennis wished he had Andy's toy in his back pocket.

Oh My God, a war zone alright. Now what? He worried Rick might have one of Andy's toys in his back pocket.

He strolled right up to the end of the bar where Dennis and Bokker were propped up on their red vinyl stools.

He extended his hand like they were long lost buddies. "Hey, man, sorry for all that crap, I was loaded and I thought you deliberately slammed the door in my face."

"No, that was purely an accident. The spring on that thing is so freakin' tight, you let go and bam it jerks back halfway instantly. Yeah, sorry for all that horseshit too, that was just a big fuck up. Good thing we didn't kill each other. "

"God knows, we tried," Uleson said. They both laughed.

"Lemme buy ya a drink, buddy," Uleson said.

"Sounds like a winner to me."

He was at Bolton's Bar on Livernois Avenue, not far down the line from the University of Detroit. The place was frequented by more than students, obviously. Thus the two-way mirrored entry door. And the piece in Andy's back pocket.

Turns out, that guy would cause another riot in Detroit in the not-too-distant future when he blew an African

American kid away in the parking lot of his bar. The cops found a screw driver next to his dead body. People had been breaking into cars in his lot. It was self-defense, Andy said.

The whole neighborhood and hundreds and hundreds of others who turned out in the streets with rabid and violent intentions disagreed.

~ ~ ~

There was Heckle and Jeckle.

There was Pixie and Dixie.

And then there was Jerry and James.

James claimed he was Reverend James, and although nobody knew which congregation was his – he claimed he moved churches a lot, sort of like a roving minister, because everybody needed his help – but he claimed he was always at church when he wasn't at the plant.

So why would anybody want to screw with the preacher?

Who knows, other than perhaps because it was great entertainment.

At least once a week a guy named Jerry – Jerry the Janitor they called him, he did work for the maintenance department – would sneak up behind James and poke him in the butt with one of his brooms.

And James would fling his arms wildly in the air and knock about 30 or 40 of the small parts his machine made off of an overhead rack, hurtling them all over the place on the floor. This was the same game these guys played every week, some weeks more than once.

As Jerry stood there laughing uproariously, bending his body backward and forward while slapping his legs and stomping his feet up and down like he was at a Richard Pryor show, the Rev. James would slowly clamber down about 10 steps from his elevated press platform as if he were ninety, and slowly retrieve the parts and re-mount them on the overhead rack while everybody in the vicinity stopped to watch and crack up too while the whole line got a 15-minute-or-so smoke break while the reverend put Humpty Dumpty back together again.

As this shit show played itself out intermittently, a different contest was taking place one line over – on Dennis' fender line.

To avoid the locker room drug-and-pony show, he started stashing his lunch on the floor around the corner from the 15-foot wide monster unit he had recently been transferred to.

Everything was fine the first few days, but on Friday of the second week, he discovered his lunch was MIA.

Always striving to be a glass half-full guy, he imagined maybe the janitor moved it while cleaning and forgot to return it, or maybe the foreman thought it was discarded garbage and threw it out. But by the time his grub was gone for the fourth time in less than another week, he knew otherwise. There can't be that many rats in here, he thought.

To thwart the thief, the next day he got Jerry the Janitor to lend him a screwdriver. He unscrewed the bottom two screws of the front plate covering the electrical box on the side of his 200 ton behemoth, and then he loosened the top two screws such that the panel would open and close freely up and down.

There was space at the bottom of the box under all the wires and circuit board to stash his brown bag in there.

We'll see what happens the next time the dirty SOB tries to rip off my lunch, he gloated to himself. Maybe I'll leave the box half open and he'll see it and the a-hole will electrocute himself.

This experiment didn't last very long.

That same day – the VERY same day at lunch time he opened the box and sure enough his grub was still there and he reached inside to grab it and the next thing he knew he was lying on the ground in extreme shock and pain unable to move and very lucky to be alive. He landed about six feet away from his press. A few minutes later he knew how Andy must have felt as this time the men in white coats loaded him on a gurney and carted him off to the infirmary.

"You are a lucky man, Mr. MulQueen," the medic told him after. "That's quite a shock you survived there."

Not just the extreme voltage required to run a 200-ton press — with the huge amperage or speed of the current necessary, the juice alone should have immediately fried him.

But they said it was even more of a miracle he survived because the maintenance guys had cleaned the floor the night before and the uneven areas adjacent to his unit were littered with pools of water.

"You're lucky you're not barbecue chicken, Mr. MulQueen," the medic said. "How you reached in that box and were not standing in that water only God could have an answer for that. Your arms would have to be eight feet long. Has to be a miracle, young man. Must be a reason you are still alive. Better say some prayers now. Somebody's looking out for you."

~ 12 ~

SEEING THINGS

Oh, that industrial strength Gulden's Mustard carpet. Perfect.

Perfect for hospitals, restaurants – or the college dorm.

Perfect for any kind of spill.

Perfect for hiding everything – except the smell.

Must have happened a thousand times, he thought, as he winced at the unmistakable musty smells-like-alcohol-puke odor that greeted his nostrils that first Saturday morning in September as he walked that hallway carpet toward his new dormitory home. He just finished enrolling that morning for the new semester.

He turned the key in the silver door knob of Room 435, Phelps-Sellers Hall, and pushed the heavy green metal door wide open.

As he set his bags down on the floor in the closet to the right, he heard the sound of running water coming from the open bathroom door, steps ahead on the left. As he walked by, he saw a guy from the side in front of the mirror washing his hands in the sink. He sported dark black hair, and tan yellowish skin, like he had Mexican blood. Dennis MulQueen turned and took a couple steps toward the doorway to introduce himself.

"Hi. You must be my new roommate. I'm Dennis."

"Actually, I believe you are my suitemate," the guy said as pointed to his right toward the opposite end of the bathroom leading to what apparently was his room on the other side.

He turned toward Dennis and extended his hand.

Dennis didn't notice his hand.

His feet were super-glued to the mustard carpet now, his eyes instantly wide as teacups. He tried to speak, but the words stuck in his throat like too much French bread. Only a slight garble was audible.

He nervously cleared his throat and involuntarily let out a deep sigh that sounded more like a gasp.

"Hi," the man in the bathroom said. "My name is Bob. Nice to meet you."

"Ah, yeah, ahh, are you okay? What, umm, what happened?"

He thought his occipital lobe was playing tricks on him. He didn't know exactly what he was looking at. It appeared like he was looking right through this guy's head at his occipital lobe.

He remained standing still in the doorway, breathless now, his gaze frozen straight ahead at the man who was his new suitemate – the man with no eyes.

Where his eyes were supposed to be hung two limp eye lids, hanging like mini wrinkled curtains, sunken in and partially concealing two red and pink hollowed-out sockets. It was early September, not October 31.

"Oh my God, I'm sorry. You caught me, I was just washing my eyes."

He had a shit-eating grin on his face. Dennis MulQueen wondered how many times this had happened before. It would have been so easy to just close the door.

But no, this wasn't Halloween and this guy wasn't kidding.

Dennis noticed a clear bottle of some kind of solution on the counter.

"Yeah, sorry, I have to wash them, or they will turn yellow, and breed infection. These are my eyes here." He retrieved two round ceramic-looking orbs out of a black plastic tray at the bottom of the sink, one in each hand. The perfectly centered fake irises were a brilliant shade of slate blue.

He raised both arms in the air in front of him, elbows tucked in next to his body, like a priest during the offertory, and Dennis was afraid he was going to reach out and give them to him to hold, or, God forbid, to touch.

Maybe he was buying time to prolong the spectacle, but he repeated himself again. "Sorry again, but my name is Bob, and no, I don't believe we are roommates, we are suitemates."

He held the eye in his right hand between his middle finger and thumb like it was a large piece of hard candy as he pointed again with his index finger toward the far doorway at the opposite end of the bathroom.

"You see, we share the same bathroom, we are suitemates," he said.

Dennis was already glad they were suit mates, and not roommates.

"I met your roomie this morning," he continued. "Nice guy, his name is Jim. He left a while ago for lunch, but I'm sure he will be back soon. Excuse me while I finish up here."

He closed the bathroom door.

Hmmm. I thought blind people were supposed to have excellent hearing, Dennis said to himself as he turned to survey his new home.

~ ~ ~

"Everything is easy, " Dr. Marshall said. "If you know what you are doing."

Dennis MulQueen looked at him with eyebrows arched.

"Even double and triple integration?" he asked.

149

"Yes. Even double and triple integration."

He was a roly-poly jocular kind of guy, this professor, an egghead genius type totally above and beyond the ordinary. Dennis MulQueen's alter-ego Uncle Fester calculus professor.

Above all, he was approachable, so here Dennis was in the guy's face once again after class, begging for help for the fifth time in only the second week of the semester.

Because he needed it.

You see, he had this point to prove.

"I've got a suggestion for you," Dr. Marshall said. "Instead of coming up here after class every day, when I only have five minutes because I have to leave for another class, go upstairs to room 425 at 7 o'clock tonight. One of my grad assistants will meet you there. He's there every night from 7 to 9, mostly for my upper class students. But he will help you too. I'll tell him to expect you."

"Thanks, Doc."

And this kind of attitude from a guy that wrote the book? Yes, and other higher level treatises he also authored, even some for grad level classes.

But darn, from 7 to 9?

There went his career at Charlie's, the local pub hot spot for students. Oh well. Happy hour was now a brain exercise.

The saving grace was Doc Marshall made it worth it. By making it interesting, and fun, if you can believe Calc could be interesting AND fun. He made it – no pun intended – a no-brainer.

By the sheer force of his personality.

He was a hoot up there in front of the blackboard, a star up there performing every day for his students. He was animated, he was hilarious, he was an entertainer but he knew his stuff inside-out and he knew how to explain things. He was an absolutely terrific instructor, a great example the

150

sky's the limit if you have a modicum of talent – and gobs of passion – to be something special.

Sure enough it worked. Not to a T, though, as Dennis did have to peer at the guy's paper next to him during the final, just to be sure. But nonetheless – after five-days-a week tutoring and numerous all-nighters, he nail-gunned a solid A in first year Calculus.

Oh, that point to prove – this was Dennis' academic version of three-a-days.

And not just math. He had Honors English with Professor McDonald. She was another outstanding teacher that challenged her students to take it to the next level.

(The syllabus included Lewis Lapham, H.L. Mencken, and Faulkner, to name a few.) Students were required to read *Harper's*, an incredibly stimulating high-level magazine (Lapham was the editor, a guy with perhaps a command of the language second to none), *The Atlantic*, and *The New Yorker*, with term papers assigned for articles in all three.

Taking the cue, he pretended he was writing *Absalom Absalom* for the first term paper in her class. When she made him read that first major assignment out loud in class in front of everybody, he figured she had to be impressed with his big-time, big-word verbiage – disingenuous or not.

So if it ain't broken, why fix it?

In his next paper he used more big words and compound convoluted language in emulation of Faulkner and HL Mencken and Lewis Lapham, showcasing an unmitigated display of acumen through an erudite countenance that left her innately thrilled beyond satiety with the profundity of his perspicacity attributable in no small measure to her professorial poignance – all aimed at forcefully and cogitatively and manipulative-intent-wise, securing the grade he indeterminately deigned unmitigated insouciance about.

You get it.

But it worked.

Another A+ in the bag.

Like netting butterflies at the Butterfly Zoo.

His new found success off the field also included an A in abnormal psyche, an A in Physics and another A in Inorganic Chem from Professor Powell.

"How sweet it is," he shouted out loud when he opened the mail to see it for himself.

A perfect 4.0, the first of three in a row he nailed down in an effort that saw him rise to the top of his class.

Oh yeah, Jackie, one more for old time's sake, how sweet it is indeed.

"The Honeymooners" was his father's favorite show, with Jackie Gleason as Ralph Kramden and Art Carney as his sidekick Norton with their wives Alice (Audrey Meadows) and Trixie (Joyce Randolph) co-starring.

"The Honeymooners" was the main event in the MulQueen household every weekend.

"You're going to the moon, Alice."

"Oh Ralph, the moon wouldn't be big enough for you," Alice would respond.

To Dennis, his father WAS Jackie.

How truly sweet it was to see him belly laugh like the great Gleason and shake those hands of his back and forth like Ralph when Dennis handed him that piece of paper that day. So much for football.

He would chew on his tongue, and hold his arms ramrod straight about a foot from his sides like he was getting ready to dive off the high board or a dodo attempting to fly once more while suddenly those hands and fingers shook back and forth at gyroscopic speed turning them into whirling dervishes of happy times while his belly jiggled up and down rhythmically as simultaneously he made the coolest most indescribably cool sound like wind on Key West bristling through the Poinciana trees as all the while his lips reverberated and bubbled and hummed like he was playing an evanescent air trumpet. The original and forever George L MulQueen Jr. hand-bob shake-and-bake.

So much for football.

It felt so good because he felt like he was finally coming close to taking care of what his brilliant friend Scaboni told him that day. He was convinced that at the root of most troubles in life were conflicts with one's parents over life choices, dreams and expectations.

He took a deep breath as he recalled that conversation once again.

Ah, those points to prove. So nice to have all that mess out of the way. No sooner did he get his first 4 pointer than the NFL was replaced by the AMA (the American Medical Association). He walked in the living room and calmly announced to his parents he was going to become a medical doctor. Like a million other college students.

They bit on it hook line and sinker, announcing to the world that their son was going to be the next Albert Schweitzer. No, he wasn't going to be any ordinary physician; he was going to cure cancer and heart disease and save the world.

Or at least that's what Dennis MulQueen imagined they were saying about him.

Of course, they did encourage him, with his mother mentioning a couple days later that an uncle, who was a medical doctor in nearby Genesee County with a thriving practice, had put the word out his nephew was first in line to join his practice and eventually take over someday.

Even though he hadn't even applied yet – or moreover even completed undergrad yet. For good measure, his father informed him that his personal physician and good friend, the esteemed Dr. Stanley H. Levy MD, a renowned local internist on the faculty at Wayne State University, would also help him with letters of recommendation and assistance in navigating his way into and out of Wayne State University Medical School, a top US medical school in Detroit, Michigan, if he so chose to go that route.

The two became friends in 1958 when George L. MulQueen was chairman of the Oakland County Youth Guidance Board and Dr. Levy was a member of that body which they created to help area kids with psychological problems who were experiencing difficulties at school or at home.

Having Dr. Levy in his corner certainly would be a huge plus for Dennis MulQueen, as this well-known physician was a top notch fixture in the Detroit medical community as well as the metro area Jewish community. You could find him at Orchestra Hall listening to the Detroit Symphony or at the Detroit Institute of Arts as well as find him reading a medical journal first thing in the morning, or of course walking the halls of Sinai hospital all hours of the day or night.

This amazing man's house was like a museum. When you exited the foyer and walked around the corner of one hallway you passed a life-size artistic rendering of Albert Einstein on the way to a gallery that included huge life-size portraits of the Dalai Lama, Martin Luther King, Moshe Dayan, David Ben-Gurion, Picasso and Michelangelo, Albert Schweitzer, Rosa Parks and Nelson Mandela.

The defining feature of the house was the lower level – the entire lower level of his Bloomfield home was a library the envy of any bibliophile anywhere. His entire basement was bookshelves everywhere. He had a home library of books – 15,000 hardcover volumes in total, including everything from Descartes and Plato and all the great philosophers on to Chaucer and Shakespeare to first edition Dickens on top of every imaginable scientific and medical book on the planet. Instead of reading the sports pages, this guy would just as soon pull off the shelves of his library a volume of *The Mind*, the quarterly review of psychology and philosophy written by Alan Turing, the genius-level scientist and philosopher who first conceptualized what became the world's first computer and is the guy credited with developing Artificial Intelligence. Turing, a major codebreaker instrumental in helping the Allies defeat Hitler in WWII, was also the first to warn the world about the digital threat to the future of humanity. Dr. Levy's upstairs gallery also contained a huge framed lithograph of the "Turing Machine," considered the precursor to the modern computer.

Dr. Levy is a man who rather than read the comics would rather read the collected works of Thomas Jefferson.

George MulQueen took Chip and Dennis MulQueen to his office one day when they were little kids just to make sure they got a chance to meet this fascinating medical doctor.

In fact, Dr. Levy could be the only guy who actually knew and was friends with four Nobel Prize winners – starting with the man who was on display in one of the corridors of his house. Dr. Levy actually met Albert Einstein while an undergrad at Princeton and one time shared Passover Seder with the preeminent scientist. He also knew Enrico Fermi, another great Nobel-Prize-winning physicist who was also on the Manhattan project, whom he met at a scientific conference in late winter of 1951 in Chicago, when Fermi was on the faculty of the University of Chicago. And he also knew Linus Pauling, the only man in history to win two unshared Nobel Prizes, who he was first introduced to in San Francisco at a conference Pauling was hosting on Vitamin C. Dr. Levy would also get to know another prominent Nobel-Prize winning Physicist named Eric Cornell, who he had over to his house for dinner when he was in Detroit as a guest lecturer at Wayne State University.

So if anybody would appreciate his son's rise to academic prominence, George L MulQueen knew it would be his personal friend and physician Dr. Stanley Hurwick Levy, who he proudly informed of his invitation to dinner at EMU President Harold Sponberg's residence in honor of his son Dennis MulQueen's rise to the top of his class after three pre-med 4.0's in a row.

George MulQueen also told his friend to look for an invitation to an upcoming awards ceremony and dinner to further celebrate the occasion.

Oh, those points to prove.

To see the old man giddy with his hand bob shake-and-bake going a mile-a-minute like that, the belly laughs rolling up and down like a shook-up pot of Jell-O when he talked about his son becoming a medical doctor, oh yes, how sweet it is, Dennis MulQueen thought.

~ ~ ~

She opened the garage door and called for her son.

He was not in a good mood, or maybe he just didn't want to hear it again.

"Come on, Robert. Come on in for dinner," she said.

"Mother, what the hell, it's only four thirty, why so early?" her son replied.

They normally didn't eat dinner until after 5.

"Just put that junk away and come inside, will you please before you kill yourself out there," she said. "By the time you have everything cleaned up out there, everything will be on the table."

He didn't believe the early dinner part. She had warned him once before about his favorite hobby.

"You're going to kill yourself, I'm telling' ya, Robert."

He shouted back at her, "The sky is falling, the sky is falling. Darn, Mother, okay, I'll be in in a few minutes."

She was in the kitchen setting the table about 15 minutes later when her worst fears came to be. An enormous boom rocked the kitchen walls and shook the floor she was standing on – it sounded like a plane had hit the house.

This was no plane crash, and she knew it.

She raced from the kitchen down the side hallway and flung open the wooden door leading to the garage. She immediately started coughing and gagging. The air was thick with acrid black smoke and the bitter stench of gun powder vapors. She couldn't see three feet in front of her.

She pulled the bottom of her sweater up to her mouth as a makeshift mask and ambled unsteadily toward the opposite wall where about 10 feet in she almost tripped over her son, who was laying prone on the cold concrete floor in a pool of blood. He was completely unconscious.

She was sure he was dead.

He had deep shrapnel wounds to his head and face, his chest and his legs. He also suffered the most horrific injuries imaginable to his groin area.

But the worst injury, if you discount the fact there was nothing left to carry on the family line with, occurred to his eyes, which were blown out of his head by the blast.

He was alive – it was a miracle he was still alive – but blinded for life. And sterile.

And forever unable to explain how or why things went awry this day when he had done the same thing so many times before. This was his favorite past time – making his own firecrackers. He had done it for years. Big, impressive, loud and scary firecrackers. For all the neighborhood kids to be envious of. If not afraid of.

He had once again carefully emptied out the black powder from a whole carton of the standard-issue two-inch pencil firecrackers, just like before, in preparation for concocting the much larger custom fireworks he liked to show off with at parties and holidays. Think cherry bombs, only five times larger and 10 times more powerful.

He used the same ace of spades playing card he had used many times before to scrape the gun powder – this time enough to make in addition to a batch of cherry bombs several of the giant columnar ones he preferred – into a single pile in the middle of a small concrete slab that rested on his lap, a leftover piece of the old front sidewalk his parents had replaced years ago.

"If only I had listened to my mother," he said as he was in Dennis' room giving this play-by-play description of what happened that day that lead to him cleaning his eyes in the sink for the rest of his life.

He pulled up his left sleeve to expose a gold watch with a black band with a bronze face and raised hour and minute hands and no crystal. He felt the dial with his right index finger and started singing.

"*Oh Charlie, oh Charlie, I hear you calling me, oh Charlie oh Charlie, we love you Charlie*," he sang discordantly to his suitemate.

Charlie as in Hungry Charlie's Bar and Grill, the most popular drinking venue on the Ypsilanti EMU campus, that was also Bob's favorite spot.

"*Come on you, big lug, you ready to go? It's two-for-one Tuesday.*"

Dennis liked Bob, he wanted to go with him again. Other than a few idiosyncrasies, like taking his eyes out in front of complete strangers, Bob wasn't much different from anybody else. He was basically a good guy who like most people, made some dumb mistakes when he was young but that unfortunately, in his case, resulted in consequences almost beyond comprehension.

Everybody says and does stupid things when they are young, it's just some people end up paying a much higher price. Dennis had great empathy and respect for his suitemate, to see him out there with courage going for it could only be inspiring. If anybody, he could have easily said the hell with it and folded his tent, like so many others in his position probably have.

As far as Dennis was concerned, there could be no worse situation in life. Being paralyzed would be one thing, but blind?

And Bob was the worst kind of blind, a guy who once had sight but lost it. Bob knew what he was missing, in contrast to those blind from birth, who can't fully comprehend what they've never experienced, something that is impossible to explain to them. Ever try to describe the colors of the rainbow to a blind man?

But as much as Dennis wanted to go with him to Charlie's again, he knew he couldn't go this time.

"Sorry, Bob, I'm going to have to take a raincheck. I'm way behind in Chem, got a quiz tomorrow. Next time, okay?"

"Okay. See you again in a while, Dennis. No pun intended."

He turned and left the room and just like that he was off to Charlie's solo.

Turned out Dennis would actually hear his suitemate again, before he would see him again.

A little less than two hours later, he heard the muffled screams, then a wham, then a bang, it sounded like a freeway pile-up. No mistaking the sounds of crunched metal and broken glass.

But this was no car accident.

Dennis pulled back the drape and leaned out the open window. There was Bob, with his white and red cane and short dark mop of hair on top that made him look like Moe from the Three Stooges, off in the distance, emerging over the hill steadily trudging down the sidewalk toward the dorm complex.

Now the sirens were blaring in the distance as he watched Bob disappear under the overhang into the dormitory lobby, just in the nick of time.

A couple minutes later he heard him enter the suite.

It was the EMU landscape guys again, he explained. Another EMU service truck parked off road, they were trimming a tree in the courtyard, and Bob stumbled into the back end of their vehicle overhanging the sidewalk.

Which now needed new windows and a bit of body work.

The same thing had already happened before and Bob had complained to maintenance to no apparent avail. He just couldn't take it anymore. This was the third time.

At least being blind does have one benefit. The cops knew who did it, half the campus probably knew by now, but they never charged him with anything for his vehicular assaults.

As Bob vented, Dennis could tell by the smell he had patronized Charlie's very well that day.

"You okay, Bob?"

He ignored Dennis' question. He needed to talk about it his way.

"I am just sick and tired of running into these bastards' vehicles, why can't they have a little respect and decency and just plain old fucking common sense and not park on the goddamned sidewalk?

"I'm going to warn the other guys. Wanna come?"

"Yeah, okay."

They walked across the hall two rooms down on the left. Bob knocked on the door with his cane, now distinctly bent in a couple places with several spots of chipped paint.

James, who was friends with Bob and also blind, greeted the two of them as they walked in. They weren't there too long, with the conversation consisting mostly of Bob bitching some more about running into the truck, before Dennis told the guys he just wanted to say Hi but needed to get back to do some more studying.

As he said good bye and got up to leave the room, he opened the door, took one step outside onto the carpet, then stepped back into the room and closed the door, without saying a word.

They kept talking, with James asking Bob about a sociology class they shared together unaware Dennis was still in the room.

Dennis felt a slight rush run up and down his spine when he thought how he would explain it if either of them realized he was still there.

More talk. Nothing worth eavesdropping.

I guess they're not going to talk about me after all, or anything interesting, he said to himself.

Just as Dennis turned to reach for the door knob, Bob said, "James I'm curious what you think about my suitemate Dennis?"

"Seems all right to me Bob. Why do you ask?"

"I just wondered what you think because actually I think he's a real asshole."

Dennis' jaw dropped but he managed to keep still.

"Bob, why do you say that, I thought you told me before he is a good guy, helpful and a good attitude and drinking buddy and all that good shit. What changed?"

"Well, I lied. He's an ass and I'm going to go back over there now and tell him about it."

Dennis quickly reached out behind himself and knocked on the door from inside where he still stood, fearing Bob might run into him on the way out. Then he opened the door quickly and then closed it again without moving a step.

"Hey guys. It's me. I'm back. I left my drink here on the dresser, It's me, Dennis".

"Well, hello there Dennis," Bob said.

"Oh, okay, Dennis," James said.

"Thanks guys, see you later."

He turned and opened the door and quickly walked out into the hallway as he pulled the green metal door shut behind him.

About an hour later, he heard the far away bathroom door open and about five seconds later a human head popped around the corner.

Dennis swore Bob could see him through those glass eyes.

"Hi Bob what's up?"

"Nothing Dennis. James and I just wondered where you got that Bravura you been wearing today?"

"Huh?," Dennis said.

"Just wondered where you got that stuff," Bob continued. "Very distinctive, smells really good in his room, that Bravura cologne you were wearing today. In fact we were talking about how that scent never left the room."

There was a pause. Dennis said nothing.

"You know, Dennis, how if you trap a raccoon and drop him off across town and he finds his way back to his home under your deck? He follows his own scent trail all the way back that's how he finds his way back home. Well, it's the same with a dog, he will follow his scent back home that's why he doesn't get lost either. And you know something Dennis? That's how blind people get back home too. Because God compensates them by giving them the same kind a nose as a mad dog. You know, don't you Dennis, that blind people are like mad dogs too?"

Dennis remained silent.

"Well now you know asshole. You better hope there is no karma or you might end up smelling like a mad dog yourself."

"Sorry Bob. I just wanted to know what you really thought of me. How you talked about me behind my back."

"Well now you know Dennis."

He said nothing as he turned and disappeared back across the bathroom tile floor to his half of the suite.

Dennis turned his attention back to the stack of books on his desk. No time to dwell on every stupid thing he'd ever done. Not enough time for that. He had other things to think about.

A point to prove, remember?

Three 4.0's in a row, a really tough pre-med curriculum, and now what? Well, it was looking like things were going to be considerably different here in post-football semester number four.

Big D was now officially D +. Or at least he could be. That's the grade he got on his last chem test. The biggest test of the year so far, the last one before the final. And going into that one, with a C + average, this means he had to practically write an infallible encyclical on the final exam to even come close to maintaining his streak of academic excellence.

But chem was only one issue.

He was hitting the wall pretty much across the board.

Skinner et all in experimental psyche, he was currently running a C + in there, and the lab was about the same. Not to mention he was barely tracking a B minus in honors English.

There were two weeks left until finals and not only was another 4.0 all but impossible now, it would take divine intervention to get even a 3.0. Realistically, at this point it would take all he could do to keep his grade point from collapsing right into the gutter – along with any dreams of med school. Or grad school of any kind.

He needed a break.

Or so he thought.

~ 13 ~

LIFE IS AN ACCIDENT

The place was called Crandon Park.

Crandon Heaven – to him.

Not because of the powder blue sky and the shimmering rays of sunlight dancing on the frothy aqua-marine waves and the tall, stately, emerald green palms swaying to the soothing salty breeze with the squeaky-white sand underfoot everywhere – there was even a concession stand, and a small zoo with gazelles, flamingoes and gators.

Not because of any of that.

Because of her.

Every step of the way from the parking lot to the water he fixed his gaze on the heavenly 17-year-old in the tiny orange-and-black bikini as she sauntered across the white sand carpet in front of him to the edge of the turquoise-blue expanse extending forever in front of them.

She had the tight athletic body of a gymnast, hardly an ounce of body fat, muscular creamy white thighs, small teenage chest, a muscular and tight bottom not too small, not too big – just perfect, really, in all ways imaginable, as perfect as only God could make a heavenly young beauty like her.

From her long thin silky brunette hair all lit up with caramel lights in the dazzling sun, to the smooth china doll skin and lean sculpted alabaster nose. From her glistening blue hazel eyes to her perfect pearly white teeth framed in by gorgeous soft and full pink lips.

True beauty, pure beauty, God-like heavenly beauty – that rarest of all beauty, that which shines even brighter in the dull light of early morning, with matter in the eyes – and no make-up.

They had an unnatural connection since the first time they met two years ago just like this at a beach on his first visit to South Florida.

They stayed in touch and corresponded and he called her as soon as the plane landed. Both her parents were drunks, his parents wanted to kill him for going there, and here they were.

Suddenly, nothing mattered.

Except this.

Suddenly, everything in the world was okay now – the minute he stepped off the plane.

The surcease of all void.

The incredible, endless delight of a sly smile, a wink, a nod, a touch of skin, a hug.

Or a kiss.

The surcease of all void.

All too good to be true – everything in the world was wonderful with her standing in front of him, the ineffable pull of the purest romantic delight on earth, the unmitigated delight of the purest of passions, the young, innocent first time love standing before him. Everything in the world was okay now.

The surcease of all void.

The advent of pure happiness. He could feel it in the air everywhere.

A tightness of mind, body and spirit that was forever.

Unassailable.

Indestructible.

Unbreakable and unstoppable.

The fire within.

Right there, in his face.

Begging for a way out, into this heaven, the both of them.

The greatest of escapes, from all earthly mayhem.

The surcease of all void.

He is right, he thought, as he listened to that same song over and over again in his head. It isn't about football, or 4.0's. Now he and John Lennon both knew the true meaning of life. It is about this.

"All you need is love.
All you need is love.
All you need is love."

He wasn't at Crandon Park. He was in the Garden of Eden.

Crandon Heaven. Life would never be the same again.

In ways he never could have imagined.

If only he could have known.

~ ~ ~

This was a northern version of Crandon Park – minus the palm trees and the postage stamp bikinis.

The rock garden by itself on the short bluff overlooking the beach and the freshwater ocean that stretched 280 miles to the south east was the botanical equivalent of anything put together by any master gardener in Florida or anywhere else in the world. Even the fabled Busch Gardens in Tampa had nothing on this floral masterpiece on the lake.

The first harbinger of this seasonal northern glory coincided with the final spring melt each year as just as certain as the sun the stars and the moon the crocuses shot through the earth like tiny little white and purple doll house baby bottle brushes. Simultaneously, delicate ribbons of spring beauty popped everywhere on the lawn, tiny sprigs of greenery supporting tiny orange-and-blue bell-bottom blossoms no bigger than a pencil eraser that brought buckets of colorful beauty to life.

Then, having received their cue, like clockwork the other members of this annual spring nature show took off one by one as next it was the dollar tree plants time to show off their manna from heaven, the large silver dollar shaped seed pods providing the background for their prolific purple blooms as days later the sweet lily-of-the-valley spread their fragrant white carpet of tiny bell-bottom flowers all across the hill side leading to the water.

Next in line to show off were the signature attention grabbers of these opulent lake-front gardens – the big lilies – orange day lilies, purple and yellow hybrid day lilies, tall ever-blooming Easter white and fuchsia and blue lilies, every-color-in-the-rainbow of lily that slowly waved welcome any given summer day here to any and all partakers of the balmy summer Lake Erie breezes.

And it kept on going from there.

Petunias and portulacas, Johnny jump ups and black-eyed Susans, the yellow and red gaillardias mixed throughout an elegant smorgasbord of hostas – first the purple hosta blooms in spring followed by the white broad-leafed hostas in midsummer then the purple and bi-colored yellow and green leaved masterpieces blooming out of their minds in late summer.

And all this – if you can believe it – and you must, because it's true – all this was only part of God's nature show on Westchester Beach that was of course produced, directed and choreographed by non-other than Moms Mabley herself.

There was something for everybody here at the MulQueen family compound on Lake Erie. And not just for family members and friends and anonymously-passing sightseers on the lane and on the beach – but for the butterflies and birds, too.

The finches loved the purple coneflower seeds while the hummingbirds loved the bright red monarda and cardinal flower and trumpet vine best while the Monarch butterflies favored the purple and orange buddleia bushes and the bright orange-flowered butterfly weed.

And day after day as a kid he waited outside in the back for a glimpse of the dazzling giant sphinx moths who daily at precisely dusk flocked voraciously to glob after glob of petunias of all colors poised like plastic-wrapped bunches of tootsie roll lollipops hanging in pots off the back porch.

Not to be left out, Pat MulQueen planted something for every family member, too.

A miniature black raspberry bush for her Mickelberry (The youngest boy, Michael) carnations for Maureen and orange butterfly flower for Peggy Pumpkin and Basil and Bear's Breeches for Dennis, and a small plant with cute button-like flowers she called her Little Chipper plant named in honor of the oldest brother Chip.

The remaining exotic tossed in for effect was the cigar plant she planted at the top center of the garden in honor of George MulQueen Jr, the titular head of this gang who always loved a good cigar, the bigger and fatter the better.

This fragrance-filled cornucopia of Fantasia-like color continued up the bank, where a separate and spectacular-in-its-own-right smaller garden lie, mostly dominated by tulips, peonies and columbines that stretched about 35 feet along the back of the four-boat boathouse tucked into the bluff.

Surrounding the house was magnificently fragrant privet, miniature lilac bushes and a pink-flowered shrub and the trumpet vine especially loved by the hummingbirds.

A special garden of delightfully colorful impatiens set off the east side of the house facing the neighbors that his mother affectionately called the Griffin Garden in honor of the dear family friends who lived there.

This garden also contained a well-planted plethora of daisies and marigolds and more multi-colored petunias. Meanwhile, mock orange bushes displayed their white and orange blooms on either side of the back porch, u ball green evergreens next to them, more privet on the porch corners in front, two more miniature lilacs, two beautiful bushes with gorgeous yellow flowers in the spring, and still more petunias and impatiens and portulaca and pansies surrounded by an interweaving tapestry of violets.

Not to be left out, the back of the property was framed in by white honeysuckle while a splendid row of prized rose bushes of multiple botanical lines set off the far north western edge of the property.

Every square inch of this 600-foot long Lake Erie lot was part of the Pat Helferty MulQueen Grand Botanical Gardens.

Yes. Something for everybody.

And let's not leave out another incredible rose garden on the west side of the house, the side that had the chimney. This one was also special in its own right because it consisted of transplants from the MulQueen childhood home in Oak Park. A space of about 15 feet dead smack in the middle encompassed the entire chimney width, nothing but luscious deep red roses, their hanging huge blooms hugely overpowering the property with their sweet syrupy smells.

These were Dennis MulQueen's favorites, the roses, along with the Mexican sunflowers his mother had several patches of at various key spots on the property. The best crop of them lined the stairway he and his mother built down the right side of the front hill.

They dug out the hill, bought the one square foot concrete slab squares, small rocks, gravel and sand then mixed the concrete and built the stairway step-by-step.

This woman was talented.

And his father appreciated her talent – and the time, effort and money she put into making this place a statement destination – a show place – inside and out.

For her, it was a no-brainer.

If you loved something – no matter what it was – you just did it and all out with passion.

Life was all about doing what you loved.

That meant it wasn't work – it was fun.

She walked her own talk, this woman, and that meant every year two weeks leading up to Memorial Day weekend and two weeks following Memorial Day, you always knew where you could find her on the weekends – at her Lake Erie sanctuary, in her gardens, overlooking the beach, the Great Lake Erie, always a nice cool breeze, lots of sunshine, the waves non-stop in their infinite grace hitting the shore with that soothing swooshing rhythmic sound of the good life on the lake in action.

That would be no different this Canadian Memorial Day weekend of 1974, that's where she was once again, working the gardens, as his father supervised from his near-by chase lounge, perched at the top of the bank, puffing on his Churchill, martini in hand.

Late Sunday and the preliminary garden work was done as closing time arrived – it was Sunday, May 19, 1974 – and they weren't planning on returning to Michigan until the following morning so he made her an offer she couldn't refuse.

"Hey, Dearie, it's almost dinner time, everything is beautiful," George MulQueen said. "How about you let me treat you to a date. Let's go to Duffy's."

"That'll be wonderful, honey," she said.

They came inside the house for a quick clean-up and change-of-clothes before heading out on the road in their 1968 Galaxie LTD station wagon.

As they emerged from the house, you could see despite the movement of the calendar, he was still as handsome as she was beautiful. And they were both still doing it. The modern suburban power couple, all these years, still going at it, he still credit union president and Dad's Club and Youth Guidance Board head, she, still the publisher of seven newspapers and a stylish and esteemed modern-day socialite in her own league among women.

The modern-day power couple living large at their favorite spot on earth, where they came to chill, to relax, to have fun and to celebrate.

Now on their way to their favorite lakefront restaurant.

Since he already had a couple martinis and hadn't slept but a couple hours the night before because of his midnight gig at Ford Motor Co., he asked Pat to do the driving.

They gathered up Michael and Maureen, and off they went down Highway 18 to the well-known and frequented riverfront restaurant on the banks of the Detroit River named Duffy's.

The place was owned by a very nice couple named Zarco and Bessie. They put everything into the place, their slogan was "The Best Place on the Lake Erie Coast." And it was.

They were very nice people and they ran a great establishment. There was all-you-can-eat perch and chicken and crab legs; there was Canadian beer and drinks and a dance band banging it out all night long.

The place was always mobbed. Boaters galore. You couldn't have a better time than at Duffy's.

~ ~ ~

At exactly 11 p.m. the phone rang at 21471 Kipling Avenue, Oak Park, Michigan.

Chip answered. His sister Maureen was on the line.

"Chip, we are at Hotel Dieu Hospital in Windsor. We have been in a really bad accident. Me and Michael were in the back, we are okay, but Mom is in bad shape and they won't let me see Dad."

"How bad was Dad hurt? Why won't they let you see him?"

"He was hurt really bad, Chip. Blood everywhere, in tremendous pain."

"Is he alive, Maur?"

"I don't know, Chip. They won't tell us anything."

As it turned out, when they rounded a curve on Highway 18A at the intersection of a small side road, a tractor pulled out in front of them, a green John Deere tractor with a green John Deere trailer in tow – with no lights on anywhere. And it was dark by the time they rounded this curve, and she had no time to react as she was on top of the tractor by the time she saw it.

She slammed into the back of it and the 1968 Ford LTD station wagon spun several times in the air, flipped and careened upside down off the road past the pea-gravel shoulder, slamming into the ground on the very edge, about six inches into the swamp on the east side of the road.

Inches from filling with water and drowning, George MulQueen was trapped between the caved-in dash and the floorboard of the overturned vehicle. There was no way out.

Pat MulQueen later estimated she was going about 50 miles an hour, the speed limit along this stretch of the highway.

As soon as the car came to rest, he said, "What the hell did you hit, Pat?"

173

"It was a tractor, George. I didn't see it. He had no lights on, he pulled out right in front of us."

She was bloodied and had massive bruising, but she had no fractures or head injury. The only way out was through the back window, so she crawled back that way in the upside down vehicle and with Michael and Maureen in tow, they escaped.

Dust still hung in the air as he began quietly moaning, the shock of the collision giving way to the intense pain of his injuries.

Luckily, a police cadet drove by the scene and immediately called the accident in. In another odd coincidence, the priest at the local parish in Harrow also was driving home from Amherstburg when he spotted their overturned vehicle on the edge of the swamp. He pulled over to see if he could help and was shocked to see it involved one of his favorite parish families.

"Oh my god, George, let me bless you. Would you like to go to confession?" Fr. James Martin said.

"Hell no, Father," he said. "I went last Saturday."

Chip had immediately jumped in his father's Oldsmobile 98 with the second sister, Peggy, and headed for the border. He got to the tunnel and pulled up to pay the fare but when he reached for his wallet realized he had left it at home. His father George had a book of bridge tickets in the glove box, though, so he was able to get through the border. The customs officers did not ask him for ID.

When they got to the hospital, their mother and father were on gurneys at opposite ends of the emergency room.

Chip talked to his mother, then went looking for his dad. He was relieved to find out he was still alive.

"Chip, I think I broke my back. Can you feel along my back and see if anything is sticking out?"

"Can't feel anything, Dad."

Chip promptly asked for the attending physician.

There was no attending physician.

He called his father's Michigan physician, Dr. Stanley Dr. Levy's first question was whether his parents could be transported. A decision was made to get George L. MulQueen Jr. over the border by ambulance to Sinai Hospital in Detroit, where Dr. Levy was on staff.

George MulQueen was in rough shape. His legs were messed up. Bone on bone. Looked like he would need skin grafts, and X-rays showed his sternum was cracked. But thank God for small favors – he also had no head injury, no internal injuries that were apparent and no paralysis.

And he was alive. Everybody in the family knew the acronym for toughness in this family – GLM Jr.

~ 14 ~

THE CHICKENS COME HOME TO ROOST

Lums. A great place to hang out. Miller High Life on tap. Great music. And those kraut dogs.

And the Florida sun that was always shining through the front windows during Happy Hour. What more could you want?

Only one thing.

Her.

The hot young babe across the table. His first. His only. His everything.

And now he had her.

Life couldn't be better.

It might have been Memorial Day weekend in Canada – but there was a much better holiday going on in South Florida. This was the first weekend they stayed overnight in the same place.

Had to be karma. As they got up to leave the restaurant, their song came on the radio.

"The first time ever I saw your face.

177

I thought the sun rose in your eyes
and the moon and the stars were the gifts you gave ..."

Sing it, Roberta Flack.

When they pulled in the driveway, he leaned over end kissed her and told her he loved her.

About an hour later the phone rang.

"It's for you," she said as she handed him the receiver.

"Hello."

"We have been in a horrible accident. Your father is in very serious condition. He has a cracked sternum and his legs are real bad. He will likely need skin grafts at a minimum. You've got to come home right away."

"Okay, Mom. I'll look into flights. What happened? Everybody else okay? What about you?"

"I just have a lot of bruises but nothing broken. Maureen and Mike were okay. They were in the far back of the wagon and weren't hurt other than a small bump on Michael's head. They were pretty shook up though. Obviously. A tractor pulled out in front of us with no lights on."

"Can I talk to Dad?"

He came on the line and other than being groggy, he sounded not too bad.

"I'm okay, Son, just got racked up a little, I'll be fine."

"That's good, Dad. Hang in there. I'll see you soon."

He said goodbye and his mother took the phone back.

"Okay, let me know what flight you're coming in on, we'll get somebody there to pick you up."

"Okay, Mom. Talk to you later."

It was a subdued evening in south Florida following that call. They ordered some pizza from Frankie's, they watched a little TV, he had a couple more Millers and they went to bed.

The next morning, the phone rang again mid-morning.

"I'm going to call the airlines now, Mom, and I will get back with you."

"You mean you haven't called them yet?"

She blew up and hung up the phone.

Later that afternoon he called the hospital and talked to his father again.

He said he was getting his leg wounds de-breeded regularly and was hoping maybe he could avoid skin grafts.

His cracked sternum was painful as hell but there wasn't anything they could do about that. He just needed a little time to heal, he said. He was going to be all right, he reiterated.

His father didn't mention anything else.

"Hang in there, Dad. Talk to you soon."

"Okay, Son. Goodbye for now."

The phone rang again the next day.

A family member on the line again.

"Look, I want you to know something. You are killing your father. You have to come home. Now. This is killing him, you being down there."

He inhaled slowly and exhaled like a fireplace bellow.

"I just talked to him. He said he's not too bad."

"Yeah, that's what he's telling you."

"Do you know when you are coming home?"

"Soon. I'll be home soon."

They hung up and after that call, he dialed the number for Eastern Airlines.

Four days later, he flew home.

After they made plans for her to fly to Michigan a couple weeks later.

~ ~ ~

The shortstop threw the ball wild.

Dennis MulQueen, who was the first baseman, jumped in the air – it was about three feet over his head – and he got just enough glove on the ball it rolled dead about 10 feet behind him. The runner kept on going, as Dennis pounced

179

on the ball and threw a laser to Tom the Bomb Maloney who was covering second base. The ball missed the runners head by not more than two inches.

Maloney snared it out of thin air like Aparicio and easily tagged the guy out.

"Jesus, D. I've never seen a rocket like that before. You almost killed that guy," Maloney said afterward in the living room of their Ann Arbor apartment as he handed Dennis a cold Schlitz and a Newport, their standard after-ball-game hors d' oeuvres.

"Here you go, D."

He was roommates with Tom, along with his buddy TJ, who set up the arrangement. They needed an extra guy, and he was available, so it was working out great. They were having a good summer. It was the first week of August already.

"Nothing like a cold beer and a smoke on a hot day after a little workout," Tom said.

You could hear the collective *ahhh*. "You got that right, brother," Dennis MulQueen said.

No sooner had the after-party begun, the phone rang. Tom grabbed it and handed the receiver to Dennis.

"It's for you," he said. "It's your brother."

"Hi Chip. What's going on?"

Just like that he said it.

"Dad has leukemia."

"What? What are you talking about? Don't tell me that."

"We just found out about an hour ago."

He could feel the anger burning through the phone.

"Huh?"

"A routine blood test, it came back positive for white blood cells, they did a couple more tests and they told us."

There was a pause. His brother said nothing. Dennis said nothing. There was no talk. Because he couldn't talk.

"You might want to come and see him now."

He struggled to say something, anything. No words possible. Dead silence. The tears flooded his face and shirt. His chest jerked up and down involuntarily, like his body was trying to reject his heart.

"I gotta go now.

"Okay. "

"Bye."

He hung up the phone. The conversation was over.

He didn't even know what kind of leukemia, or any kind of prognosis. He knew all there was to know now – life is horrible.

He walked back to his bedroom, still shuddering, and closed the door. In total shock. Janey was sitting on the bed.

The tears were still streaming down his face. He sat at the opposite end of the bed. He had to. His knees were weak. His head felt faint. He slumped back against the wall.

No way. This can't be. No no no. Please tell me it's a lie. This is a screw up.

Janey tried to comfort him.

She was no comfort.

He didn't read anything into it at the time, but it was as if she wasn't even there. The complete opposite of everything up until then.

The surcease of all fantasy. Instantly over. Forever changed. Everything.

TJ knocked on the door and Janey let him in. He told him. He didn't hear what he said. It was something consoling. But he was inconsolable, and couldn't hear him anyway.

Tom knocked on the door and walked in and offered him another Newport.

Dennis took it from him. He had a very sad look on his face. Like he understood.

He was a hell of a guy, that Tom The Bomb Maloney. He even got D a job at Kroger's where he worked that summer because he knew he needed a job.

Dennis nodded at him, but could hardly see him through the watery haze. Nobody said a word. He patted Dennis on the shoulder and turned and left the room.

He looked at Janey again. He looked right through her again, still like she wasn't there, as if she didn't exist. As if nothing existed now. Except this.

The worst day ever. Period.

Forever.

It couldn't get any worse, he thought.

He thought wrong.

~ ~ ~

It was after midnight, he could barely stay awake, he was crashing hard now like a dumpster lid, he felt it coming down upon him.

Oh, the hell with it, two more No-Doz, everything will be all right, we'll get through it, two more Cokes left. One bag of barbecue Better Made's left. Gotta keep going.

He was obsessed with keeping his streak of academic excellence from collapsing. Gotta do it. Need to practically ace everything if gonna pull it off. Gotta keep it going. His streak of pre-med 4.0's was broken the last semester, but he had to get at least something in the 3's to keep the dream alive.

Med School.

A point to prove.

He had a sudden urge to go to the bathroom.

He stood up. Wait a minute, he wasn't going anywhere. He lunged forward trying to balance himself clumsily with one hand on the table, the other one behind him against the wall.

Not only did he have big-time vertigo, now ripping pain started searing right through his chest like gobs of molten lava burning and churning right through the center of his thoracic cavity.

I'm dizzy. What's this pain in my chest? Oh My God. I've got to sit down.

Now the shooting pains shot through him from his chest all the way down his back, and through his shoulders and down both arms.

He couldn't sit, he couldn't move, he felt horrible. His chest was palpitating now and he felt like he was dying.

He managed to lie on top of the table, and then he muttered under his breath, "Oh my God, no, please, now I can't breathe." He felt like a monster was squeezing his chest.

All the classic signs of a heart attack.

Yes, I'm having a heart attack. Dear Lord, please help me stay alive. Please get me to the hospital.

But there was nobody around to ask for help this Saturday night in his top floor cubicle at the EMU library shortly before quitting hour.

He was convinced he was having either a major heart attack or some kind of massive stroke. "Oh dear God," he prayed, "please save me, I swear I will take better care of myself."

After about ten minutes of this horrible pain and fear that he was dying, things moderated just enough that he could stand, the sweat pouring off of him, legs wobbly, clutching the wall, before stutter stepping, before cautiously edging his way along the cubicle walls out into the main library using the bookshelves for support as he managed to make it to the elevator and then down the hill across the street – less than a block away – to Snow Health Center.

His heart attack turned out to be a gigantic panic attack, or technically a hyperventilation attack. Basically, this kind of panic attack occurs when an artificially sped-up metabolism abetted, in his case, by mega doses of No-Doz caffeine, accelerates respiration – the hyperventilation part – which upsets the natural gas levels in the blood, and the elevated carbon dioxide levels trick the body into thinking you are having a heart attack and you suffer the same terrifying symptoms.

The doctor told him to carry a paper lunch bag with him in his wallet and if it ever happened again to breathe into the bag held tightly to the mouth for several minutes or until the calm feeling from the newly stabilized gas levels is felt.

He returned to his dorm room and slept well and everything seemed in good shape until he awoke in the morning several days later – and checked his mail box. His midterms were in, everything calculated up to the minute, and the news wasn't good.

He would have to get 100 percent on his finals this time to have any chance at a semi-decent report card. The writing wasn't on the wall; it was in his hand.

He knew he wasn't going to be able to get out of this hole.

It was over and he knew it. He picked up the phone and dialed Professor Powell's number.

Powell told it to him straight.

"You have a C-minus, Dennis. The final is one third of the grade so when all the calculations are done, including your lab scores, you will need a 97 on the final, to get a B.

"But, Dennis, certainly a B is attainable, if you flat out ace the final.

"Dennis, I know A's and B's are wonderful, but sometimes a C is okay too, you know?"

I think that's called telegraphing your punch.

He said nothing but thanked Professor Powell and hung up. He was in despair. The problem wasn't just chem. He was almost flunking physics and in statistics he was another C minus.

He had sought perfection, just like before. But this was where he was now. The opposite.

His father was in the hospital again.

He needed another break. Or so he thought.

He asked for incompletes. They gave them to him.

He could make it up later, they assured him.

He told his parents he was going to take some time off. That sounded so much better than "I'm dropping out."

Not to them.

The rest of the conversation alternated between screaming and pleading.

~ ~ ~

The following day, he met with his experimental psychology professor after class.

He told him of his plans to take some time off and take incompletes. He was supportive.

"What about, Ben," Dennis MulQueen asked.

"Ben who, Mr. MulQueen?"

"My rat. My guy. The guy I used in my experiments. He became like my pet during the semester, Dr. Nelson. My pet rat. Where does he go at the end of the semester?"

"Well, never mind about that," Dr. Nelson said. "He won't be here anymore. We euthanize the rats at the end of the year."

"Dr. Nelson, he is snow white, he is beautiful, and he eats out of my hand now. Can I please take him with me?"

"Dennis, I don't know about that. Nobody has ever asked me that before. I don't think they really make good pets, at least that I know of."

185

"But, Doc, he's cool. I'll take really good care of him, I promise."

Dr. Nelson turned and walked silently away, like he didn't hear him, but the upward roll of his eyes said otherwise.

"Thanks, Doc."

As soon as he got Ben home, he realized, "Oh Jeezus, I can't take him on the plane with me. What am I going to do with him now?"

~ ~ ~

He had already made up his mind, but he agreed to go to the Glass House anyway. Out of courtesy.

The guy made this kind of effort, at least I can show up, he thought. The guy being no ordinary guy. The guy being Ray Maly.

Dennis had to take the elevator a long way in the Glass House to get to his office.

He was one floor directly below the top floor suites where King Henry The Deuce hung his hat. Just below The Deuce's office, actually. That's how close Ray Maly was to the top of the Ford Motor Co. food chain.

He was personnel director. For the whole place. He hired people for all the plants, all the buildings.

Hell, how could he be any less? He was married to a Kennedy. His wife Rita was the brother of former New York Yankee Bob Kennedy and the reason Pat and George MulQueen viewed Chicago Cubs' games from the owner's box. Bob Kennedy was now the general manager of the Cubs.

Not surprisingly, Ray Maly had a job opening ready.

Except the job was as a chemical engineer and Dennis had to agree to complete the necessary courses that the company would pay for as part of a contract he would sign to work for them.

"You don't need the degree right now," he said. "We will help pay for your education and tell you what classes you need and bring you in slowly, Dennis. I talked to your dad, of course. He called me and I told him about this opportunity and he also thinks it would be a good fit for you. You just have to stay in school and complete the necessary courses. It's a way to get free tuition too. This would lead to a great lifetime career with good pay and benefits. This is a world-class company and this is a world-class opportunity to be set for life, Dennis. What do you think?"

It certainly was a hell of an opportunity, a great offer. But Dennis MulQueen didn't have any interest in metallurgy or anything else in that area. He knew it was a job he would hate, if he could concentrate his way through the course work.

Dennis thanked him for his help, but told him he didn't think he could do it right now, that he would prefer to wait until something else came up. He thanked him and he went back home where the next day he got another 'offer you can't refuse'.

His uncle the medical doctor called from Flint.

"Denny, you should stay in school. Once you drop out, it can really disrupt the flow. And remember, there's no pressure. I can help you and so can others. And you know you will have a job waiting for you right here if you want. I would really like you to join the clinic staff and someday it will be yours. You are family and I would like to keep it in the family. You will be set for life."

He wondered if his uncle and Ray Maly trained under the same motivational speaker. He wondered if they were Wayne Dyer fans.

The Doc invited him to dinner and a tour of the clinic the next day. Dennis thanked him and told him he would think about everything a while longer and get back to him.

After that phone call, his father sounded like a stuck record.

You have to stay in, it looks bad if you don't. Etc. Etc. And another reminder. He brought up his good friend Stanley Levy again, mentioning again that he would help out with Wayne State Medical School if he chose that route.

None of these people knew his GPA was about to crash and burn – with the rest of his life soon to follow.

He said thanks and went back to his apartment in Ann Arbor.

~ ~ ~

Three days later, the phone rang in the Oak Park house.

"Hi Mom. Just wanted you to know if you need to get ahold of me, I'm in Florida."

"Yeah, I took incompletes. I'll make it up later. Sorry, I just hit the wall, Mom. Don't worry, everything is okay. Just need a little time to recharge."

"Come on now, don't fool yourself. You certainly can't fool me," she said.

It was a short conversation.

~ 15 ~

THE YEAR WITHOUT
SANTA CLAUS

The Santa Claus light in the side window was turned back on now, finally, the signal it was time to come back inside. They had made their beverage and snack run to Lupi's Drugstore and around the neighborhood, about six times over by now, looking for Santa Claus.

You see, these things take time.

Easy to see why.

When they reentered the house and walked in the living room that Christmas Eve of 1965, there was barely space to move. There they were, in the middle of the living room – not under the tree, but next to it, taking up as much living room space as George MulQueen's "Cobo Hall Christmas tree," as his mother called the gigantic specimens the man of the house preferred.

There they were, taking up a major portion of that Oak Park living room – a glistening white, fully loaded kit, just like Gene Krupa's. A brand new four-piece Pearl drum kit, the same maple shells as Louie Bellson's. The real deal, the same Zildjian cymbals and glistening white pearl finish as Buddy Rich's. A real professional set of drums. They could

189

have been Buddy's, they could have been Louie's. They could have been Gene's.

But they were his. For a kid like him. Proof that the MulQueen spectacle of Christmas was nonpareil worldwide.

All his, because Dennis MulQueen loved to beat on anything he could find. Maybe she thought his beating on these brand new Remo skins would be better than the pots and pans, the desk top, the bed pillows, his school books, or the living room furniture.

Dennis MulQueen was in seventh grade now; he was 13. And indeed it was another Cobo Hall tree Christmas. The giant trees were probably deliberate on George MulQueen's part – not just to aggravate Pat MulQueen, but for self-preservation. The more living room space the giant trees took up, the less room for presents.

Except for the nearly thousand dollar presents Moms Mabley was prone to pick out for her favorite son of all time, Dennis MulQueen. That's almost what she paid for this kit, in 1965, including hi-hat stand, cymbals, hardware, and a throne.

She knew what made this kid tick. She knew those drums would be the gift of a lifetime.

As soon as things started to wind down a bit and the guests departed, he moved his brand new Pearl kit downstairs and put "The Little Drummer Boy" record of his mother's on the downstairs phonograph and he played that song over and over until he could play the drum groove to it perfectly on his new drums.

"Little baby I am a poor boy too,
Pa rum pum pum-pum,
I will play for you on my drum,
Pa rum pum pum pum ..."

This was his favorite song from the first time he heard it at Christmas Eve mass many moons ago, so only appropriate this was the first song he learned to play on his brand new big-time Pearl drum kit. He was living his dream.

He was the little drummer boy.

Pa rum pum pum pum, pa rum pum, pum pum, he played over and over all night long with never a thought he had to be keeping his parents' upstairs awake. And probably the Garfinkels who lived next door as well.

Nobody said anything. Of course, it helped he had cover from his brother Chip, who was still up in the living room strumming on the nice new acoustic guitar that was on top of his pile that year.

There was something for everybody. The Bobbsey Twins – his two sisters – had pink doll houses and Barbies galore and stuffed animals, and a tricycle and beach balls and plastic horseshoes and clothes and there was candy everywhere and stocking stuffers that would be main gifts at other houses.

Christmas at the MulQueen's – a joyful celebration like none other. If there ever was a contest, everybody would be competing for second place. How could there possibly be any family in the world, in any country in the world, in any continent in the world, that could top the MulQueen spectacle of Christmas?

Grandma said Pat and George MulQueen would put the Bonners to shame. (The brothers owned the legendary world famous Bonner's Christmas Wonderland, the 27-acre Christmas store in Frankenmuth, Michigan, that never closes, with Wally and his brother boasting their store is the only place on earth it is Christmas 365 days of the year.)

Just another ordinary MulQueen Christmas. And of course, as always, bigger and badder for Dennis MulQueen than anybody else.

No wonder there was sibling rivalry. It was obvious to the whole world he was his mother's favorite – and everybody knew it.

It wasn't just the drums.

One year it was a brand new Armstrong bicycle, another year it was a phonograph with big speakers, one year, an electric light organ and a pile of records, a work bench and tools to go with it, there were always books and cameras – he got the polaroid swinger one year – and more records and game upon game upon game.

Life, Monopoly, Parcheesi, Safari, Yahtzee, Risk, Stratego, a board game called Fuedal, Rock 'Em Sock 'Em Robots, Backgammon, checkers, and Tripoly, Chess for his older brother Chip, Nok Hockey for all the kids, table top hockey, a golf game and an electric football game. You name it, they got it.

Every year it was something spectacular to compete with or even top the previous year. And every year was different. And always the one big item – how could he forget the train set to end all train sets he and his brother Chip shared the one year?

Talk about a model train set. This was Lionel's best.

They had the expensive coal burning engine that emitted actual smoke from the chimney (thanks to the smoke pellets). They had the milk car that loaded and unloaded small metal milk cans, ditto for the log car with real wooden logs, the box car with the hobo on top who laid down as the train entered the tunnel, and of course there was a coal car and two cabooses.

And every year there was a new addition. The MulQueen train set eventually accrued 35 cars in total.

George made the train tables – the same ones Dennis hid under that day he broke in the side window – they took up the whole west end of the basement because they had to in order to accommodate this city-within-a-city train display with houses and factories and schools and farms and bridges and roads.

How could it be any less?

Trains were as MulQueen as Molson Canadian and hockey.

Grandpa MulQueen was an engineer with the New York Central Railway, his last run from Detroit to Toledo occurring with Dennis MulQueen driving the train. He was only a young kid and as proof Pat MulQueen saved the pic on the front page of the *Detroit News* of young Dennis "driving" the train out of the Michigan Central Train Station that day while sitting on Grandpa MulQueen's lap.

On the other side, his mother's Grandpa Farrell was also an engineer, with the Illinois Central and of course Dennis MulQueen heard this story a million times. His parents never missed the opportunity to inspire – or at least instill – if not motivation, then fear.

His mother saved this newspaper clipping also, this one on the front page of the local Owosso, Michigan paper.

Grandpa Farrell's train was hit head-on by the engine of another train going the wrong way on the same track.

Just before impact, he jumped, and ended up unconscious in the bottom of a large ditch adjacent to the tracks. An angel from God, as identified in the headline in the paper – "Angel from God Saves Man" – in the form of a passerby who was lost and not supposed to be where he was at that time on that day witnessed the crash and saw grandfather Farrell shoot like a projectile into the ditch. The passerby crawled down into the ditch and dragged Dennis MulQueen's unconscious great-grandfather up the far bank just as the leaking boiler burst and boiling water filled the ditch where Grandpa Farrell had lain unconscious moments before.

So it was trains and toys and more stories every Christmas for all of the MulQueens and their extended family, not just wall-to-wall gifts but wall-to-wall people with the aunts and uncles and grandpas and grandmas there with food and drinks and everybody laughing and talking and walking their way around the piles everywhere jockeying for a seat.

And always midnight mass followed by the annual all-night party for the kids as the parents slept, and then everything all over again Christmas Day.

And it wasn't just Christmas Eve or Christmas Day – it was Christmas season, with the trips to the Union Toy Store starting the day after Thanksgiving.

One of the highlights of the season, of course, had to involve another train – this one being the 8:05 out of the downtown Royal Oak station to the downtown Detroit station, as all the MulQueen kids played hooky that day for the chance to take a checker cab – the "American Rolls Royce" the driver explained to an inquisitive Dennis MulQueen one year – over to the Quikee Donut shop where they would have donuts and coffee before the 9 a.m. opening of the fabled downtown Hudson's Department Store, Detroit's version of Macy's or Saks.

Moms Mabley would shop her floors while the kids were cordoned off at the children's shop. Then it was off to the toy floor, the 12th floor, where Santa hung out at one end and there was a phenomenal train set up at the other end with toys and toys and more toys wall-to-wall in the middle. Next up was lunch at the Hudson's restaurant on the top floor of the iconic department store.

The day's final stop came next, either the famous Fox Theatre or the Adams Theatre or the Palm Theatre, for a matinee movie (*Poseidon Adventure*, *Mary Poppins*, *Sound of Music*, *Fantastic Voya*ge just to mention a few of the premieres viewed at one of those venues) before catching the 5:23 p.m. train back home.

So Christmas wasn't just Christmas – it was an event that defined the entire year, if not some of the very best childhood memories – and even beyond that.

But all good things must come to an end, right?

At least according to Mickey Rooney and Shirley Booth.

On December 10, 1974, Pat MulQueen was in the Oak Park living room glued to the big screen Zenith watching *The Year Without a Santa Claus*, which starred Rooney as Santa Claus and Booth as Mrs. Claus, in an animated classic depicting the year nobody believed in Santa any more, or the entire holiday itself.

If you don't believe in omens, this movie could change your mind.

December 25th of 1974 would be worse than Christmas without Santa.

The year 1974 was the Christmas without Santa – and Christmas without the Prodigal Son.

There would be no drums, no bicycle, no ice skates, and no Dennis. There would be no train ride, and there would be no plane ride – despite the fact he had made reservations.

There would be nothing that year.

Not just Christmas without Santa – no Christmas period.

Except driving around all night long wishing he was home for Christmas. Because he knew what it meant to her. And by extension, his father, also.

So he booked a last minute reservation for 8:30 p.m. Monday night the 23rd of December, plenty of time for last minute shopping and Christmas Eve the following night.

The ticket would go to waste.

He allowed his heart to be overruled.

She grabbed him, she pleaded with him, she insisted.

So instead of celebrating and presents galore, Christmas Eve and Christmas Day consisted of driving around in circles looking for a place to find some kind of Christmas dinner.

She begged him to stay, so he did. Against the wishes of every cell in his body.

After returning later that night to the apartment he had rented on Tamiami Trail, he slowly and as quietly and secretly as he could managed to cry like an infant on and off until he finally fell asleep in the middle of the night.

At least he did call and talk to everybody on the phone, but it didn't much help.

It would be the saddest Christmas of his life.

Never again, he vowed, would he ever miss Christmas with his family again.

~ ~ ~

About a week later, his heart slammed into the back of his breast bone when he saw the Northwest Metro Newspapers return address on the gray envelope sticking out of the mail box.

She always used her work stationery.

He slid his right finger underneath the back corner and ripped the flap open, exactly one day before New Year's Eve.

After missing Christmas for the first time ever, he wasn't expecting a New Year's Eve card.

It wasn't.

She wrote that she had a horrible premonition he wasn't coming home. When the Mickey Rooney movie came on TV. An omen from hell.

The Year Without Santa Claus.

She mentioned all the pleasant Christmas details, including how she cried all night long too.

She told him how much everybody missed him, but she left out the part how many exactly were saving their gifts for him.

196

Then the last sentence of the letter.

Stay down there as long as you want, but remember, when you're dead, you're dead a long damned time.
    Love,
    Mother

~ ~ ~

A few weeks later, after he recovered from the Christmas that wasn't, he caught her sitting down in the apartment hallway outside their unit snuggled up with another guy. A firsthand view, courtesy of the eye piece in the front door.

Later that evening after she was back inside, he informed her that night he was leaving. Done. Gone. Goodbye forever. He knew this wasn't right.

"Sorry. That's it. I'm gone. Bye. I'm going," he told her as he was busy packing a suitcase in the bedroom.

"No you're not," she said.

"You can't stop me," he said.

She ran into the kitchen and then down the hallway, stopping in front of the open bedroom doorway to make sure he saw the knife in her left hand.

He looked up and she turned and ran into the bathroom and slammed the heavy metal bathroom door and locked it before he could get to her.

He had never seen her cry once. He thought maybe he heard her sobbing through the door but he couldn't tell for sure, then all he could make out was the sound of running water in the bathtub.

He banged on the door. "Janey, Janey," he called out.

Then he heard her voice above the water.

"I am going to kill myself if you leave. You can't leave. I am killing myself. I'm slitting my wrists right now unless you promise me you will stay."

He pleaded, he screamed, he shouted no, and he tried to break open the door.

But the door was metal, and so was the frame. He told her he was calling the cops. He backed up and charged again, throwing his shoulder into the door as hard as he could. He got up off the floor and started violently kicking the door. Still not a budge. Then he kicked it again as hard as he could, he pounded on it, still no budge.

"Okay, okay, okay," he screamed. "Please stop, please don't do it, I promise I will stay, please open the door. Please open the door."

The water stopped.

She opened the door. She dropped the knife on the floor.

He stayed.

Like a cockatoo on his heels, paws in the air, he cried all over again, as silently and secretly as he could once again, on and off, another whole night long again.

~ 16 ~

LIFE ON THE WIRE

These people are dressed like viaduct people, he thought. Jeezus, this can't be Florida – they look like Detroit viaduct people.

A scan of the room gave him a new goal in life – to not be one of them.

Too late. There he was, in the same room, filling out the same forms, about to hoist himself onto the same white hospital table like all the others as soon as his number was called.

Just getting in a little practice.

"Now, tell me, what's going to happen? Am I going to pass out or just die?"

"I know what you are thinking," the nice middle-aged woman dressed in white pants and coat said. "No, you won't die, and you won't get hepatitis either because we use clean needles."

She said to expect a little light-headedness, to take it easy, but that was all and she reassured him everything would be completely back to normal within hours.

That would be good timing, because he certainly could use another six pack of that $1.69 Busch by then. And another bag of rice. And some more Velveeta and bologna.

So the $14 for that pint of blood was already spoken for. The $18 for the second pint of the week – the limit was two per week – well, that bonus payment would be up for grabs. On the way back home he saw her tooling down Tennessee Street in her nice new shiny candy-apple-red Ford Mustang with the white leather seats and that gleaming silver horse on the hood and the slick white walls. Sharp. Very Sharp.

So much for that Lennon lie.

All you need is love.

Just what he didn't need – love masquerading as love. Love masquerading as a meal ticket.

The grandparents had left her a nice chunk of dough, which when passed down through her father's estate translated to a nice inheritance.

He was a college student who had problems at home and most importantly no job or money at the time, and therefore, in her eyes, no future – for her.

That's all it took.

To pound the final nails into an already closed coffin.

Who could blame her, how was an unemployed struggling college student going to take care of her needs?

More than a year had passed since he found an empty house and the letter on the kitchen table after he got back from up north that day. Right after she got that money.

"You know, if my mother hadn't married my father, things might have turned out differently. She might still be alive. He might still be alive," she wrote.

He was dripping all over the paper that day. But he knew she was right. In one respect. He would have died for her.

"Thanks for everything, you practically raised me. I will always have love in my heart for you," she said in the letter.

And the last sentence.

"Who knows, if we don't end up with somebody else, maybe we will end up back together again someday."

Thanks for the hope.

Every time he thought of her he would think of Alfred Lord Tennyson's "In Memoriam," knowing the protected early years of unbelievable connection and chemistry and the sheer joy of having each other were once in a lifetime. That stratospheric feeling of goose bumps and fluttering heart that came from just being together, doing anything or nothing, talking, laughing or silent – that intoxicating happiness and security of knowing that when they were together everything in the world was okay – he knew that was a dream lost forever.

"I hold it true, whate'er befall;
I feel it when I sorrow most;
Tis better to have loved and lost,
than never to have loved at all."

For his part, he never stopped loving, or hoping, but she would never contact him again.

~ ~ ~

She tried to talk him out of it, and people all across the country heard her.

On national TV. The cameras caught the exchange loud and clear.

"Karl, why are you going to do this?" she said to her husband of decades. "You have a good reputation. You don't need to do this."

He turned his head toward her and met her gaze.

"But I have a challenge and I have to do it," he said without hesitation. "If I have no challenges and I'm just sitting home, then life is no good."

The "challenge" was the toughest feat Karl Wallenda had ever attempted to date, a stunt he agreed to perform as part of Evel Knievel's "Death Defiers" 90 minute TV special on the CBS network the night of January 31, 1977.

Not that Wallenda needed any additional pressure – it was Knievel's show – but Evel could not perform live for the cameras that night on his own TV special because he had almost killed himself the day before in a trial run.

To get everybody geeked, the producers had just shown a tape of that pre-show disaster on the show. As advertised, Knievel was attempting to jump his motorcycle over "the world's largest indoor saltwater pool filled with 13 man-eating killer sharks" at the old Chicago amphitheater, oddly enough the site of the protests at the 1968 Democratic convention.

Evel easily cleared the pool of sharks, but he appeared to turn the handlebars in midflight, and he tried to correct his path just as he was landing but over-corrected and took a hard right off the elevated ramp, and through a barrier where he clipped a cameraman, causing his motorcycle to flip.

Knievel went flying as he went upside down, everything out of control, and landed on the concrete arena floor below, in the process knocking the cameraman's eye out and breaking his own clavicle and both arms.

If that wasn't enough buildup for Wallenda's act, another performer preceding him on the show, Ron Phillips, drove a snowmobile off a ski jump and also crashed badly. Like Knievel, he too was still alive.

But unlike those two, Wallenda had zero margin for error.

If he crashes, the whole world knew it would be crash and burn. As in burn splatter.

He was about to attempt to walk across a 3/8 inch steel cable strung 17 stories high between the Fontainebleau and the Eden Roc hotels in downtown Miami Beach. At age 72.

With wind gusts up to 40 miles per hour.

At night.

A tiny mis-step on the wire 175 feet in the air – well, that's pretty self-explanatory. The date itself was eerie, with January 31, 1977, exactly 15 years and one day removed from the state fair coliseum in Detroit where in 1962 the seven-man pyramid collapsed and two family members were killed and his son paralyzed for life at the Shrine Circus that day.

The time coincided too, as at 9:30 p.m. the Great Wallenda approached the wire in Miami Beach as a very stiff breeze accelerated off the ocean between the two hotels and up Collins Avenue.

He had always said the wind was his greatest enemy. Now he was about to discover another one.

It was dead dark by now, but the blinding TV lights shone from everywhere, from the top of the buildings, from the ground up and everywhere in between.

A single blinding gigantic spotlight was focused directly on the man himself. The blinding lights prevented Wallenda from focusing on a point at the opposite end of the wire, a focus point always utilized by the high-wire maestro to help him keep his balance throughout any wire walk.

The other unsaid enemy at work this night was Father Time. Born in 1905, at 72 years old this made Wallenda far and away the oldest to ever walk any kind of high wire, let alone in these kinds of conditions.

But he wasn't about to get afraid now. Or at least let on to anybody.

As per usual, when asked by one of the show's hosts what might happen, his response was the same. "I am in God's hands," he said. "When it is my time, I go."

Many times recently though, the subject of retirement had creeped into the conversation. After all, he had been risking his life like this for half a century. Again, it was always a similar reply: A retirement only in death.

But just how much longer could the Great Wallenda continue to put off that retirement?

As the wind continued to howl and he was about to step onto the wire, the actress Jill St. John, co-host of the show with "Kojak" actor Telly Savalas, gave everybody pause for thought.

"Why don't you just take some more time," said St. John.

Karl Wallenda wouldn't have it.

Once again, like hundreds and literally hundreds of times before, without hesitation, he shot back: "The wire looks good. I go now."

Said Savalas: "Everybody wants more live TV. I think I've seen all the live TV I want to see tonight."

The time really was now, as the Great Wallenda stepped out onto the wire and the crowd buzz below immediately crescendoed and fell silent, only the whistling of the wind now audible through the microphones.

Dead silence and the wind.

Then a little mumbling, then partway across, ever the great showman (or perhaps it really was a gust) gasps were heard as he appeared to stumble.

There were more nervous sighs and gasps from the 30,000 spectators assembled on the ground to watch the stunt in person, as he stumbled twice more, the wind whistling more audibly now with unpredictable blasts of turbulent air.

Undeterred, the greatest aerialist in history continued to step slowly forward one foot in front of the other as the wire swayed, until finally to a rush of applause he finally made it all the way across to the other side, smiling broadly on national TV as he hoisted his standard double martini reward high in the back-lit night sky.

He looked relaxed and happy, having one more time made his signature statement to the world, that with determination and no fear and belief the only guiding force, the impossible is possible. Even at age 72.

And in the deep dark recesses of his mind, maybe even atonement, if that's what partly drove him to continue, for mistakes and accidents that happened many years ago on his watch.

~ ~ ~

"D, is it safe out here? Aren't there water moccasins out here? And gators too?"

The honking noise answered the last half of the question. The moccasins, they had to be lurking out there somewhere also. They were at a sinkhole, connected to another sinkhole, there was nothing but water out there – dark water, really dark-as-night water.

And just as soon as his friend popped the question – they were up to their necks in it. They were in a canoe – TJ and another buddy of theirs, Brambles. Sure enough, Dennis had to go – and as soon as he stood up to aim over the side, just like that he capsized the whole canoe and they were all in the drink.

"Dennis, you asshole, you better hope you have cat ancestry because I'm gonna kill you right now," Brambles said.

"Oh Jesus, sorry, Brams. I didn't know, what the hell."

"I think I'm gonna kill you more than once, Dennis, you dumb fucker, right now. Everybody grab the boat."

"Jeesus, can't anybody take a joke? I didn't mean it."

None of them had life jackets on, but all managed to tread water and grab the gunnels and upright the ship and nobody drowned.

Or got eaten by the gators, which had to be real close judging by how loud the bellowing and honking was. They must have had a full belly that night because they didn't come after them. And thank God, no moccasins showed up either at their little middle-of-the-night swim party.

~ 17 ~

FACE TO FACE
WITH PURE EVIL

The little bastards.

"I'll kill you, you motherfrickers."

Brambles laughed hysterically.

"Oh yeah? How ya gonna kill 'em, MulQueen? You gotta catch 'em first. How ya gonna do that, huh, big fella? I want to see that. You better just hope they don't saw that big noodle a yours off."

"They're not that tough."

At least he hoped not.

He was looking straight down, in preparation for the next wave. Instantly there was another swarm of the little devils. They were like piranhas. Maybe they were piranhas. Mini-piranhas.

They certainly bit like it, according to his bloodied arms and legs.

He wasn't used to this. Nothing ever bothered you in Lake Erie. Not even the muskies, which if they were so inclined could be like freshwater barracudas and really rip a guy to shreds, the teeth and speed and power they possess. But unlike some humans, they only attack for food.

Same with the Lake Erie pickerel, they have nice teeth also. And the true monster of the great Lakes, the sturgeon, they exceed 6 feet and 150 pounds – but they couldn't bite you if they wanted to.

They have a big sucker mouth on their underside that allows them to filter feed off the bottom. No wonder they taste so good when dipped in garlic butter at Carl's Chop House – fresh water lobster, only better.

But in this Florida sinkhole – Dennis MulQueen was the prey.

Everybody is prey down here, he knew by now. To the rattlers, the scorpions, the coral snakes, the brown recluse spiders and the gators and those lovely water moccasins too. Even Paradise has its price.

But these little predators, these fearless little biting fish swooping in like mini F-14's to bite in formation, they were the worst – at least at the moment.

But alas, thank God, multiple beers later, it got a little easier.

Or so he thought.

They moved out of the water up to the top of the bank overlooking an adjacent sinkhole.

Dennis, Brambles, Weeby, and TJ – and one beautiful blonde girl.

That was it. That was the group. A little competition never hurts, right?

Of course, swimming at night, only the moonlight to show, none of them had any clothes on. So heck, he ought to win this thing hands down.

But Brambles had a few tricks up his sleeve to distract her from what Dennis MulQueen thought really does matter – size.

Brambles had the short tight body of a gymnast, while MulQueen had the big, strong, long and heavy body of a defensive end. So he had his buddy hands down.

Or so he thought.

They shared the same objective – to impress the blonde beauty. She had China-doll skin and delicate pink lips – she was a Tallahassee Lassie extraordinaire. And she was naked, too, like the rest of them. Oh My God, was she ever a delicate flower.

But Brambles was quite the competitor, he was almost as good a hunter as MulQueen, and he was going to give it his best shot.

"See down there, guys," he said as he pointed down at the water, with the swagger of Hemingway on safari.

Sure enough, it was at least a 20 foot drop from the top of the rocky bluff they stood on, to the water's edge below. A Walden Pond scene, really, minus the piranhas, of course.

This was home field advantage for the Bramble King. He led the gang to this spot. He was a Tallahassee native, he knew the lay of the land, everywhere, like the back of his hand.

There was a rope attached to the tree just a little to the left of them, tied to a big thick arching branch extending up and out from the tree about 25 feet above them.

"Watch this, guys," Brambles said as he grabbed the rope, which had a rudimentary handle tied to it near the end in the form of a sawed-off broom stick.

He grabbed the handle and took three or four quick steps and pushed off hard from a protruding coral rock and – *vroom* – he swung out over the open water like the trapeze guy at the circus and as he let go in midair he bent over at the waist and touched his thighs with his chest in a tuck position and in an instant he straightened his body as he did a half twist and sliced into the deep dark water in perfect perpendicular form with hardly a splash like Greg Louganis off the Olympic high board.

"Jeezus," Dennis MulQueen said, "is Brambles on the FSU dive team or what?"

"No, D," TJ said, "but he was on the gymnastics team in high school. You better not try that, D."

He should have known better. Coach Rhoades had a warning for times like this. The MulQueens were up at his house in Marine City on the St. Claire river one day when coach challenged Chip MulQueen to a race down the river to a pre-determined spot. They had a case of beer bet on the match. Before the race, Coach Rhoades went to the shed behind his house and retrieved a white buoy attached to about 15 feet of line and jumped in the water. Chip was swimming on the inside closest to shore and took an early lead; he was on the track team in high school and it looked like he was going to win the contest hands down. Then Coach drifted out into the shipping lane where the current was, and with the white buoy trailing behind him in the water he smoked Dennis' brother to the finish line for all the beer.

Afterward, he said to Chip MulQueen, "Son, never try and beat a man at his own game on his own turf."

Too bad Dennis MulQueen forgot those words of wisdom.

Bramble's head bobbed up from the water momentarily, and who did he stare at as he clambered back up to the top of the bank?

"Okay, MulQueen, top that punk."

Dennis grabbed the rope and there he was, swinging like a great ape out into the wilderness, out over the water where he let go and crashed into the water below like a very large crate of cantaloupes.

Apparently, Brambles didn't want Princess Mary to have even a scintilla of doubt. By the time the Big D clambered back up to the top of the bank, Brambles was already in the tree.

He was standing up on a branch now, rope in hand, about 12 feet above the coral rock bank. He rolled the handle up the rope and – *vroom* – he pushed off with those gymnast's thighs and there he went screaming like Tarzan and – *whoosh* – he dropped straight in the water in perfect form once again although this time he landed much closer to shore because of the changes in the rope dynamics.

"Okay, punk. Top that, MulQueen," he hollered from the water.

The seven or eight Busches by now gave Dennis MulQueen all the courage he needed to respond in an even bigger way. He climbed the tree one branch higher than Brambles, he was now about 17 or 18 feet above the coral rock bank. I've got to make sure I clear that bank, he thought as he looked down. I'll just have to push off a little harder.

"Top this, Bramble puss."

He pushed off like he was firing out against Banaszak or Pureifory.

The old weather beaten handle snapped off in his hands like it was a twig and he plummeted like a lead Zeppelin straight down almost 20 feet and slammed into the jagged coral rock embankment, which he bounced off of with a splat and tumbled over the edge as he rolled and bounced off of the rocky bank down another 20 feet into the water where his momentum carried him out about 20 feet from the edge of the sinkhole.

This watering hole was spring fed and way deep from the very edge on out or he would have killed himself right then and there.

But he was still in a bit of trouble as he discovered it's not easy to swim in deep water with broken leg bones.

Lucky for him, that fool of a friend of his, TJ, leaped off the bank immediately into the water and swam out to get him and helped him back to land or he might have drowned.

When they got to the edge, he looked at TJ and said, "Now what are we gonna do?"

They both looked up. From the bottom, the 20 feet to the top now looked too close to vertical for comfort.

But TJ was strong. Brambles crawled down to help too, and between the two of them they helped get his dead weight 255-pound lineman's body up to the top again and into the car a short distance away.

"Jeezus, MulQueen, you're fucked up," Brambles said.

"Go to hell, Brambles. I can still kick your ass. Just take me home. I'll be fine."

"MulQueen, you're nuts. You can't even walk."

Brambles was right. MulQueen only protested faintly as they made their way over to Tallahassee Memorial Hospital.

The team with the gurney met them out front. The cute brunette nurse couldn't help herself as he sat there in the back seat with his T-shirt and pants draped over his naked and torn up torso.

She looked him in the eyes, barely hiding a smile. "Now, let me guess, she kicked you out of bed for eating crackers, right?"

"Oh Jeezus. Worse than that. Please don't make me tell you. At any rate, I'm dying."

It was a bitch getting out of that car onto the gurney.

Turned out even though he felt like every bone in his body was broken, he had only fractured his right knee cap and a couple toes. They put everything back together again and sewed up a couple gashes and he was good to go a couple hours later. Turned out, none of them scored any love points with Miss Mary, the delicate white Irish rose that precipitated their Olympic diving contest. What was with this woman anyway, going to a remote sinkhole in the middle of the night and getting naked with brutes like that?

~ ~ ~

The clock read 6:28 a.m. on January 15, 1978, as they were slowly winding their way back to the trailer after their all-night sinkhole party that turned into a middle-of-the-night hospital visit. TJ flipped the radio on, just as they were coming down Tennessee Street, the main drag passing through the FSU campus. There was no music though – a special bulletin was in progress.

"The murders took place at the Chi Omega Sorority House on College Avenue on the Florida State University campus. The dead women have been identified as Lisa Levy, a 20-year-old student, and her fellow sorority sister Margaret Bowman, age 21. Two other women living in the house have also been severely injured, including Karen Chandler, and an as yet unidentified fourth woman.

"Again, there has been a vicious attack at the Chi Omega sorority house on the Florida State campus. Two women have been declared dead, two more severely injured. Police say they have no suspects yet. There was blunt force trauma and strangulation and rape, that's all we know now. Oh wait, there is another report coming into the station right now, the Associated Press is reporting that another woman, identified as Lisa Thompson, another FSU student, has been injured also. She was attacked in the basement bedroom of a house she was staying in near the sorority house. She is alive at this time as far as we know."

At this exact moment Dennis MulQueen and his friends were about two blocks away from the Chi Omega House.

"Wow, do you believe it," Dennis said, looking at Brambles and TJ.

"Oh my God. How horrifying," Brambles said.

"I can't believe it," TJ said.

"Yeah, man, some really sick motherfuckers in this world," Brambles said.

"Jeez, TJ, right over there," Dennis said, "a block away or so on College Avenue. I have walked by that sorority house many times. It's on the way to the Stonehenge, I think, if you cut around from the Sweet Shop."

All they could do was shake their heads collectively as the chills ran up and down their spines. It was the creepiest, most horrific feeling ever. Dennis MulQueen felt like vomiting. None of them, nobody could possibly wrap their arms around horrific evil of this unfathomable magnitude. At their school. While they were out partying all night at a local sinkhole.

They all felt the same creepy sense of danger, for themselves, even though they were red-blooded men, but more so for all the wonderful FSU women they knew, and for all the women of the world everywhere.

"How could anybody be that sick? It's impossible to think there is somebody out there sick enough to do this to other human beings. How could anybody be capable of doing something like this?" Dennis MulQueen said.

~ ~ ~

Felipe and Dennis were in the '62 Falcon he bought from Felipe – or more accurately, the '62 Falcon Felipe gave him for just a few hundred bucks. He was a sophomore friend majoring in English and they didn't come any better as a human being.

The old vehicle didn't have much pick up, but jeez, the guy in a square-ended white truck in front of them was practically crawling. Then the guy came to a dead stop in front of them.

Then it started up again. Then it stopped again. Dennis MulQueen didn't know it at the time, but it was all according to plan.

"What is wrong with this idiot. I'll have to pass this fool."

He grabbed the black knob to downshift the Hurst unit he personally installed in the car, but before he hit the pedal Felipe warned him, "I wouldn't pass this guy if I were you. I think it's cops. Look, there are windows in the back of that truck with it looks like a metal grate running across the back of them. It could be a SWAT team, Dennis."

Dennis momentarily paused with his hand on the round gearshift knob. He noticed the aluminum doors on the back. Then they both spotted a big dog inside looking out through the narrow back window.

"No, it's not cops, Felipe. Look, it's gotta be the dog catcher," Dennis said.

He hit it and proceeded to zoom around the stalled truck in second gear.

As they drove past the white vehicle, Dennis saw the gold police badge on the driver's side door and the big black lettering across the side: Leon County SWAT.

He got a good look through the side window of two Dobermans inside the back of the truck.

The flashing lights and sirens came on immediately and an instant later a white loudspeaker mounted on the top of the cab blared at them to "pull over and stop immediately."

Dennis and Felipe could hear the two attack dogs now going ape inside the cop's truck, snarling and barking like Steven King dark woods' beasts

He hoped they didn't make him get out of the car.

A few minutes and a fat ticket later, they were on their way again. This was maybe his sixth or seventh ticket in the last couple years for an expired inspection sticker. He had lost count.

"Ahh, the hell with it. It's just like a parking ticket. No big deal," he said to his friend as he shoved the ticket into the glove box and accelerated back down the road.

~ ~ ~

Officer David Lee was on routine patrol near Pensacola, Florida, on Feb. 15, 1978, when he saw a Volkswagen driving erratically down the road. He sped up and pulled it over. He ran the plates and discovered it had been stolen.

The clean-cut guy driving the vehicle identified himself as Chris Hansen. He had no ID with him. When he was being questioned by Officer Lee, he suddenly kicked the officers legs out from under him and bolted. Officer Lee quickly jumped up and raced after the guy, twice firing shots at him.

The cop was in good shape and he caught up to the guy and brought him down with a diving tackle. He handcuffed him and arrested him.

As he was putting him in the back of his squad car, the guy turned and looked at him and said, "I wish you had killed me."

Come on, it can't be that bad.

It was worse.

Officer Lee had no idea who the guy was. Or that it would be a career-altering arrest.

He had just apprehended the most wanted fugitive in the United States, the man at the top of the FBI's national Ten Most Wanted List.

Soon after booking the guy at the station, Lee learned from the booking desk the guy matched the description of the man wanted in the Florida State Chi Omega murders, a man authorities had charged with the murder of Michigan nurse Caryn Campbell in Colorado as well as a suspect in numerous other murders of young women.

This was the same guy identified the next day by witnesses as the guy seen recently leading 12-year-old Kimberly Leach from her junior high playground to a white van that was reported stolen in Tallahassee. The little girl's decomposed remains were found in a pig pen at a Lake

County farm a short while later. She was found brutally murdered and nude with semen stains on her nearby underwear.

Officer Lee had just arrested a man named Theodore Bundy.

~ ~ ~

Bang Bang Bang.

Right next to his head.

Or so it seemed.

Band Bang Bang again. The tin can was in fact vibrating all the way from the front door down the short hallway to his bedroom. Right to where his head lay, flush with the undulating tin-can wall of the trailer he lived in. Like a bad game of bang-a-gong on his head.

"Who the heck could that be," the woman next to him in bed said.

"I don't know, Claire. I guess I'll have to find out."

He sat up in the bed. Then came the shouts and the threats concurrent with the next round of pounding.

"Come out now. Surrender immediately or we're breaking the door down right now."

He was fully awake now.

"Hey, who is it? What's going on? Wait a minute."

"Leon County Sheriff. Open the door immediately. Are you Dennis MulQueen?"

"Okay, man, I'm coming, but don't shoot me. You've got the wrong person."

He turned the silver knob and opened the door.

Sure enough, this dog-and-pony show was for real. A guy dressed in a green shirt with gold badge and beige pants with a black leather holster on his right hip ordered him to turn around and put his hands over his head and touch the outside wall of the trailer.

"What the hell is going on, officer.?"

217

He handcuffed him and said, "We've got a warrant for your arrest here, buddy, that's what's goin' on."

That smile.

A dead giveaway.

The guy must have had his ass kicked growing up – many times, Dennis thought. This must be his way of getting even. He wore a chip on his shoulder the size of the rock of Gibraltar.

He was enjoying this way too much.

"What the hell for? I haven't killed anybody. Why are you treating me like this?"

He stuck the warrant in his face.

"Thought you were going to get away with it, didn't you?"

The guy looked young, mid or even early 20s maybe, he had to be a rookie. Maybe he thinks I'm Al Capone, and he's going to make a name for himself, Dennis muttered silently to himself. All cops couldn't be like this or there would be more psychopaths out there.

It was an arrest warrant all right. For unpaid inspection sticker tickets. I guess they are a little more serious than a parking ticket after all, he found out. I guess all us young people are jail bait, he thought, at least those of us who can't afford to pay the fee at the local garage and can't afford to have perfect tires and exhaust systems and everything else the mechanics demand you pay for to get a passing grade.

"Do you have any ID on you?"

"In my room. My girlfriend can get it for me. She is inside. Claire?" he called out. "Please bring my wallet outside to me."

He had just cashed his last paycheck and he was hoping it was enough. Claire opened the door and tucked it in the right front pocket of his Wrangler jeans.

The Leon County deputy ushered him into the backseat of his green-and-white squad car and took him to the Leon County jail.

He was about to get lucky again. The total tab, including fines, was $218.00.

He was fingerprinted and the guy at the counter told him he could pay up or maybe he could write another article for his Mom's newspaper describing what it's like to be behind the Leon County green door.

He plunked all $220 from his last paycheck on the counter top in front of the desk sergeant as the cop handed him the paperwork to read and sign. When he finished reading the documents and signing everything, he noticed the desk sergeant was gone.

He looked around and realized he was now the only person in the entire room.

When he turned around the other way he noticed a row of doors lining the far wall directly across from him. Each door had a single one-square-foot window pane about eye height.

Curious, he walked about 20 feet over to the first door and he could see there was a glass wall on the other side of a small 4x4-foot booth with a brown fabric chair with chrome plated legs in it and a corresponding booth on the other side of that glass wall separating the two booths. There was a round silver disk in the middle of the glass partition about four inches in diameter with serrated edges running horizontally across the middle.

As he was standing there he heard a noise like a yawn coming from the left. He wasn't sure what it was. He turned and walked toward the second door.

Through the window he could see a guy sitting in a chair with his back to the door. He could only see the back of the guy's head. The bright lights from the booking room cast a shadow through the glass window as he stood in front of it and the guy inside must have noticed because he turned around and stared at Dennis MulQueen.

He had wavy brown hair and a thin face with pallid skin and thin lips and dark circles under his eyes, and a long, angular nose. The guy's eyes were by far his defining feature. They were beady and dark and sinister looking, the dark circles underneath and the man's chestnut eyebrows put together seeming to frame in and accentuate the dark beads jumping around inside his head like Mexican jumping beans. They really stood out, juxtaposed with his ash-can tepid skin.

Then it hit Dennis MulQueen like a bomb.

His mouth opened involuntarily an inch or so as time froze and he made direct eye contact with the guy on the other side of the glass. He momentarily stopped breathing.

Most are orange, but the guy he was looking at through the glass window was wearing a pale yellow jail uniform. In person, he looked like a paler, thinner version of the face he had seen many times in recent weeks plastered all over the local TV and newspapers in town. His face was as instantly recognizable as Hitler's.

Chills of molten lava ran up and down Dennis MulQueen's spine.

He realized he was face-to-face with pure evil.

He was eye-to-eye with the most notorious, heinous and terrifying sadistic killer in human history.

He instantly recognized the man he was face-to-face with was Ted Bundy.

Bundy had been arrested in the Florida panhandle in a stolen car exactly one month after the Chi Omega murders, and was returned to Tallahassee to face the recently unsealed murder indictments. Details of the FSU sorority house killings and the killing right after that of 12-year-old Kimberly Leach in Lake City and other horrifying murders from his past had saturated the local newspapers and TV and radio stations for weeks now.

And here he was.

Dennis MulQueen turned and looked around the Leon County jail booking room. He was still the only one there. He looked back through the window at Bundy and raised one finger in the air. "I'll be right back," he said.

He hurried back over to the booking counter. He reached over the top and grabbed a yellow legal pad of paper and a black pen lying next to it and hurried back across the room.

His heart was pounding like a runaway locomotive as he approached Window Number Two once again.

Bundy was turned the other way now.

Dennis knocked on the glass to get his attention.

Bundy turned around and stared at him again with those eyes.

"Hello, Ted. My name is Dennis MulQueen. I am a reporter for the *Florida Flambeau*. I just wanted to ask you a couple questions. Ted, why did you murder those girls?"

He inched forward, trying to get closer, his breath about to cloud the glass. Bundy said nothing.

"Ted, why do you hate women? Did they ever hurt you? What has a woman done to you to make you hate them so?"

Bundy continued to stare him down and said nothing. Dennis MulQueen felt his knees quiver as visceral jolts of nerve pain shot up and down his spine. Chills running up and down his arms made the skin on his forearms tighten.

"How many have you killed, Ted? Tell me, please, how it feels to do it. Don't you feel bad after you do it, at least a little bit? Do you have a mother or sisters? Have you ever had a girlfriend or a daughter? Have you ever loved anybody, Ted?"

The killer sat there motionless and continued to stare, remaining silent. Then he turned around the other way again. Maybe it was a matter of circulation. A reporter at the local college newspaper? Maybe if it was a *New York Times* reporter, the response would be different.

He was struck by how different the guy looked in person from what he would have expected. He looked totally different in pictures and on the TV news. The standard media reference always presented Bundy as this suave, debonair law student, the guy-next-door type who could fool anybody.

Not Dennis MulQueen.

Not on this day.

Not ever.

The eyes don't lie. He would never forget them.

The icy cold evil windows to the twisted soul of a purely evil sadistic sociopath.

A vengeful sociopath driven by the extreme anger and misogynistic hatred that fueled the sick cravings he could only satisfy by the total control and absolute power he got from sex with a dead woman he had just brutally maimed and killed.

Is it possible to be any sicker than that?

Dennis MulQueen wondered if those eyes froze his victims the way they initially froze him, if they paralyzed his victims before they could react, like the shrieks of a giant screech owl swooping in for the kill in the middle of the night.

An All-American guy that could fool any one?

Not on this day.

Not ever.

His skin was ghoulish, a wan, yellow, pale-gray mix that reminded Dennis MulQueen of the creature on the lawn that day at the Miami Serpentarium as Dr. Hass milked his venom in front of an audience. Yes, that's it. He had the skin of a trapped cobra.

But that's unfair. Even a cobra only strikes for self-preservation.

He knocked on the glass window again. Bundy turned around this time and Dennis MulQueen met those sinister brown poison amulets head on once again as they darted back and forth in his head like the eyes of a toxic serpent from hell.

"Ted, can you hear me okay? I'm a reporter with the *Florida Flambeau*. I just had a few questions for you. Will you please tell me how you respond to the murder indictment?"

The silent treatment continued.

Then, apparently, finally, the right question.

"Ted, I read in an article last week that stated that all of the woman you are accused of murdering, or the missing women you are linked to, the girls at the sorority house and even Kimberly Leach, they all had shoulder length brown hair parted in the middle that looked like your former girlfriend, Stephanie Brooks? Is that true, Ted?"

He stared at Dennis MulQueen through the glass with those cold steel orbs of terror and Dennis involuntarily flinched and froze again, like the squirrel in the talons of that screech owl as the killer opened his mouth and began to speak.

"There is no evidence I committed any crimes," he said.

The chills continued to race up and down Dennis MulQueen's spine as he heard muffled voices and a door to the booth across from Bundy opened and the deputy that had checked him in moments ago at the desk appeared through the glass in the doorway off in the distance. He stepped aside and a brown haired woman appeared from behind the deputy, entered the far booth and sat down. The deputy closed the door behind her and disappeared. As Bundy turned around she appeared to glance at Dennis

MulQueen through the glass and mumbled something to Bundy that Dennis couldn't make out.

The woman was wearing a light brown nondescript jacket, her hair was short and straight with no real style to it. He could see a plain yellow blouse underneath the coat. She looked like she could have been the cashier at the local K-Mart, or the maid at the local Motel 6, anachronistic, like Aunt Mable from the '50s. She appeared to be wearing no lipstick or makeup of any kind. She had an asexual look about her.

Bundy mumbled something inaudible to her. The woman shook her head and waved her hands at Bundy like she was the kindergarten teacher dismissing a child's inconvenient question.

She said something else to Bundy but he still couldn't make out what they were saying.

Being a journalist at heart and this being Tallahassee, and the impact of what happened on the FSU campus, he had read everything and anything about this guy. Not only was there irrefutable evidence he murdered the girls at Chi Omega, reports were streaming in from Washington and Colorado and Utah that would ultimately connect him directly to the murders of more than 40 young women.

All with a similar look topped off with the same brown hair parted down the middle.

Dennis MulQueen wanted to break the glass, rip the door open and strangle this evil sick bastard right then and there.

At that exact moment he felt a hard knuckle knock on his right shoulder, the knuckles hitting the bone like a karate artist would put a knock on a board; it was the kind of knock designed for more than getting someone's attention.

"Hey buddy, whadda' ya think ur doin'?"

He turned around and looked.

It was the desk sergeant.

He was back.

"In my other non-criminal life I am a newspaper reporter for the *Florida Flambeau*, Sarge. Just trying to get a little information here."

"Well, buddy, I don't care who you are or what you do but I can tell you one thing, if you want to end up on the other side of the glass with him, you can get a really good face-to-face interview then, and that's what you'll get if you say one word to this guy. Where in the hell have you been lately?"

"Pardon me?"

"If you are a journalist then you should know the judge issued a restraining order and nobody, that's nobody including you, is allowed to talk to this guy or interview him or give him any press whatsoever, that's the order of the court and anything against that will land you in here in contempt of court for disobeying the orders of the judge. You got that now?"

He shrugged his shoulders and nodded his head.

"Now give me my pen and paper back. That ain't your job. Your job is over here at the desk taking care of your business, okay? I don't think the prosecutor, let alone the judge, would be too happy to see or hear anything about this. In your paper or anywhere else. But nice try.

"Come on back over here now," the Leon County deputy said as he walked back behind the counter and opened a drawer and slapped a couple of one dollar bills down on the counter.

Dennis MulQueen grabbed the change and shoved it in his right front pocket.

"Thanks, Officer."

He turned and walked out the door to the parking lot, still trembling inside with each step, but a free man once again.

With a little different perspective.

Those   eyes.

~ 18 ~

THE WALLENDA EFFECT

Planning for a skywalk at the new Seahawks' domed stadium was already underway in late March when Karl Wallenda flew to Washington to personally assess the venue and lay out the specifics for stringing the tightrope across the arena.

The local radio station interviewed him as part of the publicity for the upcoming performance. Karl, what about the dangers, he was asked for maybe the 1,000th time.

"To be 100 feet in the air on the wire is to be in heaven," Wallenda said. "If you fall from 100 feet, you're dead. If you fall from 1,000 feet, you are dead. What's the difference?"

Do you have a death wish? Do people come to see you fall and die?

"No, they don't want to see me killed, but to see a man have the guts to face death," he told his interviewer. "They want to see that a man can be daring and still succeed. And maybe my act gives them a little extra courage to carry on in their own lives."

But come on, fall? This was the Great Wallenda talking. Such thoughts were out of the equation. He was considered "indestructible" by everybody he ever encountered. Karl Wallenda was not the oldest man to ever walk the high wire for no reason.

But before the Seattle skywalk across the new football stadium, there was a promotional gig he had committed to for a circus in Latin America.

While one of the Wallenda troupes he had trained was performing in North Dakota, Karl and his personal troupe were top billing on the US tropical island nation of Puerto Rico, where he had an engagement with the Pan American Circus in San Juan. After that, it was back to Seattle for the skywalk there.

In the meantime, it was back home to Sarasota for a brief stopover before heading to Puerto Rico.

Long-time *Sarasota Herald Tribune* columnist Helen Griffiths, also a long-time personal friend of the family, popped over for a visit.

Wife Helen was in the kitchen fixing lunch while Karl and journalist Helen Griffiths were in the den at 1625 Arlington this late March afternoon, in Karl's trophy room, always the gathering spot for him. The center of the room was dominated by a large glass covered table displaying his vast spoon collection from all over the world.

The walls were papered with other mementos of his life and career, pictures, plaques and awards and trophies of all kinds of different shapes and sizes.

There was even a framed 1972 letter from President Richard Nixon wishing him a speedy recovery after a fall at the Olympia Arena in Detroit, the home of the Detroit Red Wings.

There was a framed proclamation on government letterhead making him an honorary citizen of Texas, in honor of his recreation of the Seven there in 1963 at a Fort Worth circus.

He said his personal favorite was the Waterford Crystal etched compote he received in London only a few months prior, in December of 1977. Although he finished third in the

Circus World Championships held there, the judges awarded him the same trophy as the winner for his lifetime body of work on the circus high wire.

Karl was in a mood to reminisce about everything that weekend.

The newspaper columnist asked when he might finally be ready to retire from the danger, if only because his wife Helen in the other room had been trying to get him to do so for many years. True to form, he pointed out that people get killed on airplanes, in automobiles, in the service, construction jobs, sometimes just crossing the street.

"From a chair of retirement I wait for God's hand to take me?" he asked Griffiths. "When I go, I want that to be it. A retirement only in death. When I broke my neck in October, it was not my time to go. A few feet fall ... that can cripple ... a big fall I hope would be God's answer when he is ready for me."

He always had the same answer for Helen when they talked about what might happen.

"I am in God's hands. When it is my time, I go."

But despite all that talk about being in God's hands, as of late he was uncharacteristically fretting behind closed doors, something wife Helen had never seen before. But not about Seattle or anything else, she said – just Puerto Rico.

Not the actual circus performances, to be held indoors in an arena, but the promotional skywalk that was planned outdoors before the first scheduled big top performance later that day. He had been monitoring the weather in San Juan, and it was always unpredictable, and very windy at the moment.

The two Helens and his longtime assistant and business manager Stephanie Shaw took turns trying to talk him out of it.

Join My Club 1

This was a man who only admitted fear twice in his life – the Tallulah Falls gorge walk. And the Miami Beach skywalk, also equally treacherous because of the wind, but more so because of the blinding spot lights shining on Karl that night that prevented him from focusing on his landing point.

Nonetheless, the next morning, sure as the light of day, he was up and at the airport for his flight to Puerto Rico.

Once on site, he was forced to postpone the walk several times because of extremely high winds.

"Don't do it" Ms. Shaw told him again by phone from Sarasota. "Remember, Karl, you have an out clause for the weather."

He was calling daily for Helen to come to San Juan for a vacation. Finally, she relented and booked a flight and flew there the next day to be with him.

Soon after she arrived, on the morning of March 22, 1978, he personally walked the avenue between the two towers of the waterfront Condado Holiday Inn that the wire was strung between. He strode the length of the wire at street level, personally checking each guide wire.

By early morning, hundreds of people were already gathered in the streets below and in the courtyards and on the surrounding hotel balconies.

The media was everywhere, the TV cameras, the radio stations, the print journalists with their notebooks.

The wind was a steady 12 to 15 miles per hour. But occasional gusts were way beyond that, there was no official measurement, but at least 30 miles per hour or more would be a reasonable guess according to the local meteorologists.

A little after 11 a.m.with Karl's pride on the line, he gave his familiar refrain.

"I go now," he said.

Decked out in his brightest maroon pants, his billowing ruffled white cotton shirt flapping in the wind, he inched out across the wire.

The wind was steady at this point, and coming straight at him, so he made good progress in the beginning, his typical mien apparent, legs slightly crouched, the lead foot sliding ahead on the wire with the toes on either side, heel slightly off to the side on the free foot, everything looking good so far.

Shortly after the halfway point, the wind began to gust. The people on the balconies felt it particularly strong, as did the people on the ground.

Now he was not quite two-thirds of the way across, when his shirt and pants began to blow recklessly about him and he leaned forward approximately 45 degrees, as the wire began to visibly gravitate from side to side, swaying back and forth several feet now like a two-man jump rope. Now you could see his legs begin to shake, and his dark silver balance pole began to seesaw up and down from right to left.

The wind continued its merciless assault as the wire continued to sway and his legs continued to shake and he continued to struggle to stay upright.

Now he leaned over even further, about maybe 15 seconds into this death defying dance, with his upper torso now almost parallel to the wire facing directly ahead toward the tower he was aiming for. Suddenly his balancing pole began to list badly just to the one side now, to the left, and the people on the balconies heard voices shouting, "Sit down, sit down, Karl," that were coming from the circus people watching from the destination tower.

He crouched down on the wire now, ever so slowly, and as he did the 40 pound balance pole now tipped upward sharply to the right and suddenly it was touching his right arm pit while the wind simultaneously pushed him to the left of the wire and wham it was instantaneous he slipped right off the wire as he lunged at the steel cable with his right hand in a futile attempt to grab the wire that had been his life for half a century.

Now about to take his life.

He instantly plummeted toward the ground 120 feet below at an estimated speed of 75 miles per hour. About two thirds of the way down he grabbed the pole again with his right hand so he once again had both hands on it.

About six and a half seconds of eternity later his head slammed into the hood of a parked taxi cab and he almost simultaneously cratered the asphalt parking lot floor with his body.

Shrieks and sobs and a thunderous wailing pierced the air. Several spectators fainted. There was a scurrying, horrifying panic that gripped the crowd as if people were looking for someplace to hide from such a brutal spectacle of death.

He laid there immobile as almost immediately he was surrounded by hotel and event security men and in less than a minute by the local police, who picked him up and carried him to a nearby squad car. One spectator said he saw him breathing, and he shouted to others nearby that he was still alive.

He was not still alive.

The Great Wallenda, the man who once managed to stay on the wire through an earthquake during a South American performance, the man who fell numerous times and survived numerous disasters to cross Tallulah Falls Gorge, and Veterans Stadium, and the Tangerine Bowl, and too many other venues to name, the one and only Great Wallenda – the indestructible one – was dead.

The man who once back flipped on the mast of a sailing schooner, the oldest man to walk a high wire and indeed the only man to ever skywalk with a broken neck, the Great Wallenda, was dead.

Official confirmation came a short while later from San Juan's Presbyterian Hospital.

So does the show really go on?

The answer came quickly.

Three short hours later, at the Puerto Rican Circus matinee, granddaughter Rietta Wallenda, who had witnessed her grandfather's death in the morning, climbed the wire with the other troupe members and performed the most memorable high wire act of her career – without the troupe's star performer, the Great Wallenda, whose body was now being prepared for shipment back to his Sarasota hometown for burial.

Meanwhile, the other Wallenda troupe finished up their North Dakota engagement while thousands of miles across the country in California, Steve Wallenda climbed a high wire there in memory of his idol.

It turned out to be the largest funeral in Sarasota history, attended by dignitaries and politicians and, of course, all the stars of the Circus' Golden Era were there, including Emmett Kelly, "Blinko" the Clown, band leader Merle Evans, and the entire Zachinni family of circus notoriety.

In one of those twists of irony that defy explication, because of the huge crowd, the services had to be held at Robarts Arena, the very same Sarasota venue where scenes were shot of the troupe recreating The Seven for an NBC film that aired barely one month before on national TV.

The local Mayor of Sarasota, Ron Norman, said, "He was not just a great showman, but indeed a great man whose courage and will power were inspiring to all of us."

His nephew Gunther, who had retired after the Detroit disaster, said, "I worked with him for 20 years. When I think about it, if he had to go, he went the way he wanted."

Although if he were alive, Karl would doubtless deny it, his wife Helen made it sound like he pre-determined his own demise.

"All Karl thought about for three straight months before (Puerto Rico) was falling," Helen said in an interview with the local TV station. "It was the first time he had ever thought about that and it seemed to me he put all his energy into not falling rather than walking the tightrope."

She pointed out that he personally supervised the installation of the wire, down to making sure the guide wires were secure, something she said he had never done before.

When Karl Wallenda poured all his energy into not falling, rather than walking the tight rope, he was virtually destined to fall, she said.

The Wallenda Effect was born.

But he was physically gone forever, buried that warm spring day in Manasota Cemetery, in nearby Oneco in the special Wallenda plot.

"Aerialists Supreme," the giant Wallenda headstone reads.

There he is, etched into the granite, his likeness in purple pants and purple showman's vest, steady on the wire, clutching his famous balance pole.

After the graveside service was over, after most of the mourners were gone, it was time for one last move.

In fulfillment of his wishes, the cemetery workers flipped his casket so he would be looking up at the headstone and his own likeness on the wire.

His last acrobatic move.

Ever a showman, right up to the very end.

~ 19 ~

TWO GUNS TO THE HEAD

Wallenda's sudden death, plastered all over the media of his native state of Florida, made Dennis MulQueen think of his father again, who continued to walk his own tightrope up in Michigan constantly battling leukemia.

Dennis wanted to visit, but he had no money.

Another phone call from Michigan the following week gave him no choice.

"Your father is in the hospital again and his counts have skyrocketed and it's not looking too good. You might want to come home and not wait this time."

"Okay, Mom. Jeez, that is horrible. Thanks for letting me know. I'll get going right away."

The car was broken and he had little money for gas anyway, but he knew this call was different from the other calls. As soon as he hung up the phone he took a quick shower, dressed and hit the streets with two $20-dollar bills in his front pocket and the clothes on his back. And his right thumb pointed up in the air.

It was the only way.

One ride up Thomasville Road got him to Valdosta, Georgia, where after six hours standing on the shoulder of the highway he started panicking. How in hell am I going to get home, he mumbled.

Please God, for Christ's sake, please get me a ride home, he said as about 15 minutes later a tall white van pulled over and came to an abrupt stop about 20 yards past him. The right rear turn signal was flashing. The vehicle was about the size of a typical UPS truck, only this one had faded out whitewashed side walls and faded red trim.

The words "Birdsong Farms" were starkly painted in six-inch bold block letters across the side panels. Underneath, in much smaller print, read "Ocala, Florida."

As he hurried over to the passenger window, he saw two scruffy-looking guys inside sitting in black vinyl chairs that swiveled atop aluminum shafts that went through the center of black metal plates bolted to the floor. A lever protruding from the side of the chair seat allowed the occupant to go up or down, forward or backward.

"Hop in there, man. Where ya headed?"

"Oh, on my way to Michigan. Thanks a million. you guys."

"Don't kid me, man. If ya had a million ta give me, ya woont be standin' there by the side a the road all stranded in this about to be poundin' cold-ass rain with no raincoat tryin' ta' get ta Michigan now would ya now, man?"

Dennis MulQueen smiled.

"No, you're certainly right about that, but got no choice. My Dad's in the hospital dying of cancer and I lost my job and I'm trying' like a bitch to get back there to see him."

"Oh shit, man, that sucks. No problem, man, we can help ya out at least like two-thirds a the way there, okay? We're goin' all the way back up ta our homebase stables. We's from Bird Song Farms in Ocala an we're headin' ta the home ranch way up in the northeast of the good ole blue grass state, good ole home sweet home Kentucky."

One look around the van confirmed these guys were indeed horse men. There were shoes lining the back walls, hammers and nails and all kinds of tools, saddles and blankets, bottles of what looked like medicine with white typed labels and jars of vitamins and god knows what kinds of supplements. Looked like they did it all. Smelled like a horse was hiding out somewhere in the van, too.

He told the guy the whole story of his father and his cancer and how everything in life pretty much sucked these days. "I hear ya there, man. But don't ye worry, okay. We're all in it together there, buddy." The driver told him his father had died when he was young.

"Don't worry, we'll get cha' up there in plenty a time. 'Scuse me a minnit. I jess gotta ring on my upstairs phone."

He extended his right arm slowly toward the dash, as he made a four-finger fist and rolled his wrist to the right and stuck his thumb upward and out like he was getting ready to hitchhike himself. Then he jerked his arm with his hand and upright thumb in the air up and down like he was pointing at the sky with his thumb.

"Okay, good news, the Guy wanted me ta tell ya he's gunna be there a good while yet, I mean ur daddy, ur gunna git there in plenty a time. So jus' don't you worry now there anymore, good feller."

He continued.

"And need be I must say it. Ya gotta stop worryin' urself to death now, buddy. It's writ all over yer face like greasepaint, and the Man on the big line in the sky tells me ur daddy is gonna make it through and live fer a good while yet, okay? Say a prayer to ur Maker and now let's jess have a li'l faith an' carry on cuz it ain't over till the fat lady sings and she ain't singing anytime soon, ya got that now? We'll be doin' the singin' round here, okay?"

"Oh jeez. Thanks, man. I really appreciate it."

"Besides, we're all only here temporary anyway, like we'll all be meetin' up agin' in the end so jess try an' live the right way an' let the chips fall where they may becuz we can't do nuttin' better anyhow, ya hear? If we keep worryin' 'bout when it's all over, well, we jess might fergit we got another day called today and it jess might be the best one ever and we don't wanna miss it now. And oh, by the way, I'm Johnny an' that dude over there is my pardner Jeremy. You can call him Jer fer short."

"I'm Dennis, John. Thanks. Sure as heck am glad to meet you guys."

"Jer, I reckin' we could all use a little pick-me-up 'bout now, don't ya think?"

Jeremy nodded in the affirmative. "Yep," he said. "Sure could, boss."

Just as Johnny finished talking, he slid a metal ashtray out of the dash and passed Dennis the fattest joint he had ever seen. It looked like a Swisher Sweet.

"Now you light that up," he said as he reached back with a plastic lighter in his hand. As Dennis lit the joint and inhaled, Johnny flipped the channel button and spun the volume dial up and sure as heck the Fifth Dimension flooded the car with "Let The Sun Shine In."

They passed the joint around, and then it was Simon and Garfunkel's time. "Bridge Over Troubled Waters" filled the car.

Dennis had stopped going to church a long time ago. But that song – his father's all-time favorite – coming on the radio at that exact moment in time struck him as if not spiritual, then at least some kind of karma from somewhere inexplicable.

"How ya feelin' now, buddy?" Johnny asked as he turned around and saw Dennis in the backseat making the sign of the cross.

"Oh, just sayin' a li'l prayer, I see. Sorry for interruptin'. Who to might I ask? Anybody in particular?"

"Well, ah, yeah, actually, to a guy named Martin, St. Martin de Porres."

"Oh yeah, well who in hell might that be? Some preacher was he, huh?"

"Well, actually, he was a guy that lived back in the seventeen hundreds. I believe, he was an illegitimate kid whose dad was Spanish and his mother was African and some Native American. She was a former slave, so he had a tough life from the start and especially after his dad abandoned him when he was two, and you know how people are, even the people in the Dominican religious order where he was a lay brother mocked him. You know how human beings are, they called him half-breed, bastard slave boy – hey, blackie, that kind of thing."

Johnny laughed loudly as he turned toward his buddy in the swivel seat next to him. "Sounds like he coulda been raised in Kentucky, eh Jer?"

"So what'd he do, donate a lot of money to the church or something? Isn't that what ya had ta do to be a saint in that there Cath-o-lic Church? You gotta pay ur way into good graces, right?"

It was Dennis' turn to laugh.

"No, he was poor as hell, but he did manage later on to start an orphanage for kids and a hospital for sick kids. And at the hospital some unbelievable things happened. My Mom told me about it."

"Oh yeah, like what kinda shit was that s'posed ta be?"

"Well, he was amazing. People, more than one, it was documented by many people, they would walk in on him in his room and the guy would be levitating clear off of the floor and the room would be filled with light, a blue light would fill the room when he prayed. And then, it was also documented, miracles, people that were dying and on death's doorstep he would reach out to them and bless them and they were miraculously cured.

"Now I'm not religious, I don't go to church or any of that crap, but who am I to challenge other people's beliefs? I mean why wouldn't it be possible? I definitely do think there are some special people on earth. It sure is ironic he turned out to be my Dad's favorite spiritual guy because he was the patron saint of people of color and a great advocate for social justice.

"He was of Spanish, Native American, and African descent like I said, and that's a tough go in this world as bigoted and mean as people can be. But how neat this guy stood up against all that and became the patron saint of Vietnamese and African people and Native Americans. Now that's what you would call apropos because he was the illegitimate son of a Spanish nobleman and a freed slave. Even his own people, the novices at the Dominican friary, they too called him a mullato dog and didn't want him to be a priest."

"Well, well, there ya go. You keep on prayin' then, don't lemme interrupt and maybe yer daddy'll get a miracle there too, Dennis. The important thing is you have ta believe in 'em in order for one to happen, right? We all better believe cuz sooner or later, if we live long enough, we all better jess believe in miracles cuz we all might need one sooner or later."

It wasn't long, with the combination of the weed, being on the road, just being with these guys, a sense of peace and relaxation descended over Dennis MulQueen in the backseat.

They sang songs to the radio, chatted some more, and he mostly slept on and off for the next several hours. They stopped for lunch, and then got right back on the interstate.

He was beginning to wish Kentucky was at the north pole. He was very comfortable in the backseat of the Bird Song Farms' van rolling down the highway.

The ride through Georgia and Tennessee and the Smokey Mountains brought back memories of the old family Florida trips. On the road again. The soothing sounds and feelings of being on the road again. Soon he was so relaxed he fell asleep. He awakened moments after the lumbering hulk of a vehicle coasted to a stop again.

He sat up and took a look. They were in a gas station parking lot. Still half asleep, he didn't know where they were.

"Hey there, Dennis. Ya musta been real tired, ya slept mosta da way back there. But we're here now, at the crossroads, at the end a this here part a da journey. We have ta go east here now, over thataways, and you wanna keep on goin' straight north here an' on through Cinci ta git to Detroit. So we gotta part now, buddy, until the Good Lord brings us back together agin' someday. Great known ya, man. If ur evers near Bird Song Farms, why you jess pop on in and holler hello now, okay?"

"Oh my God. Wow," Dennis said as he looked at Johnny, then Jeremy, then out the window. He opened the backdoor and then he knew he didn't want to leave this guy's van. A burst of cold air hit him in the face.

"Man, it's damn cold for April, isn't it?"

"Yeah, can feel it, huh. Feels like a big ole cold front done busted in on us up here now, all the more colder I reckin' cuz we're all used ta dat Southern-fried-chicken weather."

The actual air temperature felt like it was in the low 40s, but with a gusting wind it felt like it was going to snow any second.

Dennis MulQueen hesitated a minute with the van door open, wishing now more than ever he didn't have to get out of that van. He wanted to stay there forever.

"Jeez, I wish I didn't have to go, John. Can't thank you enough."

Then he felt his heart beating, up high like it was in his esophagus, like he was going to have another one of those moments.

Johnny leaned forward in his seat at that very moment and reached into his right back pants pocket. He turned around and thrust a wad of bills in Dennis' right hand that he had extended toward Johnny to shake goodbye with.

"Here, man."

"No, Johnny, I appreciate it but I can't take your money."

"Yes, you can. Ya have ta. It's only fifty, but it'll git u some grub an' a place fer a night if ya git stranded, but I don't see that happening whatsoever. And now don't you worry, we're gunna say prayers fer ya and yer daddy too, aren't we, Jer?"

"Oh yeah, man. Right on," Jeremy said.

Dennis hoisted himself out the open door and stood up in the howling cold air.

"How do you know I don't have a million dollars in my pants," he said.

"Man, I already told ya I know you ain't got no darn million dollars standin' out on the road back there."

Dennis laughed, thinking out in the cold now he might need the money after all as he only had a thin cotton shirt on.

As if the guy was reading his mind, Johnny hollered, "Hold on a minnit now," as he whirled around on his vinyl seat and got up inside the truck and grabbed a green military style coat off a hook on the back wall, jumped out of the truck and grabbed Dennis' right hand and pulled his arm out from his body and laid the jacket across his outstretched limb.

"Here ya go, man. You might need this."

Now Dennis was trying not to cry in front of the guy. But he couldn't help it any more than he could believe it.

The jacket looked brand new. It was crisp and bright olive-green with great big square pockets on the sides and lots of insulation inside – a long and heavy coat.

"No, man, No. Oh my God," he said.

"Now put it on. Try it on right now, man."

Dennis put the coat on.

It was a perfect fit.

"See, there ya go. That coat is meant fer ya, man."

"And now listen here," Johnny continued. "I wanna say it again. Don't you worry. The Good Lord had a plan fer us all, so don't fight it. We jess have ta trust in it. Everything's gonna be all right. And I think you'll be glad you got a nice coat now, buddy, cuz look out there, the wind is howlin' and it's as cold out here as a well digger's ass in January, so you git you a bowl of hot chili at that li'l diner over there ta warm ur tummy and git back on da road an' you'll need this here army issue green coat. It's a nice one and it'll do the job real nice fer ya. There's a roll-up hood in back an' you'll probably need that too 'less a cute chick recognizes ya and picks ya up real quick and offers ya a warm shoulder. And she's be a fool not to, won't she be, Jeremey?"

He guffawed and Jeremy shook his head and Dennis smiled, as he moved his head slowly from side to side.

"Or somethin' else, if yer real lucky."

Johnny turned, slid the back door shut, opened the front door and jumped back in the driver's seat, pulling the front door shut with him.

"An' one other thing," he said "You take this too, and if yer ever passin' thru Ocala, Florida, why you stop in and say hello now, okay there, man?"

He reached on the floor between the two seats into a tan cardboard box and pulled out a red-and-white baseball cap. It was a very unique hat. The front and back panels of the hat were white, and two side panels were fire engine red. Across the front white panel in small black letters the name and city were screen printed: "Birdsong Farms. Ocala, Florida."

Now he really couldn't believe this guy.

"Didn't we just meet? Hey, man, you're wrecking all my preambles. I mean, my previously conjured up preconceived notions about the world."

"What's that, spit it out, man. What exactly did ya say there?" It dawned on Dennis that he was speaking Hondeau-ese to the guy. That was the term he coined for his friend Bokker's older brother for his occasionally hard-to-interpret philosophical meanderings.

"What I'm trying to say,' Dennis continued, "is I can't believe we met like this, only this morning. And you doing all this for me. A perfect stranger. I mean, this is amazing. I mean, you are amazing, Johnny. I can't tell you how much this means."

"Hey, buddy, like I said, we're all in it together. We're all gunna meet up agin' someday. Jess tho' don't let's be in no hurry to rush things, okay now, man?"

Dennis reached inside the truck and shook Johnny's hand like he was going to never let it go. He didn't want to let it go any more than he wanted to get out of that van.

"Now git outta here. Now git on yur way, don't you git all broke up on me now er I'll have ta go outta this here truck an' horsewhip the hell outta yer ass clear across the great state a Kentucky. Okay now, ya got that, my friend?"

It worked. They were both laughing hysterically now.

They looked each other in the eyes one last time, like two strangers passing in the night, two people randomly meeting on a roadside in Georgia, like blood brothers from a past life coming together for a reunion, a magical moment in time where two complete strangers came together to make a statement – that no matter what, we are never alone.

He couldn't explain it if he had to. All he knew is he felt it in his heart, and that was all that mattered.

He put the hat on and then buttoned his new coat up to the very last button.

As if acting on some cosmic cue, as if to certify some unknowable force in the universe that doles out hope in these most unlikely of moments, as if to affirm a connection beyond themselves, they simultaneously saluted each other at the same exact moment.

"Onward, Pixen; go get 'em, Vixen," Dennis MulQueen said as he turned and walked away.

The van took off and he turned to run after it, but it was too late.

He realized he forgot to get the guy's phone number, last name or address. He didn't know if he would ever make it back to Birdsong Farms, if he would ever see the guy again, but he knew one thing for sure – he would keep that hat and coat forever.

~ ~ ~

It was dark now, and one short ride and several hours later, he was still stranded in Ohio north of Cincinnati at the same spot on the side of I-75. He was starting to wonder how he was going to make the final leg home. He was in the middle of nowhere, and it was a good thing he kept the coat because it was damn cold out there now.

Oh wait, this guy's stopping.

Oh my God, it's a cop, he realized.

This is odd, he thought. He's on the shoulder, he's driving right past me. About 10 yards down he screeched on the brakes and switched the blue lights on.

A trooper jumped out and hurriedly strode towards him with his hand on his gun holster, which he appeared to be fumbling with. Jeez, this doesn't look good.

It wasn't.

Less than three feet away now, the cop screamed "freeze" as he freed his weapon from the holster and pointed it at Dennis MulQueen's head. As it turns out, if it had been a clean draw Dennis would have been dead. The fumble gave Dennis MulQueen the split second he needed to throw his hands in the air and shout, "Don't shoot don't shoot. I'm on the way home to see my parents."

"What is that in your pocket." the obviously flustered police officer said.

Dennis MulQueen glanced down and sure enough he could see protruding about two inches from the right pocket of his newly bequeathed green lantern jacket the black end of what appeared to be a long handled, large-toothed black comb.

"Officer, this guy that gave me a ride felt sorry for me, so he gave me this coat when he dropped me off. He didn't want me to freeze. I think it looks like the handle on a brush or a big comb, officer. I know what you are thinking. I swear it's not a gun. I have never had a gun, I never will."

"Lift your right hand in the air slowly and then with your left hand slowly unbutton the coat and without moving your right hand slowly pull the coat off of your back and drop it to the ground. One wrong move and you're dead."

Ahh, that coat. His talisman forever. Nobody harms me when I'm wearing this coat, he said to himself. But just to be sure, he did exactly as he was told and dropped the coat on the ground.

"Now take ten steps backwards and stand there and don't move."

He took 10 measured steps backwards and stopped.

The cop walked forward to where the coat was on the ground and bent over with his gun still pointed at Dennis and removed a long flat black comb from the right pocket.

"Where is your ID"

"In my back pocket officer, in my wallet."

"Okay, now slowly like real slow get your ID out for me. Again one false move and I will blow your head off."

"Officer, I'm going to turn slowly to the right now and extend my left hand out front so you can see it and I'm going to slowly turn around so you can see my wallet in my rear pants pocket okay? I'm just hitchhiking home from Florida."

He slowly extracted his wallet and extending it out from behind his body, he slowly turned around and took his license out and offered it to the officer in his right hand. The cop reached out and took it from him with his gun the whole time still pointed straight at Dennis' chest.

"Officer, please don't shoot me. I'm just on the way home to see my Dad. He has cancer and is dying in the hospital."

"Stand right there and don't move. I'll be back in a minute." He walked backwards about five steps before turning around while still looking behind him at Dennis as he returned to his patrol car and got back in. Dennis figured he had to be running a LEIN check on him. Jeez, I hope I have no more inspection sticker tickets out there, he muttered to himself.

The all clear must have come through as the Ohio State Trooper got out of his car and walked back to Dennis MulQueen and gave him his license back.

"Man, you have no idea how close to death you just came. If my holster hadn't jammed on me there you would be dead. That's never happened to me before, it must have happened for a reason. Because we just had a cop shot just down the road 20 miles from here by a tall white guy dressed up in military gear. And here you are just down the street, on the very same freeway in a green military coat with a shiny black object sticking out of your pocket that I was sure was a murder weapon. All I can tell you is this is your lucky day. It is an act of God you are still alive.

"But let me tell you something else. You might not be so lucky with the next guy that comes along, there are cops out here everywhere. This psycho is still on the loose and we are going to find him. So I advise you to leave the green coat off and get the hell off this road. You better get the hell out of here just as soon as you possibly can."

He turned and started walking back to his patrol car.

"Thanks, officer. Thank you for saving my life," he called out.

The cop took about two more steps toward his cruiser, then he straightened up and stopped in his tracks. He turned around and looked back at Dennis MulQueen.

He walked several steps back toward Dennis MulQueen and stopped again.

"You know what, you wear your heart on your sleeve there, young man. I believe you are telling me the truth about your father, I could see it in your eyes. There's a truck stop up there at the next exit, it's about five miles away. Come with me. I'm not supposed to do this, don't you dare tell anybody, but I'll drop you off up there and maybe you can call somebody or get a ride up there. Otherwise you're going to get killed out here like this."

He thanked the cop as he bent over and picked up his green coat and draped it across his arm as he followed him back to the squad car and hopped in the backseat. What a treat to be in the backseat of a cop car and not be under arrest, he thought. The trooper took off like a bat out of hell as the radio was blasting alerts with numbers and cities and coordinates he couldn't make sense of.

He told the cop he was sorry about his colleague. The Ohio State Trooper said thanks as they pulled off of the freeway at the next exit down. He brought his cruiser to a stop at the top of the ramp and looked right, then left, then turned to Dennis MulQueen and said, "Now you get out here. And be careful, you have to walk across the bridge here and the truck stop is on the other side. See there across the road that big red ball with the 76 on it. That's the truck stop.

"You best get a ride outta there, young man. You'll definitely be a lot safer there than standing on this freeway. Good luck to you and I hope your father gets better."

"Thank you, officer. Thank you again for saving my life, God bless you, officer," he said.

He got out and just as the door shut the cop made a left turn and roared off into the night. Dennis could see him tearing back down the I-75 South ramp heading back the other way. Okay, so there goes Cat Life Number 6, he said to himself. And still counting, thank God.

He was still a bit skittish when he got to the truck stop and walked up to the first big rig he came to at pump number 1. The place was packed with long distance transport trucks everywhere, must have been 25 or more of them on the grounds. This was a truck stop all right.

He wondered who dressed this guy, as he watched a swarthy-looking guy in a red flannel shirt with a red kerchief around his neck and a square-brimmed red baseball cap with his jeans tucked into his cowboy boots descend from the cab of a fire-engine-red Peterbilt.

Dennis MulQueen wondered if the guy had red underwear on too. Better not ask, he chuckled to himself.

As Dennis walked toward him, the trucker began unscrewing the cap on his diesel tank. "Sir, don't mean to interrupt," Dennis said, "but I've gotta catch a ride back to Detroit. Could you possibly help me, my Dad –" The guy cut him off in midsentence like a slammed fist on an oak table top.

As he began to speak he raised his right hand in the air like he was pledging allegiance to the flag or swearing in a new witness in the court room, as he blurted out, "No, pal, you best get ur ass outta here right now. You see, I don't like strangers walking up to me in parking lots, you see, unless it's a pretty woman. You ought to know even though this job is killer sometimes, you ought to know better no trucker in the world is gonna risk his job and give you a lift to nowheres. It's against the rules, man. I'd be fired just like anyone else if they got caught."

"Sir, I've got 50 bucks here and my Dad in in the hospital right now."

"That's what they all say before they get in your cab and shoot and stab you and steal all ur money and whatever else they can get from you. Boy, don't you listen? I said get the fuck outta here."

Dennis wondered if he detected something in his voice, or his eyes, but whatever it was, as this gruff-acting, gruff-looking guy put the aluminum-handled pipe in the gas tank hole and squeezed the lever tight he stopped and turned around and looked at Dennis again and said, "You said you're headed to Detroit, right?"

"Yes sir, that's correct."

"Well, I'm headed south. But I can tell you the only way a trucker is allowed to give a ride is if it's to another trucker who's broke down. That would be okay and might get you a ride home. Good luck to you."

"Thank you, sir," Dennis said. "Sorry to bother you. Thank you, sir. Have a good night."

He walked past the guy's rig and on toward the main building.

He walked through the double glass doors and he couldn't see an open seat anywhere. Is this Bingo night at the Legion or a truck stop, he wondered?

To the left against the wall there was a row of booths and the center of the joint was filled with white linoleum-topped dining tables surrounded by chrome-legged, red-backed vinyl chairs. All of the booths and tables were occupied by at least one person.

There were several women in the crowd as well. They didn't look like truckers. Maybe trucker's assistants.

The smell of coffee and bacon grease mixed in the air with reams of steadily swirling acrid yellow-and-white cigarette smoke.

Over against the right wall just inside the door about five feet in was a platform two feet off the ground with a partially glassed-in front top. The center window was open and there was a guy in a cowboy hat sitting in there quietly overlooking the whole scene. He held a silver microphone in his hand that he used to communicate to the truckers the numbers of open pumps, or to let so-and-so know his itinerary was ready or he had a call waiting or his vehicle repairs were finished and he was ready to fill up and get out.

He also handled reservations for the repair garage out back but also a small row of trailers on the far end of the property that were for those looking to bunk cheap for the night who didn't have a sleeper cab. He also collected all the tab money from everybody including the diners. There was a small green cash register on a wooden shelf off to his right.

So this is what a real truck stop is like. The mother of all truck stops.

As Dennis approached the booth the guy with the silver microphone leaned forward in his chair and said, "Lane 10, lane 10 is now open." His voice boomed out over the loudspeaker.

He looked at Dennis MulQueen and said, "Yeah, man, what can I do for you?"

Dennis cleared his throat. "Hey, my rig broke down, down the road. They are sending a crew out, but I need to get to Detroit. They got another load for me ready to go. Time is money, you know. Do you happen to know anybody going to Detroit?"

He retrieved the microphone that he had returned to a plastic stand screwed to the countertop and pushed in a small black rectangular plastic bar on the side in the middle as he spoke into the aluminum ball again.

"We've got a trucker here who needs assistance getting to Detroit. He's broke down and needs a ride to Detroit. Anybody going through or near Detroit, Michigan, please approach the booth."

Not a minute later a lanky guy with matted-down greasy black hair with a thin scraggly salt-and-pepper bandito mustache sauntered up to the booth with a listing gait, like a rodeo rider who had taken one too many bull rides. His thin slitty eyes with beady small dark-brown irises combined with his greasy-matted hair and dangling toothpick to make him look like a cross between an old matador and an inner-city hitman.

"This is the guy here," the guy in the booth with the yellowed suede cowboy hat and the big jowls said as he pointed his stubby fingers at Dennis.

"You the guy? You need to get to Detroit?"

"Yeah, man, I do. I'm stranded here.

"Where you outta?"

"Detroit."

"Well, we're in Ohio. Aren't they gonna send somebody out for you, or get you somebody local even?"

"They can't get to me till tomorrow so they said to get back if I can and they will send somebody for the rig. We don't know what's wrong with it, if it can be fixed or not. I think the engine is blown. They don't want to take a chance on me missing my next run out tomorrow morning at 6 a.m. They asked if I could get back ASAP on my own. They've got another truck loaded to the gills ready to go out and they need me."

"Okay. Follow me. I'm gonna pay first and then we'll take off shortly. I'm out back on the side. I already gassed up. My name is Curtis, by the way."

"Thanks. I'm Dennis."

"Here you go, Lenny," he said as he handed the guy in the booth his white receipt and a $20 bill. Dennis followed him out the door, down the parking lot to the right to a big flatbed parked at the rear of the restaurant. There were three large circular items flat on top as wide as the flatbed itself underneath three separate black tarps. The three of them took up the entire flatbed. He could see under the front of the first tarp, something shiny and battleship grey, must be steel coils he surmised. He had seen them come into the Rouge many times before.

He climbed up the ladder steps on the right and opened the door and hoisted himself into the passenger seat. Curtis was already in the driver's seat.

Curtis slowly eased the lumbering red colossus out of the parking lot and turned left and went across the bridge and made a left onto the north ramp of I-75 toward Toledo.

At first when they got on the road it felt to Dennis MulQueen like they were riding a giant roller coaster where you feel the vibrations and a little clanging jolt as the metal box passes over every single annoying joint on the track, or crack in the road as it were here.

But as they got rolling the bumps and dips and potholes on the road made this multi-ton behemoth lurch and sway and jump all over the road more like a beached whale.

This was a rough ride period. The road was rough, the vehicle suspension was rough. The seat he was sitting on was rough. And the tires that were supporting tons of this steel, he knew they were rough too as he almost jumped out of that seat through the window as one blew with a very loud boom not long after they left the truck stop. The sound and a simultaneous jolt of vibration telegraphed the disintegrating rubber as Dennis saw large black ribbons of tire careening off the edge of the road through the round silver ball at the bottom of the foot high outside rearview mirror.

He understood why these guys wore kidney belts. Once they got going to about 50 miles per hour, the roller coaster motif gave way to a new level of vibrating discomfort that made it seem like he was now trapped inside a giant paint mixer. This thing sure wasn't going to win any races. He glanced over and saw they were now only going 45 miles per hour even though with the vibrations it felt like 95.

"You got a heavy load, eh?" he said.

"Oh yeah. Coiled steel. But not only that, on this run and as bad as this road is, I've got to be extra careful because I'm not attached."

"Pardon me?"

"I mean I've just got a couple lines, one on each side, but they are not fastened down. So I only roll about 45 to 50 depending cuz you can feel this thing shake, and I don't want nothin' rolling off of here. That wouldn't be pretty."

"One of these babies cuts loose, the car over there next to us would be like a giant recycled tin can that King Kong just stepped on, you got it? I mean thin as a Necco wafer, you got that? I mean not as thick as one sheet of the rolled steel I got on there and that would include whoever's in the vehicle as well."

He must have sensed Dennis was about to ask him then why in god's name aren't the steel coils 'attached'.

He said, "I'm doing a short automotive run to Detroit from the plant in Tennessee. It's much easier doing it this way rather than taking hours to chain up and unchain all that crap with those heavy-ass fuckin' winches. You see, time is money and I can't afford to waste all that time on these short runs and cut my profit way down, so as long as I don't go over 50 and don't hit no big holes, I'm good. If for some reason I do get stopped by one a them flat asses they won't know no difference."

"That's good to know. Hey, it's been quite an ordeal. Mind if I take a little nap?"

"No, go right ahead, man. I'll wake you when we get to Detroit."

About an hour-and-a-half later the truck hit a pothole and a violent thud jerked him alert again.

He thought maybe they had hit something.

Turned out, it was just another blown tire, this one much closer to the cab judging by the thunderous noise.

"Don't look so scared, man. It's okay. Just lost a li'l rubber there, we're okay. That's why we got 18 of 'em.

"So, hey, man, when are they coming to get your rig?"

"Oh, sometime tomorrow."

"Well, here, okay, I know you said you got a run at 6. I got a few here to keep ya company, make ya feel a li'l better."

He reached in his right pocket and extended his hand out toward Dennis, slowly turning it over, uncurling his fingers enough to reveal a hodgepodge of about maybe 20 to 25 pills of every shape and size and color you could imagine.

"The pink and black ones, they are the best. They will give you a hell of a nice buzz and give you at least a day, and so will the reds, man, they are real nice too. You ever had any of these? They are awesome."

"No, I haven't."

"How long you been drivin'? A guy has to have some help in this business, especially cross country. You done any cross country man?"

"Oh, I'm pretty new at it, only a couple runs for me."

"So, tell me man, what happened there with your rig, man?"

"What do you mean, Curtis?"

"I mean your rig. What the fuck happened there, man? Where'd you break down?"

"Oh, really close to the Kentucky border. Not really sure what happened. I'm not too mechanical. She just quit on me."

"On the highway, without warning?"

"Yeah, she just lost all oil pressure and that was it. Seized right up. No compression, nothing."

"What kind a rig you got, man?"

"I got a Peterbilt."

"Oh yeah. You got toggle switches on yours? What kind a set up you got?"

He hesitated a minute before answering.

"Well, ahh, yeah, I got toggle switches."

"You got extenders on 'em? What kind you got?"

"Oh all kinds."

"Who installed em? You installed 'em yourself?"

"No, mine came with them."

"Oh really, never heard a that. What was you haulin?"

"Oh, I had a load of ball bearings."

"Really, where from?"

"Oh, I'm coming from Florida."

"Oh yeah? What company?"

He hesitated a few seconds again, then blurted out "DAB Industries," the only name he could come up with because that was the name of the company his brother Chip was currently an executive at.

Curtis suddenly eased off of the slow lane onto the shoulder. The entire rig, coils and all. As the truck coasted to a stop on the side of the road, Dennis MulQueen noticed Curtis lean to his right and put his hand inside a small pocket lining the right side of his seat as he started talking.

"Look over there to the right, what is that?" he blurted out. Dennis looked to the right and before he could see or say anything he heard the click and saw the glint out of the corner of his left eye. He slowly turned his head 10 degrees to the left and there six inches away pointed directly at his head was a fat black handgun in Curtis' right hand.

"You so much as move and I will blow your motherfucking head off. you ignorant lying cocksucker. What kinda' low life criminal are you? There ain't no Peterbilt in the world that comes with toggle switches, they have to be added on custom.

"And I'm a steel hauler and there's no goddamned ball bearing factory in Florida and DAB industries they are a supplier but they don't make no fucking ball bearings. Now you just get the fuck outta my truck right now before I blow your motherfucking brains out. What kind a criminal are, you mother fucker? You know what I do to people that try and rip me off? I kill 'em, man."

"Hold it, hold it, hold it. I mean no harm. I'm not going to rip you off, Curtis, I promise. I'm just trying to get to Detroit."

"You lyin' son of a bitch."

"Curtis, my dad is in the hospital dying from cancer. I just need to get home to see him. Please don't kill me. I tried truckers before you and they told me it's against the law to take hitchhikers. Only broken-down truckers. I'm sorry."

"Yeah, that's what they all say, asshole. Open the door slowly and slowly get out a my motherfucking truck right now while you're still breathing."

"Right here?"

A state trooper had just passed them on the side of the road. But he had enough sense to keep his mouth shut about that.

"That's right, motherfucker. Get out, motherfucker," he said, and as he waved the gun in Dennis' face again he jumped out and landed on his hands and knees on the ground. He forgot about the ladder steps.

Thank God, there was an exit ramp about a quarter mile up the road as he managed to scramble up the bank and make it to other side of the service ramp undetected by any law enforcement. He was just outside Toledo. He went straight to the pay phone at the gas station there and his sister answered and agreed to come and get him for the final leg home.

He asked for an update and she told him their father's counts had been sky high and he had developed an infection. But by the time Dennis and his sister got back home to Oak Park, he was on antibiotics and one of his father's doctors, Dr. Voravit Ratanatharathorn MD, had jumped him to the head of the line and got him on the leukapheresis machine at Harper Hospital and gradually his numbers were declining.

~ ~ ~

George MulQueen was sent to Harper and referred to Dr. Voravit by his head oncologist, Dr. Prem Khilanani MD, who he had met through Dr. Gerald Levinson, DO, an associate in Dr. Levy's Detroit office. Like attracts like, as these guys were all top-notch physicians. Voravit and Khilanani were cutting-edge hematologists and had bailed out George MulQueen many times already. They really knew how to manage these kinds of life and death situations.

About three days later George MulQueen was back in his internist Dr. Levy's office in northwest Detroit on 7 Mile Road seeking clearance to go back to work.

He decided to pop the question. "Dr. Levy, how long do you think I have? Tell me the truth."

Dr. Levy looked at him with that air of confidence he had about him and said, "George, we got the first five in, now we're working on the second five. Okay?"

"Thanks, Dr. Levy."

He was back to work the next day. Dennis said his goodbyes and hopped a Greyhound back to Tallahassee. An advertised 20-hour bus ride turned out to be 28. But he didn't care. He was back on the road again. With his green lantern jacket in tow.

~ 20 ~

THE PRODIGAL SON

The guy in the black cowboy hat told him to go in the cooler and get the two aluminum racks of chicken parts cut up and packaged and stock the counter with them.

He followed Dennis MulQueen into the giant walk-in refrigerator and as he walked to the back and bent over to remove the aluminum pans from the shelves, Dennis MulQueen heard a drawling voice from behind say, "Now that's interesting. You trust me enough to turn your back and bend over in front of me in the cooler like this."

Dennis recognized the voice of the guy in the black cowboy hat behind him, one of his bosses, before he turned around to face him. He was a rough-talking individual, with Brylcreemed dark thin hair and buck teeth who usually wore that black cowboy hat and a bolo tie with a silver steer head and a nasty attitude to complete the look. He was scrawny and wiry too. He was the assistant market manager, his name was Wilbur. Dennis wouldn't trust him as far as he could throw him.

Dennis didn't get along with the guy. He didn't like Dennis, Dennis didn't like him, so he generally tried to avoid him. But the last few days it was as if Wilbur were stalking him. It was the second time this week he followed him into the cooler and made a snide remark.

But Dennis wasn't afraid to talk back to this guy because he was the head meat market manager's pet and he felt safe. The market manager, who was named Ralph, and Dennis were tight as beads on a string and got along great.

Normally, he just ignored Wilbur, but he had had enough lately. "Why is that, Wilbur? I shouldn't turn my back to you because you might stab me in the back, is that it?"

He didn't look at Dennis. He just chuckled a nasty guttural sound with that same sneer on his face Dennis had seen so many times before.

The following week, Ralph wasn't at work all week. Dennis walked up to a nice guy named Ray Burnley who was busy cutting up some scraps and throwing them in a grey plastic tub on the counter. "Hey, Ray, where's the boss? I haven't seen him all week. Is he on vacation or what?"

"The boss is over there in the backroom right now, Dennis."

Ray was a really short guy. He wore the funniest high-top black faux-leather boots, chukka boots Dennis called them. He most often wore either a faded flannel shirt or a thinner solid color shirt with short sleeves, that he sometimes alternated with T-shirts with the cigarette pack in the front pocket.

Ray could have been a great greaser, but he didn't know quite what he wanted to be. He had his hair slicked down with Vaseline hair tonic. Dennis recognized the clear plastic bottle with the black-and-white-and-red label with the yellow liquid inside that he would occasionally pull out of his locker to apply to his greasy mop after lunch. He was a total nerd but a super nice guy.

"Ray, I just passed through there a little while ago, but I didn't see him over there."

"Well, I just came through there to get these tubs and he's there now sitting at the desk," Ray said.

Dennis MulQueen walked back across the meat room and stuck his head around the corner and sure enough there sat Wilbur at the old scratched up black desk in the corner. No Ralph anywhere.

He walked back over to Ray who was at the giant grinder machine now getting ready to make hamburger.

"He's not back there, Ray. Wilbur is over there."

"Like I said, Dennis, the boss is sitting at the desk. Ralph was fired last week. I thought you knew that. Wilbur is the man now."

~ ~ ~

The little flying wasps – they were his pets – thanks to Brambles.

Brambles showed him how to train them.

You find some string, preferably kite string, but you could use twine or even an extra-long blade of wild grass, or almost any filament. The longer, the better, for the dramatic effect. But first, you had to recognize these critters in flight, on the way back home.

If you didn't keep a close eye and catch them re-entering the nest it was game over because when they landed they were gone in a millisecond down under and you'd never find the front door because the holes were so small and usually concealed under a leaf or a board or a tree branch or something.

You had to look for the small hole under that leaf or in the middle of a pile of twigs or next to a clump of wildflowers, and once the lair was discovered you drop the line into the hole and slowly withdraw it and voila, there is one of these cool wasp-like creatures attached to the end of the string and *vroom, vroom, vroom*, round and round and round they fly in the air in a mad circular dash to nowhere.

They won't let go of this mortal threat they perceive in the thread, or string, or whatever it may be, as they hang on for dear life and fly incessantly in circles in hopes of carrying the imaginary enemy off to some other place and time far away from home sweet home.

Or at least that's what world-renowned entomologist Dennis MulQueen surmised was going on.

Even though they were identical in appearance to the northern wasps, these guys didn't sting. Brambles called them mud daubers.

A smaller version of the blue crabs, he laughed out loud as he recalled a recent St. Georges Island crab hunt with Claire that ended with a memorable skinny dip with a group of other students around a giant beach bonfire.

Brambles taught him this form of entertainment as well. Except for this sport you needed something better than a little string. These guys did bite. Hardware store twine was best, but even a couple long shoelaces tied together would work.

You just tie a piece of bologna to the end of the twine or shoe laces and walk out into the gulf and once the water gets waist high or better you drop the string into the warm gulf waters away from your body and within a minute or less you just pull it up. And have some kind of basket or burlap sack or some kind of bag handy – if you wanted a delectable dinner in the making.

On the end of the string would be a blue crab, just like that, and even though the bologna may be gone, the crab refuses to let go of the string. That simple.

A giant marine version of the mud dauber. But with a much more delectable outcome.

In the bag he would go, then you rip the string out of his claws. You could get an unlimited supply this way.

Anything for entertainment – and a great meal at no expense to boot.

Speaking of which – now it was time to go get the keg and stop off at Spears Seafood to pick up the oysters for a different kind of entertainment.

Saturday night home entertainment.

Dennis and TJ were putting on a party and they expected a decent crowd.

After the beer got going, everybody got going – and since there were no suitable trees or sinkholes nearby, it was time for Brambles to challenge Dennis to a push-up contest in the living room. Brambles got all the way to 39, and dropped mid 40th.

Amazingly, Dennis duplicated his effort to a T. Thirty nine and bust.

You couldn't script it any better.

Ray Burnley from the meat market dropped by in the middle of it all, and he didn't disappoint. He was again one of the nicest – but nerdiest – guys ever. He always had those shiny black faux leather chukka boots on, rain or shine, work or party. He had a big pointed nose, gaps between his front teeth, and he was dressed as always that night like a train hobo, the same blue janitor's pants with a solid colored thin-ply short-sleeved shirt. Dennis couldn't help but make fun of the guy; it was almost like a sport.

But at least he mocked Ray in ways he was sure he didn't catch on.

TJ took it all in, only subtly shaking his head with a wry grin telegraphing that he got the joke. But he was too classy to join in.

TJ invited an African American buddy named Michael from work to drop by. He was a cook at the cafeteria but an even better cook outside of that limited student menu. He treated everybody to some outstanding soul food; it was the first time Dennis had ever had real chitlins and hog maws and black-eyed peas, all good, but the greens stole the show.

Another friend of TJ's named Helen was there, but she didn't have too much fun. Late into the evening's festivities, she wandered into the back bedroom to see their cat Bambi who had just given birth a couple days ago. They probably heard the hysterical shrieks 10 miles away.

Helen discovered two little runts in the litter dead on the bedroom floor. So much for the party atmosphere as Helen ran out the front door hysterically screaming and hollering like Karl Wallenda's daughter that day in the hospital lobby.

"You murderer," she screamed at Dennis at the top of her lungs as she ran out the front door of the trailer.

The party was over.

It was 3 in the morning and about quitting time anyway.

The following Monday Dennis MulQueen strolled into the the market at 8:30, a.m., exactly one half hour past his scheduled arrival time.

"Late again, huh, MulQueen," Wilbur said as he passed him on his way to the time clock. "You seem to be making a habit of this, aren't you?"

"Sorry, Boss."

"Now there is a new schedule up there that starts on Thursday. Make sure you look at it."

Odd, Dennis thought because the new schedule for the following week had always been posted on the previous Thursday, which coincided with pay day.

He rounded the corner on the way to lunch and checked it out. His new starting time starting Thursday was 7:00 a.m.

~ ~ ~

Two nights later, the wind came in gales, the rain fell from buckets in the sky, and sure as the dirt in Tallahassee is red, the power flickered like a dying candle.

And out went the lights.

Along with the heretofore trusty alarm clock his mother had given him, unbeknownst to him, in the middle of the night, in the midst of a sound slumber. The big neon green block numbers were flashing 12:00, on and off every half second in his face when he awoke in a fit on his own.

He jumped out of bed and grabbed his wristwatch from the top of the dresser.

The rain was gone and the sun was peeping gently through the bedroom window blinds and he thought for a second maybe he got lucky.

Almost.

The silver arms read 6:48 a.m. He threw a pair of jeans and sneakers on, grabbed his black Wizard T-shirt and raced out the door pulling the shirt over his head as he ran down the driveway and across the street toward the store only a block away.

He punched his card. The small purple numbers read 7:06. Whew. Just barely made it.

He threw his white coat on and headed to the cooler to get his chicken boxes out for cutting, but Wilbur intercepted him at the swinging aluminum doors leading into the cold room.

He had that shit-eating grin on his face again, little dried white saliva bits in the corners of his mouth.

"MulQueen, that's really not necessary now, okay?" he said as he stepped in front of Dennis and extended his left arm like a traffic cop blocking his path to the cooler. "Come with me, I need to talk to you."

He sat down in his brown wooden swivel chair in the corner and tilted it back so his feet were off the ground. "Sit down MulQueen," he instructed.

As Dennis sat down in the black wicker chair on the other side of the old weather-beaten desk, Wilbur leaned forward and reached down to his right side and took his key ring off of his belt and used a small gold key about the size of a Master Lock key to open a drawer to his left.

He removed a blue metal rectangular box that looked like an old fisherman's tackle box and opened it. The lid was opened toward him, so Dennis couldn't see what was in it.

Wilbur set a small wire brush on the end of a single stranded aluminum shaft down on the table to the right of the box. Then he removed a small two-inch bottle of light blue liquid. Next he took out of the same box a small orange bottle with a white cap on top.

"Remember, what I told you a few days ago?"

"What's that, boss?"

"Well, let me refresh your memory. I said three strikes and you're out, partner. You are late again, Dennis. I told you not to be late again. We got a business to run here."

"Wilbur, I punched in at exactly 7:06. You know there was a really bad storm last night. My alarm shorted out and didn't ring but I still woke up and punched in at 7:06. That's hardly late is it, Wilbur? You're not really going to fire me for being six minutes late, are you? On a night with a storm like that?"

Wilbur removed his right hand from behind the box as he closed the lid with his left hand to reveal a large black handgun with a long barrel.

He picked up the brush and opened the bottle and dipped the brush inside the bottle.

"Let me refresh your memory again, Dennis."

He slid the brush down the barrel of the gun and moved it in and out as he spoke.

"I told you two days ago, one more time and that was it. So you don't need to punch that clock anymore."

There was a moment of stunned silence.

"Now, you're not really going to fire me for being five minus late, Wilbur, are you? The alarm cut out because of the storm. And I still got here within five minutes of start time. Hey, I am getting a wind-up clock today for backup so tomorrow I'll be a half hour early if you want. I really need this job, Mr. Dudas."

"That won't be necessary. Sorry, you're out of chances, MulQueen."

Dennis jumped up and walked to the far wall and pulled his card out of the aluminum rack next to the gray and white time clock.

He walked back up to Wilbur's desk and flicked it on the top.

"Take a look. Right there is says 7:06. You are really going to fire me for being six minutes late? You have got to be kidding me."

"Hey, pal, sorry, but you are not six minutes late. You are an hour and six minutes late. Over an hour late. I had to have Willie fill in for you, he's got most of your chickens already cut up and in the case."

"Huh?"

Dudas pointed to the schedule on the wall next to the clock.

"An hour late? No I wasn't. I start at 7, it's on the schedule."

"You better take another look, pal."

Wilbur really had that shit-eating grin going now, like that day in the cooler, only this time as wide as Emmett the Clown.

Dennis walked over to the schedule on the far wall and looked. Next to his name in pencil was scribbled 6:00 a.m.

He turned around and looked at the blue metal box on the table and the black gun in his boss' right hand. He wanted to grab the gun out of the jerk's hands and pistol whip him with it.

"It's your responsibility to check the schedule," Wilbur said. "You were supposed to be here at 6 today."

"I did check the schedule a couple days ago. It said 7:00 then, Wilbur."

Wilbur turned the gun over in his hand and moved it back and forth in the air like a windshield wiper, as if the gun was saying, un, uh, I don't think so.

"Then you musta read it wrong. Had to pull Willie off of pork to have him do your chickens, and now he's behind on the pork counter. We're way behind today cuz of you, MulQueen. See you later, MulQueen, time to move on."

Dennis straightened his arms and pushed his chair back from the desk and leaned forward like he was going to get up, but then he leaned back again and stayed seated.

He thought about it twice and gingerly stood up, turned and walked out of the store for the last time.

There was no Amalgamated Meat Cutters Union in this town. And he couldn't afford a lawyer and that would not have helped anyway.

This wasn't Detroit.

This was Tallahassee, Florida, where indeed the dirt runs red.

~ ~ ~

He recognized her immediately. The same plain Jane androgynous-looking woman he saw a few weeks ago at the jailhouse sitting across from the wavy-haired demon with the scraggly lower teeth and the cold black beads for eyes.

The same woman sitting across the glass from the monster a couple weeks ago chatting it up like they were at the local Dairy Queen.

There she was, on local TV, telling everybody what a great guy Ted Bundy is. How innocent he is.

She was identified as a woman named Carole Ann Boone, who at one time sat right next to Ted Bundy in an office in Seattle and witnessed him help people and save lives

The same brunette he saw at the Leon County jail. She had worked with Ted Bundy at the Washington State Department ofEmergencyServices hotline in Seattle.

She came down to Tallahassee to visit her old friend and stick up for him. He is innocent, she protested vehemently. He is being framed. No way he did any of this. He is a really nice guy, there is no way he could have done any of this he has been accused of.

She was acting like he was her husband.

So this is love.

Or this is massive Stockholm syndrome.

No, that's different, that was Patty Hearst, forced and cajoled and influenced into becoming one with her kidnappers.

This was voluntary. Ted Bundy married Carol Boone a few weeks later in a carefully-orchestrated courtroom ceremony reciting their vows in front of an astonished judge overseeing his murder trial. Bundy, who was in law school for a time, put that knowledge to use, knowing that vows recited in a courtroom in front of a judge are valid and legally binding.

Not surprising. Remember Eva Braun? Hitler had lots of girlfriends too, Dennis MulQueen recalled.

~ ~ ~

They were at the shuffleboard table. He slid his left foot forward on the carpet to get in better position and just at that moment, snap, he heard it, a sound like a toothpick snapping in half, just a little ping.

He felt a sharp jab in his left big toe. What the hell did I step on, he wondered.

He lifted the foot in the air and grabbed it and twisted it counter-clockwise to get a better view.

He saw nothing.

He dropped down on the floor on his bottom and twisted the foot counter clockwise again with both hands this time. He barely noticed a tiny pin prick of blood in the middle of the toe.

Nothing came out. No bleeding. Just a tiny spot.

He pushed on the spot with his right index finger, and it hurt. Uh-oh. He knew something was in there. He could almost feel it. He got a small anxiety twinge in his chest, he worried he might push it in deeper. He didn't want the darned thing traveling, whatever kind of sliver it was.

What was that about being luckier than good?

Claire had great eyes and she was already bent over on the floor with her head low to the shag carpet trying to see what was going on.

She ran her hands along the surface of the carpet and squeezed her left thumb and forefinger together, then she held it in the air, and titled it toward the light, a tiny metal shaft, he recognized it as the head of a sewing needle.

You could see the eye at the end. She dropped it in her outstretched right hand and it appeared about a little more than an inch long – meaning there was probably at least another good inch of it missing in his foot.

"Let me see your foot again Denny."

She pressed her finger lightly on the pin-head crimson spot and he flinched.

"Oh my God, I think it snapped off in your foot."

She got the tweezers and another needle out, and half an hour later it was time to give up. They both knew this thing wasn't coming out without help.

"It's in there pretty deep. I think it needs to be lanced by a doctor," she said.

He hoped they weren't going to amputate – she drove him to Tallahassee Memorial and he found himself laid out on a white table feeling like a sacrificial lamb on the altar led to slaughter, surrounded by a half dozen medical personnel all garbed up in green scrubs with powder blue masks and there were flashing lights on colorful screens and white-paneled boxes on tables and tubes everywhere, attached to poles all around with big gray metal machines on either side with aluminum flex-tubes with metal tools dangling from the end and metal shafts like mini steel beams connecting one another and the lights were big and round and blinding. He was wondering if they had him confused with somebody else. Is this going to be a simple needle extraction or a quadruple bypass, he said to himself.

He was always a little afraid of hospitals, ever since that time when he was a kid and the guy got stabbed in the Providence Hospital triage unit one curtain over from him when his parents took him in there after he fell off his bike and hit his head on the pavement.

The main feature of this room was an X-ray machine with a long cyclops-like multi-hinged metal arm that the doctor was directing by hand at Dennis MulQueen's elevated foot.

They started digging, and they kept on digging – to the tune of more than 20-minute's worth of digging. That felt like two hours' worth of digging.

They started X-raying, and they kept X-raying. The damn machine was humming and honing in and out every few minutes like a skipping record.

"Hey, guys, did you get to China yet?"

Nobody laughed. They even switched up the head digger with another digger – still nobody could find the darned thing.

He couldn't believe it was taking this long.

Jeesuz, more X-rays, are they going to fry my foot right off of my body? He felt like Puff the Magic Dragon, he was afraid to look, he was afraid his foot was neon green by now.

At a minimum, he knew his big toe was hamburger.

An eternity later – in reality it was a little less than a half hour total – the room broke out in cheers and clapping like the Seminoles had just won the national championship. A short Caucasian doc held the prize aloft in a pair of large bent-end tweezers that at the moment seemed more like hedge clippers to him.

The thing was over an inch long. But still, you're talking a needle in a very small haystack. This wasn't even his foot, it was his big toe.

"Yeahhhh, all right, we got it, Dennis."

Apparently, they knew what he was going to be in for a short while later.

They wrote him a prescription for Dilaudid 2 mg pills.

The pharmacy did not have 2 mg Dilaudid, only one milligram. Claire drove him back to the ER to get the scrip rewritten.

She got back in the car and they pulled out of the parking lot – just in time for the Novocain to wear off.

By the time they got back to their house, he wanted tree trimmer clippers so he could cut the darned thing off.

He couldn't believe a toe could hurt that bad.

About an hour and a dose of Dilaudid later, it wasn't so bad anymore.

~ ~ ~

A couple weeks after the toe incident, she walked into the living room and told him what he knew was coming but didn't want to hear.

She had hinted several times in the last few weeks. But it still knocked him on his duff.

"Denny, I have decided this isn't the place for my future, or our future. It's time to go, Denny."

He sat there with his head in his hands.

"Denny, I love you and I would like you to come with me."

He sat there and looked at her with his eyes as wide open as his mouth, contemplating what she just said.

Even though he knew this day was coming sooner or later, he was still in shock about what he knew her departure would mean for his existence.

"Denny, do you want to come with me? I would really like you to come with me. It's a really nice place. I already told my aunt, she said you are welcome to stay with her as well. You could have a spot in the basement, she said. Of course, I would have a bedroom upstairs, but maybe I could sneak down in the middle of the night."

Then came that sweet cackle again, the one he knew he was going to miss real bad.

"But really, Denny, it would be a chance for us to start all over again in Colorado. You know there's lots of jobs there. Things haven't exactly been working out for us here. We have to do something, I am going to go, probably I'll be packed up and ready to go by the coming weekend."

He couldn't lie. He wanted to go. She was his best hope – his only hope.

The only thing between him and that viaduct.

She always had a job. She was very good to him. She loved him like no other.

But he couldn't lie to her.

He loved her just enough, he had to let her go. Not enough to keep her. He had to be honest. He knew she wanted to marry him. She wanted children with him.

In his heart he knew he couldn't give her that. He couldn't make a commitment like that. And he couldn't string this special woman out forever. It wasn't fair to her. The truth hurts. She deserved better.

She had graduated from FSU in May, now summer was starting.

The thought kept running through his mind. Where and when are you ever going to meet a gal like this?

She had two degrees now, the FSU paper on top of a degree she had already earned from the University of North Dakota.

And she had a face like Cheryl Tiegs, and she took care of him like nobody ever. He knew how much she loved him.

"Claire, I love you too, you know I do, honey. I would love to go with you. But I just can't right now.

'I'm just not ready right now, Claire. I, ah, Claire I love you, you are a beautiful human being, but I can't give you what you want, what you deserve. Unconditional love and marriage and children and a great life. That's what you deserve. I just can't do it for you now. I'm so sorry. It's just bad timing. But maybe in a while –" His voice trailed off into the distance like the whirr of a spinning top disappearing around the corner into another room, another time.

She rushed over to him and put her hands around him and hugged him tightly to her chest. He felt the tears drop on his shoulder like that night in the kitchen with his mother. Hopefully he wouldn't have the same regrets.

"It'll be okay, Denny. Don't worry. I'll do the worrying for both of us. I am going to worry so much about you, Denny. Promise me you'll be okay, that you'll come up when you can, things will be so much better by then."

They hugged each other for the longest time.

They spent their last weekend together that first week of June; she said she was leaving the following Monday morning.

She had purchased a fancy new-looking metallic royal blue Buick Century with white leather interior with money her parents sent her so she could make her great escape safely.

She left him the old green beat-up Catalina that was on its last legs and a couple hundred dollars.

He stood in the driveway and waved and kept waving for the longest time that day, long after he could no longer see the shiny chrome bumpers disappear down Leon Street.

He realized people might think he was nuts standing outside by the street waving at nothing. I hope she doesn't turn out to be the only girl who ever loved me, he said as he slowly turned and walked back up the driveway to the apartment.

~ ~ ~

Claire was gone but he still had his Dilaudid to keep him company. And by extension, John Reimer, the carpenter guy who lived behind him, who knew about his foot injury – and his Dilaudid.

He came over begging one night about a week after Claire left. He was in construction and told Dennis he would help get him a construction job. But first he needed a favor. The real reason he came over.

Dennis found out Reimer knew about more than carpentry. Dennis relented and gave him a pill. "Let me show you something," he said as he set the pill on the table and walked over to the dish rack next to the sink and grabbed a tea spoon.

"Now this is what you do," he said. He placed the tiny orange pill onto the spoon and crushed it with the square head of a carpenter's pencil he took out of his back pocket.

He took a small rag out of his other back pocket and tied it around his arm just above the elbow. He poured a very small amount of water from a plastic bottle onto the crushed

273

orange powder on the spoon, then he took a Bic lighter out of his pocket, flipped it on and moved the flame back and forth underneath the spoon. Then he took a small syringe out of his breast pocket and drew the liquid out from the spoon by drawing back on the plunger.

"This is what you do, baby. Now we're gonna float to heaven."

He didn't look at Dennis MulQueen when he spoke – he was totally focused on the task at hand. He straightened his arm, stuck the needle into the bulging vein on his upturned forearm, and slowly pushed the stopper in.

Then he handed the syringe to Dennis, who was careful not to get stabbed with the darn thing. He knew about hepatitis. His father warned him about drugs.

"Okay, now it's your turn, Dennis. Get another pill out, you saw how I did it. I can help you but I'm not gonna feel like. Ahh. Oh man. I'm like. Right now, oh baby. Love you, man, thanks so much, man."

Before he could finish the sentence he sat back in the vinyl kitchen chair, smiled, and tilted his head back. Like he really was in heaven.

"Oh baby," he said. "I love you, man. Thank you, thank you, thank you."

Dennis recalled his father's words from long ago. "The junkies, they kill themselves all the time. Don't ever do it, Son. All it takes is once."

He couldn't do it. For once in his life he listened to his father.

"No thanks, John. I'm just going to take a pill straight up."

"Take two," Reimer said. "It will be incredible."

Dennis decided to take one and a half.

A little while later, he told Dennis to call a cab and about five minutes later they headed off to their favorite watering hole across from FSU, Poor Paul's Pourhouse.

The pills hadn't fully hit Dennis yet. He ordered a shell from Tony the one-armed bartender who plopped a glass of cold frothy Busch on the bar in front of him.

"Tony, hope you don't mind me asking, what happened to your arm?"

"Oh, we were all fucked-up last year, we were out driving back from a sinkhole, I had fallen asleep, I was in the front passenger seat, my buddy Hank, he was driving, he was all fucked-up too. He couldn't see the road, I guess. I was passed out in the passenger seat with my arm hanging out of the window. He drove too close to a sign, goodbye arm. He was going about 60, that thing sliced my arm off like butter. They couldn't even find it in the dark for almost an hour, you know, the cops and the paramedics. Hank drove me to the hospital, thank God, and here I am."

"Sorry to hear that, Tony, but you're a hell of a bartender. Never had a better beer in my life."

Right about then the drugs and the half-a-glass of beer started hitting him. He remembered the first part of his father's lecture, but he forgot the last part about never mixing pills of any kind with any kind of alcohol.

Then the mix really hit him. He sat there about five minutes more before he stumbled to his feet and out the back door. He didn't know where John was, he didn't hear Tony hollering after him for the buck and a quarter he owed him.

He barely made it past the parking lot to the alley before collapsing on the ground underneath a tree. Who knows how much urine or vomit he might have landed on there, but he didn't know or care and it wasn't going to matter.

Must have been hallowed ground.

Because he was lucky.

He puked like a madman right there on the ground or he certainly would have been dead right then and there.

He was so messed up he couldn't even crawl if he had to, let alone get up and find his way back home. He just lay there, beside the road under the tree in a pile of puke next to a line of cars, behind Poor Paul's Pourhouse, like he was dead.

The good Samaritans must have had the night off or they gave him up for dead already as one after another they paraded past him until the bar was closed and all the cars were gone and the sun was coming up.

Good thing he didn't take two or most likely he never would have awakened underneath that tree. Nobody even so much as called the cops.

Just one more viaduct person on the streets of Tallahassee, Florida, they probably figured.

~ ~ ~

Certainly looked impressive, the tool belt and the big authentic framing hammer dangling back and forth from the metal ring holster as he strutted around like Thor, prancing up the hill towards the job site. With the shiny aluminum Stanley tape measure tucked in the same belt off the left hip. And the flat pencil tucked behind the right ear.

Very authentic looking. The old man always said walk in a room like you own the place and they'll think you do. It also helps if you can fake it with a tiny bit of authenticity, too.

Bust ass as much as possible. No matter, sometimes it's just not going to be enough by itself. You have to know a little bit of what you're doing.

In his case that little bit was electron microscopic.

He was the saw man, and in no time, just to keep the crew supplied with boards he was slashing and hacking irregularly cut 2 x 12's like a drunken fool with Skill saw in hand.

He was responsible for cutting enough wood in exact lengths for the floor foundation to keep the whole crew pounding away.

Not even an hour into the day and *wham*, the freaking saw flew out of one of the boards like a missile, narrowly missing taking Dennis MulQueen's head off.

In his haste to keep up, he badly pinched one of the 2x12's. David, the foreman, came over and pulled his jean shorts up to reveal a nasty eight-inch scar on his right quad that showed a nasty inch-and-a-half indentation.

"This is no paper cut, Dennis. You see what happens when you don't know what the hell you are doing out here. That happened on my first day on the job too.

"You told me you had experience doing this when I hired you.

"Now listen, the owner just got here so we've got to change things up. He can't see all these shitty cut boards that don't fit right. I've got something else for you to do. See that pile of trusses down there at the bottom of the hill. Bring those up here while we finish putting up the floors and walls here, okay?"

Never-say-die Dennis MulQueen proceeded to shock the hell out of everybody on site, himself included, and single-handedly complete a job that would be performed by a large back hoe on any other job site.

By himself, he moved an entire pile of trusses one-by-one up a steep hill from the street at least 200 yards from the building under construction. This was a big two-story colonial house under construction and these were big trusses and his back was killing him after the first couple but he kept dragging them up the hill like a possessed fool.

As he was walking back down the hill for the last time after quitting time, he felt a hand and arm wrap around his shoulder. It was Dave.

"Sorry, Dennis. Listen man, I gotta tell you something."

They stopped and looked at each other. "Dennis, if I'm on the *Titanic*, I want you on the ship with me, okay? I love your attitude and your grit and determination. I can't believe you carried that wood up here. Do you know what you just did? You're making it really tough on me, Dennis. I mean, Dennis, I can't believe what you just did. You can tell your grand kids about this. Those are 40 footers, Dennis, and each one weighs about 300 pounds. I thought surely you would give up and quit. That was a super Herculean feat you just pulled off.

"But, Dennis, this ain't the *Titanic*. Look, I'll tell you the truth, I didn't want to fire you, that's why I told you to do that. I thought you'd make it easy on me. I know you're a really good guy. John told me that and that's why I hired you.

"Plus you're funny as hell man. But, Dennis, this ain't no *Titanic*, I can't let this ship sink. I got a lot on the line here and a lot of other people to think about. Did you see that guy in the blue golf shirt in the morning? That was the buyer of this particular house. And the guy in the tan hat with him, he's the developer of this whole subdivision."

He waved his arm in the air like he was trying to shoo an invisible fly away.

"And those guys notice when they see how raggedy ass those cuts were. Man, I want to thank you for your effort, there is no quit in you. Your determination is dynamite but you almost fell off the top of the other building yesterday; that's why I grounded you on the saw over here today with this crew. John told me you really needed the job, but then today when you almost decapitated yourself with the skill saw, Dennis man, I can't let you get killed out here and not one of your cuts was within 15 degrees of straight. I can't have shit fucked up out here. So man you've got find you something else you can do and I recommend it not be construction, you know, just for your sake alone, okay?"

Dennis thanked the guy for giving him a shot and headed back to home sweet home, the apartment on Leon Street he had recently rented, to ponder his next move as the summer continued to roll on downhill.

~ ~ ~

He was out of work more than two months now, since he lost the last job at Jax Liquors after a few sodas showed up missing on the inventory sheets. Claire had sent him $200 from Colorado, but he used that up in a hurry and now he was behind on the rent again, two months now, and he didn't know what he was going to do this time.

That's when he heard the knock on the door and he answered and of all people it was the guy he made fun of just like everybody else because he was such a nerd.

Ray Burnley walked in and sat down on the black couch in the living room and the short little nerd grabbed his right foot and positioned his right leg across his left leg just behind the knee and Dennis could see he was wearing the same fake leather vinyl chukka boots that he made fun of him for at the house party. Dennis sat down in the chair in the corner.

Ray was still working for Wilbur at the meat market.

Dennis offered Ray a glass of water. He said no thanks.

"How ya doin', Dennis?"

"Not too bad, Ray. Considering I'm losing my ass here with no job and no food and no friends. And I ran the only girl that ever truly loved me out of town. Other than that I'm great. But seriously, not that bad. I could be dead. Actually, maybe." He stopped and grinned at Ray.

"Oh Jeezus, Dennis, I thought you were gonna tell me you were outta beer. Or something serious," Ray said. "Then it would be really bad."

God love the short little nerd. They laughed their asses off.

"Besides, you got me. I'm your friend, Dennis. Something told me things might be a little rough for you. I knew since we last talked your girlfriend had left town and you were out of work again so I thought you could use a little cheering up."

He reached into his front shirt pocket and retrieved a folded-in-half envelope and handed it to Dennis.

Dennis unfolded it, ripped it open at one end and reached inside. He counted seventeen twenty dollar bills and one $10 bill. Exactly $350. The sum he owed for back rent plus $30 left over for food and more $1.29-a-six-pack Busch beer on sale at Sara's mini-market across the street.

"Jeez, Ray, I can't believe it. So big of you. Oh my God, you don't have to do this. Ray, this is a lot of money and I don't know when I can pay you back."

"Don't worry about it, Dennis. Everybody has ups and downs. You know what I've gone through with my divorce and everything, you were there for me and listened to all my problems. And now I know what you're going through. I know how I was when me and my ex split up and I lost my job. You were there for me, Dennis. I know you're in bad shape right now too. I want to help you. You are a really good guy."

"Oh man, Ray. Thanks, man."

"You're welcome, Dennis."

No more words. Time to water the grass again. This is unreal.

I'm gonna really miss this guy someday, he said to himself.

Another teacher.

No more making fun of Ray Burnley, that's for sure.

~ ~ ~

Desperate times call for desperate measures.

Another month had passed since Ray bailed him out and still no job.

It was into September now.

"Anything at all. Please. Anything. I would appreciate anything right now."

The guy just stared at him and said nothing. He got in his car and shut the door, his face a blank canvas. He betrayed no emotion, nothing whatsoever. He wasn't sure if the guy thought he was a liar, just a basic con man, or otherwise too pitiful to be bothered with.

At any rate, he didn't as much as shake his head, in either pity or disgust, he just bent his knees and slid silently into his car seat, nonchalantly almost as if he thought this young college guy didn't even exist, a phantom in the night.

So now it was off across the street from the Golden Arches parking lot to the Howard Johnson's, in that glassed-off space just outside the hotel lobby, where the cigarette machine is located.

Smokers have to feel guilty, they have to be more compassionate than your average burger guy.

Good luck with that.

They looked and stared and kept walking, like he was the guy in the freak show at the carnival.

~ ~ ~

The phone rang the next day.

"Hi, Denny. It's your mother. Your father asked me to dial your number and see if you are home. He said he wants to talk to you."

There was a pause on the line.

"What? He has never called me before."

"He just said out of the blue he wants to talk to you. Hold on a minute."

He heard her call out.

"George, he's home. He's on the line."

There was a pause of about a minute.

"Hello, Son. Is that you?"

"Yes, Dad, it's me."

"How's everything going down there. How are you doing?"

Another pause.

"Bear, are you there? It's your father. Just wondered how things are going. Your mother is worried about you. What's going on down there. How are your classes going? "

"No good, Dad."

"When are you coming back home?"

Words would not come.

Nothing.

He tried to, but he couldn't.

"Sss. Sarrr."

Another pause.

"Sorry."

He finally got the word out.

"Never."

Then pure emotion poured out of him involuntarily.

"Sorry, Dad. I'm never coming home. I mean never. I can't come home. I'm never going to see you again, Dad."

Then he screamed it out loud.

"I'm done, Dad. I'm never going to see you again. Any of you."

"No no no, Son, wait a minute now. Don't talk like that. Listen, Son, it's never that bad. Listen, come home right now, everything's okay now, get home right now, Son, everything will be all right. You'll get a nice job, everything will be good."

"Thanks, Dad. I've gotta go now."

"Wait a minute, wait a minute."

He handed the phone back to his mother. He could hear his father saying something in the background.

"Denny, come home, please. All is forgiven. Your father wants you to know everything is okay now, if that's what you want. Bring the girl home with you if you want. He said now everything is okay. Just come home."

Too late for that.

He never told them all that was over a long time ago.

"Your father just went in the other room to get the check book, he said to send you some money. Please use it to buy gas and food and come home."

"Thanks, Mom. You don't have to do that."

He added, "Remember Fr. Polakowski, Mom, at U of D High? Remember I had him for English class?"

"Yes, he loved you, Denny. He told me you were brilliant, he said you were a great writer, but you were a little lazy."

She chuckled.

"Yeah, Mom. Father Polakowski made me read my paper in front of the class. It was about *Look Homeward Angel* by Thomas Wolfe. You know what he says in that book, Mom? You can never go back home again."

"No, that's not true, Son. Of course, you can. Come home. You'll see. Your Dad will have the – He has..."

He cut her off.

"Okay. We'll talk. Thanks for the call."

He hung up the phone and he wished he had jumped off that parking deck a long time ago. It would have been so much easier.

Two days later, a check arrived in the mail – air mail. It was for $200.00, and included a note.

"We are anxiously awaiting your arrival. We will have the fatted calf ready. Don't delay, Denny. We can't wait until the Prodigal Son returns home.

Love, Mom."

Below her signature was his father's.

The only letter he would ever receive signed by his father.

~ 21 ~

THE MIRACLE OF LIFE

When he looked down in the morning light the red welts that covered every square inch of his legs from his toes to his knees made him think of what happened to Dostoevsky after he had become a huge literary sensation in his homeland. He could never forgot that scene, in Siberia, the military prison at Omsk, where the great Russian writer was exiled in the mid-1800s for his political activity.

So dark, so dank, so cold, and so desolate, he described the place in a letter to his brother in 1854. He was all alone, a condemned man, no contact with the outside world allowed, with no hope for survival, his health deteriorating, "stinking like a pig" and gagging from the stench of the "wooden trough for the calls of nature," sleeping frozen stiff on a wooden board with no blanket and only bread and cabbage soup for food, as all the while "the fleas, lice and other vermin by the bushel" attacked him morning, noon, and night.

The bigger they are, the harder they fall.

Yes Fyodor, I can relate, he said as he swatted again his legs covered like candy dots with the welts from the huge Florida black fleas that incessantly swarmed and attacked him the second he stepped in the apartment he was too poor to have fumigated.

As if she was feeling his angst, his baby strolled over and made a concerted effort to lie down at his feet. It took her several seconds and carefully selected maneuvers to make it all the way down. She sensed his anguish – maybe shared it would be better – because although he was sure she was his soul mate and came over to console him, the truth was Bambi, his oversized black and white cat, was probably looking for comfort for her own fat, pregnant, flea-bitten self.

And she certainly needed it, the poor thing. Of course, he couldn't afford to get her spayed and now she was full-blown pregnant again and about to drop at any moment. Maybe she just knew he would make a better mid-wife the second time around.

"Oh baby, we gotta get out of here, don't we? Me, you, and the babies. Before we all starve to death and die from these fleas. But wait a minute, you've got a flea collar I gave you. I hope it's working, dear Bambi."

He reached down to pet her.

Big mistake.

She bit him good, even drawing blood. Pregnant cats apparently don't like being petted.

But they needed to get going. He needed to get going while he still had some of the money left his parents sent him to come home.

He walked outside and looked at the Green Giant in the driveway. No, the wounded warrior would be a better name. It looked like a combat vehicle for sure. The rear right fender was smashed in, the all-black, almost-bald fat tires leaked, and the North Dakota license plate was expired. And had an expired registration in the glove box in the name of a woman named Claire.

On top of everything, the tail lights were shot. The left one wouldn't light up at all, and the only way to keep a rear light on at night was to depress the brake pedal just enough to get the right rear brake light to come on, but the trick was, not enough to have the brakes actually engage and melt the pad to holy hell. If he didn't push it down enough, there were no tail lights at all, light switch on the dash pulled out or not.

Not to mention, his driver's license was expired, and he had no proof of insurance, because he had no insurance.

And he was a young-looking college student with longish hair.

About to test his luck one more time.

There's road kill, and there's road prey. And there was Dennis MulQueen, on this ultrawarm September day in 1979, probably both – prey about to be the kill for the first cop that spotted him in this banged up illegal and dangerous unroadworthy jalopy with everything expired. And he sure as hell wouldn't be able to blame the cop.

But he had no choice.

He was out of chances.

It was now or never.

At least he tried. He stopped by the Secretary of State's office in the morning and learned he couldn't do anything about the expired tag and registration because he had no bill of sale to prove he owned the vehicle his departed girlfriend left him. At least, he was able to renew his license. A quick stop at the local mechanics and he learned he needed more than light bulbs – the electrical system was fried and needed some kind of new harness that cost way more than he could afford.

When he got back to the house, he immediately balled up all of his remaining clothes in a sheet and threw them on top of the tan back seat, the purple and grey and black wool tweed sport suit his father bought him years ago at Art Knitting Mills on top of the pile. Then he placed a cut-out cardboard box on the passenger side floor in back, with a couple of nice cotton towels lining the floor of the box. He put two bowls from the kitchen on the driver's side back seat floor, one for water, the other for the small bag of dried Purina Cat Chow he placed on the floor next to the bowl.

In between, he placed another small cut-out box filled with cat litter. He went back inside and packed a small worn-out beige suitcase with all of his letters and a few toiletries and that was pretty much it, except for his prized Puka shell necklace, a nice souvenir he got from Hawaii that was loaded with turquoise chunks throughout.

He threw the suitcase in the back seat next to the wool sport coat and he tossed the puka shell necklace with the giant turquoise chunks, along with $100 in the envelope with the letter his mother sent him, into the glove box. The remaining $70 he kept in his right front blue jeans pocket.

The only thing left to do – he had to figure out how to get his buddy in the car.

He knew it was going to be a battle but she was a good girl, and no way was he going to abandon her.

He loved her.

Sure enough, the first couple attempts to move her were like guerrilla warfare. She hissed and snarled and clawed the hell out of him. She was pregnant to the nines and hurting and very uncomfortable and she didn't want to move. But he managed to hang on as she only got him one really good rip with her hind feet before he got her to the car. Thank God it was only a 10-foot walk or it would have been worse. He dropped her in the box with the towel and she calmly laid down like she knew this was her new home – her only home.

He closed the doors and cranked the old beast up, said a prayer and pulled out of the drive headed down Leon Street.

He took a circuitous backroad route out of Tallahassee, thinking if he could just get past the college area and the Capitol District, and make it to Thomasville Road, he would have a chance to at least make the state line before going to jail.

He deliberately left at 2:30 in the morning, thinking night time after quota time, on a Monday following a weekend that hopefully met quota, would give him his best chance. But really, what are the chances of making it all the way to Michigan like this? Less or more than making it through another month in Tallahassee?

Case closed. He was already on the road now anyway. If his timing was right, by the time it was light he would be going through Atlanta about rush hour, which he figured would give him his best odds of making it through undetected in the middle of traffic.

Sleep would be no problem, as the one thing he did inherit from his father, and his mother also, which his years of midnight shifts and all of her newspaper deadline all-night Tuesday sessions evidenced, was the ability to function at a high level for long sleep-deprived periods.

The one thing he couldn't forget was the brake pedal. He had to be constantly vigilant, he had to push it down just enough to make the one rear tail light come on at night but not enough to actually engage the brakes. He smelled a burning smell at one point in the middle of the night so he knew at that moment, despite his best efforts, he was burning the pads somewhere.

Overall the first night was a success, he made good time, it was past dawn already and he was approaching Atlanta, right on schedule and with that biologically inherited immunity to sleep deprivation he decided to keep going, thinking the heavy rush hour traffic would be at least as good a cover as the darkness with only one tail light.

He deliberately skipped the business loop, which would have taken him around the city where he would be more visible and opted for the main artery through the congested downtown.

Even though it was September, in downtown Atlanta on this day you could fry an egg on the front seat, it was so hot. The temperature was listed at 93 degrees on a billboard he passed, unseasonably hot, even for Atlanta, but it felt like 120 on the stop-and-go freeway.

As he was approaching downtown, in the heart of the heat, he spotted a guy on the right shoulder who looked like he was dying on his feet. His tongue hung out of his mouth like a sick dog. His hair was greasy, and long as it was unkempt. Amazingly, he couldn't believe that in the heat of that moment in time the guy was wearing a red flannel shirt, although he did have it halfway unbuttoned down the middle and both sleeves were rolled up. He had the shiny greasy skin to match, long scraggly sideburns, and faded blue jeans that were bleached white in spots that looked not too bad compared to the rest of him.

There he was, standing dead still in all his ignobility with his thumb up in the air holding a simple cardboard sign with the words RIDE PLEASE scratched out in black ink. He was standing near the exit ramp just after entering the downtown area.

With Dennis momentarily stopped in the traffic, the guy must have sensed a sucker come to save him as he hurried over to the mean green machine like it was the last chance saloon.

"Oh thanks, man, I thought I was going to die out there."

Dennis let him in.

"Yeah, I can see that. Where you headed?"

"I don't know, for sure. I'm thinking up north, somewhere, anywhere really to get out of this heat and maybe find me a job of sorts up there."

"Well, you can take your pick. I'm going all the way to the Canadian border, if I make it that far. Should be cooler there."

"Oh, great, man, let's do it."

Dennis MulQueen explained it would be an unconventional route – what with all of the exacerbating vehicle conditions, the expired license plate, and the cat in the back, they would be traveling mostly middle of the night and rush hours. The guy was cool with that.

~ ~ ~

Uh-oh. Here we go. Off to jail.

Everything had been great so far driving mostly after midnight through rush hour, sleeping upright in the car for a couple hours at a time, on the side of a side road, anywhere he could find a spot that seemed off the beaten path just enough to not raise any suspicions or be spotted.

Until the next day when they got to Loudon County, Tennessee, and it was just like that rock and roll tune that perfectly captured the terror of seeing those blue lights flashing in the rear view mirror.

Sure enough, he went too far into the day as they stopped for gas and a cold drink and as soon as he pulled out of the gas station the bubble lights from behind filled the car and he pulled over not a hundred yards from the freeway ramp. Should have never picked this guy up, Dennis thought to himself. They probably think I'm with him, the number two profile, two young white down-and-outers in a down-and-out looking vehicle.

Too late. The cop was already out of his vehicle and Dennis MulQueen could see in the outside mirror he was the prototypical southern state trooper. Burly, just enough of a potbelly, gruff-looking, salt-and-pepper mustache, he had the Mountie hat on and everything. Tan outfit, black boots, the rigid military walk. Hand on his piece as he approached the Green Monster. He swore like a trooper, too. He had the police persona down to a T.

"Now just where the fuck do you think ur goin' there, pal, with this smashed-up hulk and an expired North Dakota license plate, coming thorough my county of all places. Just who the fuck do you think you are, buster?"

He told him the truth. In a roundabout way.

"I'm just trying to get home. My girlfriend loaned me her car. My Dad is in really bad health."

The cop cut him off immediately with a look that said he was ready to arrest him on the spot for daring to be so stupid.

"Listen here, man, I don't wanna hear all your lame horseshit. Now give me ur driver's license and ur proof of insurance and ur registration."

He handed him his Florida driver's license, and opened up the glove and handed him the registration and old insurance document that was in Claire's name. He removed the envelope with the money and the note from his mother inside from the glove and folded it and put it in his back pocket just in case. He could only hope the $150 he had left would cover his bail.

"Jeesus Christ Almighty, I never seen anything like this in my life," the cop muttered under his breath as he walked back toward his cruiser when about halfway he spun around and march-stepped back to the Green Monster.

"Hey, you there," he said pointing to the guy in the passenger seat, "gimme ur ID."

He handed the cop a piece of rumpled up paper, no telling what it was.

Then he ordered Dennis to get out of the car and come with him.

He opened the back door of his patrol car and ordered Dennis to get in.

Okay, this is the part where I lose my freedom for sure, he thought.

When they were both in the car, the cop turned around towards Dennis and looked him in the eye with that squinted-up, gnarled-up facial expression cops have when they are really pissed and ready to beat the crap out of somebody.

"Now, buster, I wanna know who the fuck do you think you are coming through Loudon County like this with an old beat-up jalopy with expired plates and an expired registration and expired insurance. Now nobody comes thorough Loudon County like this, you understand me, man? This is my county, and just who the fuck is that grimy derelict in the car with you? How do you know this guy, how are you related to him ? How long do you want me to put you in jail for?"

"Officer, I am really sorry. I swear to you I'm a really good person and I have a perfect record. I have cops in my family who would be mortified at this, so you know I would never be doing this if it wasn't an emergency. My Dad is really sick with leukemia. He's not doing well, and I am just trying to get home, I'm just trying to get home before my Dad dies. I have no money left, I got laid off my job, I just want to get home to see my Dad before he dies, and get a job and start all over again."

"Yeah, and the bum in the car with you?"

"Officer, I swear to god, I was coming through Atlanta, and this guy was standing there on the side of the road, the traffic was stopped up, it was a hundred degrees, this guy was just standing there by the side of the road panting with his tongue hanging out, I felt really sorry for him, he was carrying this sign that said PLEASE in all capital letters. He walked over to the car and he said he was trying to get up north to get out of the heat and look for work up north. I don't know anything about him, I don't know who he is, I don't know where he came from, I know nothing about him. I don't even know the guy's name."

The trooper, obviously exasperated, let out a big sigh. Dennis was sure that wasn't a good sign.

"Buddy, you better be telling me the truth. So help you God."

"Officer, I swear I am telling you the truth. I never met this guy, I don't know him from Adam. He is obviously a big hardship case."

The trooper instantly turned his head around and looked at Dennis again.

"Yeah, and you?"

Dennis exhaled himself now and his head dropped a bit forward. He reached in his back pocket and pulled out the envelope with the money in it – and the note from his mother.

He handed it to the cop.

"Officer, please take a look at this. You'll know I'm telling you the truth."

"Jesus," the cop said as he snatched the envelope out of Dennis' hand. Dennis prayed in silence for about one eternal minute as the cop took the note out and looked at it.

"Jesus Christ Almighty," he said. "So you're the Prodigal Son, huh? I guess I don't want to go to hell. I can't believe I'm doing this. I could make my quota for the month off of you, buddy."

He got out of his vehicle and walked around the back and opened the rear passenger side door and handed Dennis back the envelope. "Okay, now get out and listen to me carefully."

Judging by the pained expression on the cop's face, he was more inclined to shoot Dennis MulQueen and throw him in the ditch than let him go.

308

"Now I don't know why I'm doing this. I could send you to jail right now but I'm not even going to write you a ticket. It would take me all day to write you up the number of statutes you are in violation of here and I don't have that much time. I've got to get back to work. Now I'm going to let you get back in that junk heap of yours over there and against all better judgement I'm going to let you drive off in that junker on two conditions.

"One, that you swear on the Holy Bible so help you die, that you will keep driving and not stop until you are plum out of the state of Tennessee and furthermore that you promise you will keep that grimy bastard with you in the car until you are over the Tennessee line, so help you God. And also you have to promise me after I'm giving you this break of a lifetime that you will get your act together and get a decent car and valid plates and insurance and never drive through my county ever again like this or next time I will lock you up for a very long time. Do you understand?"

"Yes, officer. Thank you, officer, I swear I will get him out of Tennessee and I will never drive like this again."

"Now, good luck to you, and good luck to your father. Now, go on and get the hell outta here right now, okay? And good luck to you the rest of the way."

"Thank you, officer."

Dennis MulQueen jumped back in the Green Monster and off the Prodigal Son triumphantly went in a cloud of dust and a pile of crap, with a feeling like he had just won the lottery. Which he actually had better odds of accomplishing than getting that cop to let him go that day without even a single ticket.

He could not, he would not, ever believe the guy let him go without a single ticket. And all the money still in the envelope. Now if his luck could only hold out through two more states.

~ ~ ~

When they got to Ohio, it was time again to pull into a gas station for a refill. Not too far from the spot where not too long ago he almost got his brains blown out if not for another good cop's jammed holster.

"After I fill it up I'm gonna go inside and use the rest room, and maybe grab a couple bags of peanuts and a drink or something. Want anything?"

"No thanks, that's all right," he said.

When he returned a little while later with a brown paper bag and opened the car door and jumped back in that's when he realized his hitchhiking passenger was no longer in the car. Dennis went back in the store and looked around, he checked the bathroom, he walked around the exterior of the building, he couldn't find him anywhere.

He went back in the store and approached the clerk.

"Excuse me, did you see a guy with a red flannel shirt on?"

"No, I didn't see anybody."

He went back outside and got back in the car. He turned around and looked again out the back window to look for the guy.

That's when he noticed his suit coat and shoes were gone from the back seat.

He reached across the seat and opened the glove box. The Puka shell necklace with the giant turquoise rocks was gone. Thank God, he had taken the envelope with the cash inside to pay for the gas.

He jumped out of the car and ran out back behind the store. Again he looked in all directions and saw nothing. He went to the other side of the property where there was a ditch. Nothing there. He ran across the street and looked over there. He looked up and down the road. Nothing. Nobody. Anywhere to be found.

He finally gave up and got back in the car and headed south again on I-75. At least, I was able to keep one promise, he said. I got him out of Tennessee.

He would never know for sure where the thief went. But down the road a ways it dawned on him.

He never thought to check the dumpster out back.

~ ~ ~

He heard the squeals coming from the back seat.

He had to pull over. They were just outside Toledo, where he almost got his brains blown out a second time that day in Ohio by Curtis the steel hauler with the toggle switches. He was convinced it would have happened, if not for his green lantern jacket. The military jacket from Birdsong Farms, which he thankfully had rolled up in the sheet in back.

Thank God, the good luck charm that saved his life twice was in that sheet or the grimy bastard would have assuredly stolen that too. No wonder the Tennessee state trooper made him promise to get that sleazebag out of his state. Like a good journalist, a good cop can read people like an open book. As much as he knew Dennis MulQueen was telling him the truth that day, he knew that guy was no good.

As he brought the lumbering green giant to a stop on the shoulder at the top of the exit ramp, he recalled how that song about "four dead in Ohio" played in his mind that day he almost got killed twice in the Buckeye State.

Now the words were transposed. This time it was four born in Ohio. He got up on his knees and turned around and looked over the seat at the box on the passenger side floor.

Holy mackerel, he said.

Four new members of the family.

The miracle of life.

And speaking of miracles.

311

A little more than an hour later, he put it in park on North End Avenue, across the street from the childhood bungalow at 21471 Kipling Avenue, Oak Park, Michigan. Hey Thomas Wolfe, who says you can't go home again.

~ 22 ~

LIFE IS A MULQUEEN
HOLIDAY

"Goddamn it, stop it right now. Cut it out, get down off of there right now, you little bastards."

No doubting the source of that refrain – George MulQueen had just walked in the living room as all four of the little darlings frantically clawed their way up and down the brand-new nylon shears that adorned the living room full-length 18' x 7' picture window. These recently installed see-through curtains, the pride and joy of the home's decorator, Moms Mabley, were already ripped and frayed in several spots.

About a minute later came a loud sustained knock on their master's bedroom door.

"Jeesus Christ, rise and shine, will you? Let's get the show on the road. Get up outta the bed and get going. Jesus Christ Almighty, you're not going to get anything done lying on your ass all day."

Dennis MulQueen's father said nothing about his darling little kittens destroying the brand-new living room drapes.

"Okay, Dad," he said. "I'm getting up."

"Come on, Son, you can't be unemployed your whole life. Get off your ass and get a job."

He jumped out of bed and threw on a rumpled shirt and pair of pants he grabbed off a chair in the corner.

His father was back in the kitchen by now rifling through the refrigerator for some leftovers. That was his routine, he had just returned home after working all night at his Ford Motor Company job where he was a safety engineer. It was Saturday morning, so he was off from his other job as Job Upgrading Coordinator for the Detroit Public Schools.

But he was soon off to help out with the football team at St. James before returning home for a little sleep and then he would start all over again with a little dinner and the half-hour ride back to the Ford Motor Co. complex in Dearborn by midnight for a weekend double.

How he did it was a mystery. Nobody ever saw him sleep more than a few hours at a time.

But when he got needled by friends and family for his workaholic ways, he was always quick to reply. "Hard work never killed anyone," he would say.

But what about the stress of being married and raising five kids in a three-bedroom bungalow – and four newborn kittens?

That question didn't need answering.

He was sitting at the head of the kitchen table when Dennis walked in a few minutes later.

"Jeesuz, Son, look at you. You can't get a job dressed like that. For starters, you need a sport coat. Remember what your grandfather said? *Vestis virus facit*. An old Latin phrase, Son. The clothes make the man. And it starts with your shoes. You're only as good as your shoes. You can have a thousand-dollar Italian silk suit on, but if your shoes aren't shined, then you might as well be naked, let alone wearing filthy tennis shoes like that, Son."

He looked down. His Converse black tops had seen better days.

His father got up from the table, walked to his bedroom at the end of the hall, opened the closet door and returned to the kitchen holding a shiny black pair of old-time leather-soled wingtips in one hand and a tweed sport coat in the other.

"Here, start with these. See if you can get your big dogs in these. And here's a coat. See if this fits."

"Thanks, Dad. I'm sure I can fit in them."

He would quickly recall another of grandpa's sayings back from his days playing hockey on the frozen Ontario ponds. "You are only as warm as your feet. Keep your feet warm;
 if your feet are cold, you'll be cold all over."

Well, Grandpa Helferty, you could have added a third foot adage, you could have also said wear the right size, because if your feet hurt, you will hurt all over. Now he knew how the Chinese women with bound feet must have felt. He reached down and pulled the laces undone and slid out of his new shoes a good two sizes too small – once in the car. He was on his way to apply for a job at the *Oakland Press* in downtown Pontiac, Michigan.

The shoes – undersized or not – did the trick.

They hired him, as a stringer. A reporter who would cover stories and be paid on a piece-by-piece basis. A non-staff member (read: no benefits) who could nonetheless appear in the paper with his or her own byline as many times a week as the city editor decreed.

His first assignment: a school board meeting in Milford, Michigan. Go cover it, MulQueen, were his marching orders. We want to see what you're made of. And so he gladly did. Hurt feet and all.

Can't wait to get that first paycheck, he thought as he pulled in the parking lot at City Hall. It's already spoken for. Tom McCann Shoes, here we come.

Then the drape store.

~ ~ ~

Appearances belie.

The middle-aged guy propped up on a wooden stool near the front wall wore dark brown glasses with large roundish aviator-type lenses, a green-and-white checked thin-ply plaid shirt and plain navy slacks. His shoes were black leather, round in front with no design to them and slightly scuffed, shoes like the school janitor would wear, or maybe the FedEx guy.

He looked like he could have been anything average. A clerk at the auto parts store, a small-town minister, or maybe a desk sergeant at the local police department.

A light-stained acoustic guitar rested on his lap, and he started strumming it as soon as Dennis MulQueen walked in the local downtown Pontiac joint that the guys at the *Oakland Press* told him you had to be at for happy hour.

The guy had a round, jocular-looking face with a disarming, almost absent look about him. He didn't look like he belonged on stage.

Until he opened his mouth.

Appearances belie.

He tilted his head forward a few inches, toward the microphone, and the words flowed forth smooth and effortless like a delicate Irish brook over cobblestones.

> "*I had five strong sons, who fought to save my*
> *jewels,*
> *They fought and they died, and that was my*
> *grief, said she.*"

Now his head moved gently from side to side as he sang, his forehead creasing with the words, his lips slightly aquiver.

You could tell he was singing this song from his heart, as if he had some personal attachment to the story he was telling.

A guy to his left played the accordion, and another guy on the right strummed a banjo, but you had to force yourself to notice them. It was clearly the guy in the middle's show.

> *"Long time ago, this proud old woman did say,*
> *There was war and death, plundering and*
>   *pillage,*
> *My four green fields ran red with their blood."*

Appearances belie.

Now his whole body swayed back and forth as he sang, a tender barely audible wail underneath it all. Invisible, yet palpable, everywhere he filled the room with his presence. The place was packed.

> *"What have I now, this proud old woman did*
> *say,*
> *I have four green fields, one of them's in*
> *bondage,*
> *In stranger's hands that tried to take it from me,*
> *But my sons had sons, as brave as were their*
>   *fathers,*
> *My fourth green field will bloom once again, said*
>   *she."*

Dennis MulQueen found himself standing still in the middle of the bar, staring at the guy, transfixed like he was at a U-2 concert instead of a local bar gig with an unknown guy up there holding him in the palm of his hand.

I think he's going to cry, no, jeez, I'm going to cry, I better get out of here, he thought as he turned and walked about 10 paces the other direction and took a seat at the far right end of the bar.

317

He knew how to stop such sentiment in its tracks.

"I'll have a Harvey Wallbanger please," he called out to the bartender.

The old guy behind the bar served it up to him in a tall frosted daiquiri glass with a couple long skinny black straws.

"Man, that ole guy can really bring it, can't he?"

"He ain't old," the wavy-haired guy behind the bar said. "He's just had a tough life." He smiled and chuckled.

"All of us," Dennis said as he broke out in laughter the bartender didn't hear as he was already on the way down the line to the next cocktail.

The place was called the Mill Street Inn. This was as good as it got in Pontiac, wall-to-wall people for a Friday night Happy Hour celebration.

The police, the lawyers, the sales people, the government workers, and, of course, the journalists – they were all there.

Thank God for the wingtips. He was now one of them, formally on board as a stringer, hoping he could build some trust and get more important assignments over time from the *Oakland Press* editors and ultimately win a staff job with benefits and a nice steady salary.

So here he was, an unknown among the town cognoscenti, at the head of the bar.

Another banger and a couple more Irish ballads later, he turned to the left to survey the crowd, and he caught the guy lumbering across the room in his direction.

Dennis turned back around to face the bar. He heard a *clunking* on the floor gradually get louder. With each step, he heard another *clunk*.

He turned around a second time to look. It wasn't exactly a limp, but the guy had a plain black cane in his right hand and he seemed to be dragging his right foot a little bit.

Dennis quickly turned back toward the bar; he didn't want to appear to be staring. It was the singer, heading straight at him.

Seconds later, he heard a voice from behind him.

"Hey there, what's going on?"

Dennis said nothing; he wasn't exactly sure who the guy was talking to.

Then he felt a sharp elbow knock him on the side of his left arm.

"Hey there, I said, what's going on up there?"

Dennis turned around and his jaw involuntarily dropped and froze open a good inch.

It might have had something to do with the optical effects of the glasses, but the guy had astronaut eyes coming at him through those aviator lenses that looked like they could see right through him.

"Yeah, I was just wondering, what's going on over there with you?" he said.

Dennis didn't know what to say. This guy, a total stranger, caught him totally off guard.

"Aw, nothin' man, just been hanging out here, trying to get on staff at the local paper downtown, you know, the *Oakland Press.* They hired me as a stringer, I've gotten some good ink over there so far, I'll see how it goes."

He pulled out the stool next to Dennis MulQueen and sat down

"I see," he said. "Now what's really going on?"

"Huh?"

There was a slight awkward pause.

"No, I mean, see that?"

He raised his cane in the air and pointed to the mirror.

"Well, I look over here from my vantage point over there and your big round face comes across the room clear as a bell and says you've got something on your mind. So I just wondered, if there's anything I can help you with."

Dennis MulQueen was flabbergasted at this total stranger coming up to him out of nowhere in a crowded bar like he was some kind of telepathic mind reader.

"I just moved back from Florida," he said.

"Oh, Florida, what part?"

He told him Tallahassee.

"Oh, so are you friends with Ted Bundy?" he asked as he broke out with a sheepish sly grin on his face.

"Well, actually, he is an acquaintance of mine," Dennis said. "I have been out with him."

"No way, I know you're kidding me."

"No, I'm not kidding. I've been out with him all right. At the local jail."

The singer scrunched his eyes in disbelief.

"What? Oomph. No way. You don't look like a jailbird. Tell me about it."

Dennis proceeded to tell him the whole story about their encounter at the Leon County Jail after they brought him in on a warrant for no inspection sticker tickets – the day he came face to face with pure evil.

"Darn, things could be worse. We could have been related to some of those poor girls," the singer said. "Now that's what is horrible in life, that is the worst, coming face to face with evil like that and having no choice in the matter. It's just hard to imagine people choosing to be that sick and that evil. But at least, well, thank God they finally got him."

"Yeah, that's for sure," Dennis said.

Bundy was convicted during the summer, on July 24, 1979, and the judge gave him the death penalty without blinking.

The singer wouldn't give up.

"So when did you come back from Florida, and why did you come back? Your buddy Bundy's in jail, the weather is great, and the women are even better, right?"

He gave in. To a total stranger he just met in a bar with a funny gait and a ridiculous, impossible-to-figure-out-who-he-really-is countenance.

"What's going on? Why did I really come back from Florida? Okay, I'll tell ya. No real reason, other than I get to watch my father die."

"Ooh, my, that's terrible," the singer said as he scrunched up his mouth this time. "Sorry to hear that. What happened?"

"Well, he got in this horrible accident, about seven years ago, he and my mother were on the way to a restaurant over in Canada on the Detroit River, a tractor with no lights pulled out in front of them, they hit the damned thing. My mother was driving, she was messed up but nothing as bad as my Dad. The station wagon flipped, my dad was pinned in there no way for him to get out, so they cut him out of it with torches, they sent him to two different hospitals, both of them took full body X-rays. He was a medic in WWII and that's all he did all day and night during the war, was give guys X-rays, they were in the same room back then, the combination of all that radiation and the trauma of the accident. He ended up with leukemia shortly thereafter.

"He's battled it for going on seven years now, but these days he can't even take a MulQueen Holiday."

"A what? A MulQueen Holiday? What the heck is that?"

He explained how his internist Dr. Stanley Levy forbade his father to drink any Guinness or martinis, but on special occasions, once in a great while, his dad would break the rules and cheat with what he called a MulQueen Holiday.

"But he's had a bunch of bad spells lately, so no holidays on the horizon. Jeez, I hope he makes it a while longer, but it's not looking too good right now. I'm Dennis MulQueen, by the way."

He extended his right hand.

"Nice to meet you, Dennis. I'm Roger McCarville," he said as they shook hands. "And that's my band you saw up there, the Irish Wakes and Weddings Band. I have a transportation company on the side."

He rubbed his hands together.

"*Hmm*, MulQueen. That's a nice Polish name. Now I see where the holiday gets its name." He smiled a weak quiet smile that nonetheless spoke clearly to Dennis through the smoky bar room chatter. That this guy was different from ordinary people. He immediately knew that much about the guy. That he cared, and he must be clairvoyant as well, Dennis thought, to sense out of nowhere across a crowded smoke-filled bar that something was amiss.

He focused on Dennis again with those penetrating blue eyes, pursed his lips, and then looked down again and shook his head slowly back and forth a couple more times. "Well," he said, 'I know one thing. Everything happens for a reason. Of course, we will never know the meaning of some of it, like your Dad's accident. But that's only in the beginning. In the end, we'll know everything."

He paused. They stared silently at each other some more, like some kind of cosmic connection was being cemented as they sat there together at that bar. Neither of them said a word for about 30 more seconds.

Then he started up again.

"Me, I'm here because I've got a beautiful wife and six beautiful children to love and take care of. But the most important thing I've come to realize is above all I'm here because that Guy in the Sky wants me here to take care of business," he said as he pointed toward the white ceiling with his black cane. "He carries the big stick that stirs the drink for all of us. He's got things for me to do, things for all of us to do. Or we wouldn't be here."

He pointed his ebony cane up in the air again for emphasis.

"Speaking of which, the main thing I think he wants right now for us is to be happy. I think it's time for a MulQueen Holiday."

He bent forward in his elevated barstool chair, and reached down on the right like he was fumbling with his pant leg. Dennis tried not to stare and look straight ahead.

Then he peeked out of the corner of his eye and now Dennis MulQueen's jaw dropped about three inches.

The guy named McCarville sitting next to him pulled up his right pant leg and unstrapped a prosthetic leg from the stump where the bottom of his right leg used to be.

With the black shoe still attached to it, he hoisted his artificial leg in the air, in the packed bar, in front of everybody, like it was the Stanley Cup.

"Stan the Man, get over here right now and fill it up," he shouted. "We need Guinness. We're ready to celebrate. We're on a MulQueen Holiday." Everybody in the vicinity had raised eyebrows, he heard a couple "Oh my God's," but he couldn't tell where they came from.

The guy behind the bar with the curly brown-and-gray-streaked hair strolled over carrying a full pitcher of dark frothy draft, and leaned over the bar like he was seriously going to pour it in the top of Roger McCarville's hollowed-out fake leg.

"I'll fill that baby up. Let me have it," he said.

The bartender laughed as he leaned back and reached underneath for two pint glasses which he slapped on the bar counter in front of them and promptly filled with the pitcher in his right hand.

323

"Stan, I want you to meet this guy. He's the new reporter down at the *Oakland Press*, Dennis MulQueen. Dennis, this is Stan Stevens – he owns this joint. Stan pour yourself one too. We don't like to drink unless we are alone or with somebody, right, Dennis?"

"Got that right," Dennis MulQueen said as he reached out and shook Stan Stevens' hand.

"Sorry, but if you're a friend of his I'll have to charge you double," the owner said as he looked at Dennis and nodded at McCarville.

"Now watch out for him," the bar owner continued. "Another Guinness and he'll be passing that leg around like it's the collection plate at Sunday mass."

He turned and walked away as the singer named McCarville bent over and strapped his right leg back on, then he leaned back and knocked on it with that same multi-purpose black cane of his, like he was knocking on a hollow wooden fence post.

"Miracles happen, Dennis. Don't ever forget it. I'll say some prayers for your Dad. Believe me, I know, this one's plastic, the other one is like a piece of wood. They sewed it back on crooked and it hurts like hell," he said with a grin as he pointed to his left leg.

How appearances belie.

He proceeded to tell Dennis of that day they were out on the water on his best friend's boat celebrating, how when they were cruising along somebody on the boat hollered "Turn here," and the driver made a sharp turn to the right and Roger McCarville who was sitting in the bow was thrown from the boat and run over by the boat as the propeller cut his right leg off completely and nearly severed his left leg.

He said as he laid in the water bleeding to death, he looked up through that tunnel to the sky and he prayed and prayed – please don't let me die, please let me live Lord –

and his friends on the boat acted quickly, a couple were paramedics, and they acted quickly and got him out of the water and put tourniquets on him and an ambulance rushed him to the hospital and he did live, then as he laid in the hospital he didn't know how he could continue to live, he couldn't make it like this he said, he didn't know how he would make it, what was he going to do with a house full of young children and a wonderful, beautiful wife and no job he could work anymore. He was a traveling salesman for Dixie Cup; how on God's earth, he asked himself, am I and my family going to survive, over and over he asked himself as he lay in that hospital bed.

Then a friend visited him in the hospital during his darkest hour and gave him a book and a medal.

The title of the book was *The Porter of St. Bonaventure*, he said.

He paused and looked Dennis MulQueen in the eyes. "You ever heard of Solanus Casey by any chance?"

"Who is that, some religious guy? Then no, I don't believe in any of that stuff, I haven't been to church since high school, unless you count Christmas time and Easter when I have sometimes gone to humor my parents. Sorry, I don't believe in all that religious stuff, it's not for me."

"That's okay, it's not about religious stuff – it's about Solanus Casey the man. And his mission here on earth. And what he did here on this earth.

"Fr. Solanus Casey, he was a friar around town, and like I said everything has a reason – this guy's reason was saving people like me. So look up this guy, will you? If you are ever in trouble, please say prayers to this guy, for your dad, for yourself, and me too while you're at it. Even if you don't believe me, because you will see, you will come to know things you didn't know before, all you have to do is open your heart up, okay?

325

"Dennis, I see the way you're looking at me. I understand, it's like trying to describe the color blue to a blind person. If they haven't experienced it they'll think you're crazy, they'll never understand what you're talking about.

"Just trust me though, remember that name Solanus Casey, okay? Bring it all in, let it all out, and you'll get there and you'll be lucky enough you'll have the same quandary someday.

"You won't be able to explain it either, but you'll know just like me, just as sure as the sun and the moon and the stars, we're not alone here, Dennis."

He clambered down off his barstool.

"Now excuse me please, it's hard work, but somebody's gotta do it."

They laughed simultaneously as he drained the rest of his Guinness and clumped his way back over to the stage, his divining rod in hand, that black cane, conducting traffic every step of the way.

A couple songs later, in the middle of "Seven Drunken Old Ladies," Dennis noticed the statuesque blonde at the far end of the bar staring at him. Make that staring red-hot laser beams at him.

She didn't have big penetrating eyes like the singer, she had little darting slits. Powerful in an entirely different way. She had Swedish blonde hair and China-doll skin and with the smoky eyes and the red lipstick to go with her unbelievable body she looked like Jayne Mansfield. She was wearing a satiny white blouse and tight black jeans. This woman is Hollywood material, he muttered to himself as he got up to go to the restroom.

When he returned a few minutes later, he had company. She was sitting in the chair immediately to the left of his, the seat that had been vacated by Roger McCarville.

She was fumbling with her glass as he sat down. She stirred her drink with her fingers.

She turned to him right away.

"You don't know me, do you?"

"Well, no, I don't, but I have to say I wouldn't mind knowing you," he said. "Who are you, I might ask?"

"My name is Buffy. I know you."

"Oh yeah, how's that?"

"I see you drive by almost every day the last couple weeks. Where I work. Two streets over, in the corner building. You stop at the light, I see you coming by in your red AMC every day and I thought, look at that guy in the red AMC, he is a handsome boy, would I ever like to meet him someday. And I walk in here tonight and here you are. I assume you are going to work somewhere in the morning."

Sure enough, he did drive by there every day on his way to the O.P. office. This was getting scary – and more interesting – by the moment.

"Yes, I just started recently at the *Oakland Press*."

He looked and she wasn't wearing a wedding ring. "I'm curious," he said, "exactly what a woman of your stature is doing out here unaccompanied on a Friday night like this? Could be a little dangerous, don't you think." He smiled his own best Hollywood smile. "If you need a bodyguard, I'm available."

He signaled to a young lady behind the bar who was helping the owner out to bring her a drink. She trudged over and grabbed Buffy's glass and tipped it over into the sink below.

You could hear the ice cubes clink against the stainless steel as Buffy jumped up on the chrome railing on the bottom front of her chair and leaned over the bar and looked down. "Oh no. Wait, my glass," she said as she pointed downward with her right index finger.

She laughed a nervous cackle as the barmaid reached down in front of her and held up in the light a gold wedding ring with a small diamond that she had fished out of the bottom of the stainless steel sink.

"My lucky night. Look what I found," the barmaid said. Buffy moved her head sideways and grinned a very strange nut-casey kind of a grin. The barmaid looked over at Dennis and smiled as she reached out and dropped the ring in Buffy's outstretched hand.

He would have liked to get to know this woman under different circumstances, but notwithstanding her beauty that was pretty much the end of that conversation. He swigged the rest of his Guinness, said goodbye and got up to leave.

Before he could get out the door, Roger McCarville interrupted a chorus of something about Thompson guns and "off into the green, into the green," to shout in his direction.

"Friday and Saturday night. See you soon," he said, waving at Dennis.

"Hey, everybody, look over there, there he is, Senator MulQueen is leaving the building. Hurry up, ladies, before he gets out the door, his speaking fees are very reasonable. He's going to be President someday. If you don't make it in time, that's okay. Just give me your number. I'm his booking agent. I'll contact him for you."

The door slammed behind him and in a hot minute he was back on his way down Woodward Avenue toward Oak Park.

~ ~ ~

Victory isn't everything, it's the only thing.

No, that's not Churchill, or Roosevelt. Or Patton or MacArthur.

That was a football coach. Vince Lombardi.

But it could have been him.

In fact, that was him.

George L. MulQueen Jr.

He thought the same way as the great generals, who thought like the great football coaches. Like Woody Hayes and Lombardi. And his best buddy Coach Rhoades.

Like those guys, he was also a great student of history. He earned his masters at U of D in history. No wonder he loved to coach the game and thought like those guys.

And talked like them sometimes, too. Much to the chagrin of Pat MulQueen, his beautiful and esteemed wife.

Or didn't talk.

Dennis MulQueen had heard it many times at home.

Loose lips sink ships.

He assumed that was a Navy thing (George MulQueen Jr. was a medic on the *USS Gosper* in WWII).

But certain things just weren't talked about around the house.

Like the family history in the Old Country.

Maybe he wanted to protect the kids, to keep them from hating, to keep them from reverse bigotry.

But they heard the stories anyway. Through the grapevine. Through eavesdropping on the late-at-night conversations in the Oak Park living room, or downstairs at the cottage on the lake.

Of their women, raped, and their heads stuck on posts in the town square. How their family farm in Askeaton, thousands of acres, was taken away from them and cut into small little partitions leaving the MulQueens only a tiny fraction of what was originally theirs. How the great potato famine happened under British rule resulting in thousands and thousands upon thousands of the Irish starving to death.

And the MulQueen family was lucky to end up with sixty acres out of the whole mess.

It wasn't talked about much even though the family was heavily involved in the Irish community. George MulQueen Sr. had been a long-time president of the AOH (The Ancient Order of Hibernians) in Detroit in the 1930s and 1940s. There were many events and fundraisers held. But again, not much said.

But the younger MulQueens couldn't help but take notice when on August 27th, 1979, news of the latest carnage in the Old Country's Troubles percolated throughout the American media. And the late-at-night MulQueen household. He heard them talking. The IRA had scored their biggest propaganda victory yet in the centuries-old war for Irish independence. The British war hero, statesman and member of the House of Lords, Lord Louis Mountbatten, was assassinated by a bomb planted on his 30-foot boat just off the coast of Ireland as he was out tuna fishing.

Mountbatten usually holidayed there at his summer home, Classiebawn Castle, in Mullaghmore, a small seaside village in County Sligo, Ireland. And apparently, his whereabouts were no secret.

The IRA immediately took credit for the bombing and issued a statement saying, in part, "This operation is one of the discriminate ways we can bring to the attention of the English people the continuing occupation of our country. The death of Mountbatten and the tributes paid to him will be seen in sharp contrast to the apathy of the British government and the English people to the deaths of over 300 British soldiers and the deaths of Irish men, women and children at the hands of their forces."

Sinn Fein's vice president Gerry Adams said of Mountbatten's death: "The IRA gave clear reasons for the execution ... What the IRA did to him is what Mountbatten had been doing all his life to other people. And with his war record, I don't think he could have objected to dying in what was clearly a war situation."

But that wasn't all.

Later the same day, just after 4 in the afternoon, IRA fighters also killed 18 members of the notorious British Parachute Regiment, (the same regiment that carried out Bloody Sunday) in a bombing attack known as the Warrenpoint Ambush.

In this revenge attack, IRA guerrillas ambushed the British Army with two large roadside bombs at Narrow Water Castle on the Newry River, which separates Northern Ireland and the Republic of Ireland.

It was the deadliest attack yet on the British Army during The Troubles.

War – past and present, never ending war – that was the history of the MulQueen family growing up in Ireland, that was the continuing history of Anglo-Irish relations to this day.

Never Ending War. The Anglo-Irish wars, a microcosm of the history of mankind.

And a microcosm of George MulQueen's family history, and his personal history too.

A war with no end, going on seven long years now, fighting his own personal war every single day, against an enemy as feared as any ever faced on the battlefields of the world – cancer.

So seven long years into his personal war now, about a month after the Warrenpoint Ambush and the Mountbatten killing, on the occasion of George McQueen Jr.'s 57th birthday, his son knew what he wanted to give him. He went to the Little Professor Bookstore in downtown Oak Park and personally picked up a copy for him.

"Here's a little light reading, Dad, just to keep you focused," Dennis MulQueen said as he handed a 1,200 page hardcover manuscript to his father in a small paper bag. "Remember, Dad, it's all about victory. It's not *everything*, right, just the *only thing* like you like to say. Here's to your continuing victory, Dad."

"Oh my God, Son, it's heavy. What is it?"

"The ultimate war treatise, Dad. In every bloody detail."

"Is it about Detroit?" he said, as he laughed that contagious belly laugh of his, a laugh forever inimitable, always enchanting and mesmerizing, as his belly shook and the walls vibrated.

How sweet it is.

Dennis MulQueen was glad to be back home again. In the vicinity of that laugh again. In the same house as that laugh again.

Oh Jesus, not again, he had to turn and walk out of the room.

His father opened to where Dennis put the bookmark. He took it out.

It was a bookmark shaped exactly like a shoe. An old brown leather shoe.

He inscribed it himself.

> *Dear Dad,*
> *May you live long enough to finish this book. And long before the devil knows you're dead. And my new shoes are worn out. Enjoy the read, Dad, and thanks again for the shoes - and everything else.*
>> *Love,*
>> *Your favorite #2 son,*
>> *Dennis.*

It was only apropos that on October 2, 1979, his Dad's first birthday with Dennis MulQueen back in the fold (still – despite the cats destroying the house), he had just handed his father the ultimate historical war tome, indeed a very light read, all 1,200 pages.

War and Peace, the greatest book ever written, by the great Russian master nonpareil, Leo Tolstoy.

~ 23 ~

IT'S NOT YOUR TURN

It didn't take long for them to find out what he was made of.

His radar was impeccable. He could find a rat in a hay stack quicker than a barn owl.

He knew something was up before he got inside the building. There was no place to park.

He circled back around the school and parked on a side street two blocks away.

Enrollment was great. Finances were good. The football team had been on a tear, victory after victory. A league championship run.

So why all the cars?

He was going to get a quick answer as a slew of angry faces greeted him in the foyer of Pontiac Catholic High School that night for what he thought was going to be an ordinary school board meeting.

The pinched noses and downturned lips and squinty eyes dominated the cramped hearing room down the hall because that most remarkable championship football season in school history was for naught – completely wiped out, in fact.

All those victories nullified by the league because several star players had transferred in that year and played for the school – even though they were ineligible to play.

According to Catholic League rules, students transferring from another district were required to sit out a year if they didn't live in the new district. The players were mysteriously provided addresses of houses they didn't live in, but which they used on official school paperwork. However, somebody blew the whistle on this scheme. Rumor was, it was a player who had lost his playing time to one of the transferees. Or the player's parents.

The Archdiocese found out and the suspensions and invalidated wins were a done deal, it was revealed at the meeting. A great season was ruined amid humiliation and embarrassment.

What wasn't revealed was who was responsible.

The angry mob wanted answers – and scalps. The meeting immediately devolved into a who-done-it, he-said she-said shouting match. Some tried to blame the students and their parents, while the school principal blamed it all on the athletic director who blamed it all on the coach.

"How could you do this to our school? How could you let our students down like this," an angry mother in a powder-blue pantsuit shouted out of turn at the principal seated at the head table.

Another parent rose and said, "Those kids worked their tails off for those wins. You have taken our proudest moment ever and turned us into the laughing stock of the entire league. You should be fired for this."

The school principal quickly rose to defend himself.

"I knew nothing about this," Principal Joseph Duby said. "This was the responsibility of the athletic director and the head football coach. I have relieved them of their duties. They are no longer with the school."

Standing in the far back of the room against the wall, Dennis MulQueen's radar lit up like the sound board at a Bob Seger concert. And when his antennae lit up like this, there was usually a very good reason.

He just didn't believe the guy.

Time for a little digging.

At the end of the meeting, as everybody filed out of the school, and after he was done interviewing parents and school officials, he walked back down the hallway to the drinking fountain. He lingered outside the trophy case embedded in the wall, stalled in the rest room for a bit, grabbed another coffee at the little table in the corner of the lobby, then took a walk down another hallway.

Soon the building was empty – save Dennis MulQueen and a couple of janitors. He looked down the long corridor and saw nothing as he walked past the lavatory and the snack table toward the main entryway.

He made a left at the panel of aluminum doors which comprised the main school entrance and stopped in front of the first door on the right.

This polished oak door with a natural finish immediately adjacent to the main school doors had a brass plaque at eye level which read on top: "Principal" and beneath that in smaller letters, "Joseph Duby."

He tried the doorknob.

Locked.

He heard noise, it sounded like it could be coming from the next room down the hall. He quickly removed his journalist's notepad from the left inside pocket of the sport coat his father had given him and hurriedly scribbled a short note which read:

Dear Mr. Duby,

This is Dennis MulQueen, a reporter for the Oakland Press. Please call me. I have some important information for you regarding the athletic scandal. Please call me as soon as you get this message,

    Sincerely,

    Dennis MulQueen.

At the bottom, he printed the main number of the newspaper.

As soon as he completed the note and ripped it out of his spiral reporter's notebook, a middle-aged maintenance guy in a royal-blue shirt with dark navy pants exited the classroom two doors down pushing a yellow barrel on wheels with his right hand and lugging a cylindrical gray floor vac with his other hand.

Dennis approached him immediately.

"Hi there, sir. My name is Dennis MulQueen. I am a reporter with the *Oakland Press*. I was here tonight to cover the meeting and I have a very important message for the Principal. If you don't mind I'd like to leave it on his desk to make sure he gets it. The future of the school and everybody's job is at stake, sir. I want to make sure he gets it first thing in the morning."

"Well," the janitor said as he rocked backward a bit on his dark black leather work boots. "I don't see no harm in that. I was just making my way in there shortly anyway," he added as he looked down and removed a large ring of keys attached to his belt by an aluminums hook. He quickly found the one he was looking for and opened the door.

"Go ahead, there you go."

Dennis walked over to a large wooden desk near the far wall and placed the piece of paper on top of the desk.

He turned and walked back toward the doorway and as he was exiting the room the janitor turned to walk the other way and as he did so, Dennis reached behind the door and turned the brass bar above the doorknob counter-clockwise as pulled the door shut.

"Thank you very much, sir. You have a good night now, okay."

"You too," the janitor said as he pulled the yellow barrel and the floor vac with him as he entered the room immediately adjacent to the principal's office.

Dennis stood there immobile in the hallway silent as a church mouse for about 30 seconds. Then he spun around on the balls of his feet, reached out and turned the brass doorknob to the right, opened the heavy oak door with the brass plaque on it, and quietly re-entered the principal's office.

He gently closed the door behind him and walked around the large wooden desk and tried the center slide-out drawer.

Locked.

He tried the other desk drawers.

All locked.

He walked over to a file cabinet against the wall. Also locked. He walked back around the desk and noticed a silver wastebasket off to the side next to the wall. It was full to the brim.

When he walked over to the wastebasket and looked down, he noticed small pieces of torn paper resting on the top layer. He saw part of the letterhead of the Archdiocese of Detroit on one fragment.

A loud *clunk* made him flinch as something hit the shared wall in the room next door. He bent over and one-by-one hurriedly removed the paper scraps from the top of the waste basket and shoved them in the inside right pocket of his sport coat. He stopped just inside the door and made the sign of the cross before he turned the brass bar above the doorknob clockwise before he gingerly turned the knob and exited the office, pulling the door shut behind him. He tried it. It was locked again. He looked to the right just as he heard the rattling wheel sound of the yellow barrel. Dennis hurried around the corner and exited the main doors of the building and headed toward his car.

Once back at the *Oakland Press*, he sat down at a desk across from the city desk and immediately began rearranging the paper fragments on the desktop.

He had retrieved every single one of them.

He perfectly reconstructed a letter from the head of the Catholic League from early in the school year reminding the principal that students transferring to his school from a recently-closed Detroit high school were ineligible to play athletics in the current school year without permanent residence within the Pontiac Catholic district.

This was a big scandal now. And Dennis MulQueen's first scalp.

He made several calls and spent the rest of the evening and on into the wee hours of the night writing an article exposing the school hierarchy's full knowledge of and full participation in the school's playing of the ineligible students and the subsequent attempt by the school principal to coverup his participation in the scam by shredding the evidence and throwing it in a wastebasket.

He got the head of the Catholic League out of bed at 2.a.m. for comment. The *Oakland Press* editors ran his piece as the lede story with a banner headline across the front page of the next day's *Oakland Press*.

The principal was quickly fired that same day joining the AD and the head football coach on the unemployment line.

Dennis MulQueen was on his way with his first big scoop.

How sweet it is.

He left the office the next day at 6:30 p.m. after filing a follow-up piece on the firings.

On a whim, he decided to drive down to Dooley's, an old haunt on Grand River Avenue in southwest Detroit, to have a beer and see if he knew anybody there to celebrate with. He had been in there before. Some of the U of D guys would occasionally pop in there. The joint was also a favorite gathering spot of his father's and his football coaching buddies.

Well, there's at least one person I know here, he said as he pulled in the parking lot and saw the big blue Olds 98 right smack in the middle of the lot. His father's unmistakable big boat.

He walked in and there he was, holding court with the boys at a table in the center of the bar. George MulQueen was busy bragging about all the money he had in the bank and how his wife Pat and all of his kids were taken care of for life with the settlement he got from the accident when his son sneaked up behind him.

"I thought the Beatles said money doesn't matter," Dennis MulQueen said.

His father turned and looked.

"For Christ's sake, forget about those mop heads. Your mother sent you down here to get me, eh?"

"No, Dad. Actually I haven't been home. I came straight from the paper. I got my first front page bomb today so I thought I'd go out and celebrate a bit. I had no idea you would be here.

"I just had a crazy hunch, I drove here like subconsciously. For old time's sake, I guess, I remembered being here with you and coach Tobin and Rhoades a long time ago when you brought me here. I didn't expect you to be here today."

"That's interesting because I haven't been here myself in a long time," his father said. "I haven't been here in at least a year but I decided to stop by today. It's this guy's fault. He called me up today outta the blue to see if I could make it down today and I'm glad I did."

He pointed across the table at his good friend Jack Griffin, the same John M. Griffin who owned Griffin Bros. Construction Company in Detroit, who lived right next door at the lake.

Dennis MulQueen showed his father a copy of the paper and his expose laid across the top of the front page.

"It's the shoes, Dad. Like you said. A guy has to have a good pair of shoes to go with that Italian suit."

His father's face lit up like a Christmas tree.

"And a good cold draft. Sit down, Son."

He unfolded the paper and held it up for Jack Griffin to see.

"Nice job there, laddy," the Westchester Beach neighbor said.

"Nice, Son, very nice. I'll be darned, you are your mother's son. "

"Don't be so humble, Dad. Don't you have a master's degree and just half your thesis away from a doctorate?"

"Yeah, but she wrote all my best papers," he said.

They both laughed again.

"Now that you're working, it's your turn to buy a round."

He didn't say anything. He was looking for a rock. As a stringer he only got paid once a month and it was near the end of the month so he only had a ten and a couple singles in his pocket and he didn't want to embarrass his father in front of his friends because there were about a dozen at the table.

His Dad read his look and slipped a $20 to him under the table without saying a word.

"Okay, guys. It's my round. Everybody in?"

A surly-looking guy at the end of the table glared at Dennis and shot back, "Yeah, asshole. What a ya think ya cheap fucker, you trying for a light pot?"

He was drunk, and he had on a white T-shirt and a black leather jacket with black hair slicked back like the Fonz. Dennis didn't recognize this guy as being one of his father's crowd.

He wasn't.

Apparently he felt he had to act like this to justify dressing like a cheap imitation. This drunken idiot had just come out of nowhere and sat at the end of his father's table.

The guy wasn't done. "You're an asshole, too," he said. "You must be his father, you fat fucker." He pointed at George MulQueen. "You're both assholes," he said.

After not being there to defend his father at the AOH that day, not being there when he had the accident that day, after quitting college football that day, after quitting on the Ford Motor Co. career offer that day, after quitting on med school, after quitting on Christmas that year – finally he had a chance to show his father he wasn't a quitter.

He jumped up out of his chair like he was shot out of that cannon at the circus that day, but before he could defend his father's honor by beating the shit out of this punk – heck, before he could even straighten all the way up, his father grabbed his right arm and tugged him back down into his chair.

He leaned over and whispered, "Son, let it go. That guy's an obnoxious drunk and he's not worth it. You would kill him and for doing the right thing you will get arrested and he'll come in here and cause another riot tomorrow. People like him just aren't worth it. Don't get your hands dirty on white trash like that."

Dennis couldn't help it. His guilty conscience was hard to tame. He wondered if his father secretly thought the guy would kick his ass.

He said nothing and paid for the round.

The shell was going down smooth a few minutes later when a guy wandered over from the pool table and announced to the whole gang he was looking for a partner to play doubles with him. Dennis raised his hand immediately.

"I'm in," he said.

"Great. Let's go, pal. It's our break."

The jukebox was blaring "Rambling Gambling Man" by Bob Seger and these guys were knockin' 'em down. The pool balls – and the drinks. The other two guys – and Dennis' partner – they could all play. Less than two songs later, it was Dennis' shot at the only ball left on the table.

The 8-ball for game.

The joint quieted as all eyes were on the pool table now as he got up off his chair to shoot for all the marbles. Before he could take two steps toward the table to chalk up, the booming voice from behind rattled the bar room air. "It's not your turn. It's your partner's shot. Sit back down."

Dennis straightened up and stopped dead in his tracks. His partner got up from his chair and started walking to the table with his stick.

Dennis MulQueen raised his left hand at his partner in the form of a stop sign and turned around and stared at his father.

"No, it's not. It's my shot."

He turned and resumed walking toward the table.

"We don't care which one of you shoots," the top guy from the other team said. 'Just one a ya all shoot and miss so we can win the game."

The bar was dead silent now as Dennis chalked his cue while examining the layout. It was a bare angle near full-length corner shot, there was nothing in the way, but lots and lots of green in between the two balls. This wasn't a 9-foot Brunswick gold crown, but it wasn't a 6-foot Valley either. This looked to be an 8-footer, a standard table for most league play.

The solid white ball at the near end sat not more than two-and-a-half inches from the rail about a foot over from the near pocket, while the 8-ball was about six inches past the center line of the table, about three-and-a-half-feet from the far corner pocket – but a slight five to seven degree angle off of straight center into the pocket. One of those not quite straight-in full table shots with the cue close to the rail. A tough shot for most league players, a for-sure tough shot for most bar room players let alone the very occasional pool-playing Dennis MulQueen.

As he stepped up to the table, he felt the silence in the room grip his throat like a hungry panther. He knew one thing for sure: the way these guys played, he had to make it or it was over.

He leaned over the table, then he straightened back up, tilted his head back about three inches like he was going to look at the ceiling as he closed his eyes and took a deep breath and slowed everything down to a crawl and pretended he was on top of Mount Everest looking down on the world.

That was the zone he knew he needed to put himself in if he was going to pull this one off.

He wanted it bad and he knew the only way was to transport himself to that special zone of intense inner relaxation which forms the core of all focused concentration. He instinctively let go and allowed himself to feel the absolute relaxed exhilaration that came over him as he visualized the snowball-white cue ball striking the jet-black 8 with an authoritative crack as it zooms straight into the hole.

It was working as he felt a beautiful rush of excitement course up and down his spine. He actually felt high as a kite as he leaned over the cue ball and stared the 8 down, and in that moment of sublime concentration he saw, felt, and heard only those two balls in perfect alignment with one another and the hole as he hit the cue strong and true and relished that crack he had imagined as the two balls collided perfectly and the black ball with the number eight on it rolled straight as an arrow dead center into the back of the far-left pocket.

He turned and looked directly at his father, and continued looking at him all the way back to the table.

"Like John Wayne said, eh, Dad, under pressure it's not always the guy that shoots the fastest, it's the guy that shoots the straightest, right, Dad?"

He looked and sounded like he was pissed when he made the comment.

For sure it escaped him at the moment, he wouldn't figure out until many years later where his father was coming from when at the tensest moment of the match he announced to the whole bar that his son was shooting out of turn. But he knew one thing for sure at that moment: he was damned glad he made that shot.

Points to prove, what a beautiful thing.

"Nice shot, Son," his father said.

A few rounds later they were out the door and down Grand River in the big blue monster, Dennis behind the wheel. His father said they would come back later for Dennis' AMC wagon.

They pulled in the Oak Park driveway about 15 minutes later.

Before either of them exited the vehicle, his father started talking, out of nowhere.

"Yeah, Son, his kid, he just keeps fucking up, getting in trouble with drag racing, getting kicked outta school, it is tearing Barry up inside. I mean, this is his son. So he gets real pissed, he smacks him when he probably shouldn't, he doesn't mean it. But, Bear, the thing is, he's really hard on his son, but there's just nothing as important in a man's life as his son, and seeing the pain he goes through, it's just something ..."

His voice trailed off and Dennis MulQueen couldn't make out the last words. His father opened the passenger side door and they started walking together side-by-side the few steps toward the house and for once it felt like the old days again, just the two of them, out on the town together, just like the old days like after being out on the lake alone together half the day catching fish after fish, just the two of them, like that day after that ballgame at the Dairy Queen together after Coach MulQueen's son broke up Elliott Blumberg's no-hitter in the seventh inning, like that day when he would find years later copies of all three of those 4.0 report cards secretly filed in a manila folder in his father's dresser along with the letter of commendation from the university president, and that football game picture he would find in the file cabinet in his father's room of his son in his game-day uniform with all those future NFL players on the same field with him, just like all the good old days he wished could last forever and ever until the end of time.

~ ~ ~

"TJ, did you see that on the news? Big Brother finally admitted it. Perfect timing, eh? Just in time for Thanksgiving. The bastards finally admitted they drowned our own guys in Agent Orange. Our own men, poisoned to death with that vile shit. Either that or burned to death with

331

napalm, if they weren't maimed by IED's or shot to death. But we had to stop those big bad commies from taking over Viet Nam, right?"

The guy in the car with him didn't even flinch. His buddy had the patience of Job.

"Turn right here, D. I think it's a couple blocks down."

Anti-war, anti-government, anti-evil, anti-everything. After a dozen years of hanging around together, he was habituated to his buddy's rants by now.

He had to be – or there would be no friendship. But it went both ways. TJ could get off on some pretty good anti-establishment soliloquies of his own.

But the difference was Dennis MulQueen couldn't help it. This was a guy that when he was a youngster in early spring used to sit outside in the yard and cry as he watched the last snow of the year slowly die off in the ground before his eyes as the sun and the warm spring air did the final melt of the year and he vowed to move to Alaska someday, or the Yukon, or Greenland, or some place in the world where the snow didn't have to die every year.

"Corporate warfare is wrong, TJ. Eisenhower had it right. He warned us to beware the industrial military complex taking over the country. But it's too late now, isn't it? The greedy war mongers are fully in charge now. That war was nothing but a proxy war against China for control of the cheap labor and resources and arms market of Southeast Asia. That's how the world is going to end. Buried by the greed and the stature that only the power of money can buy."

"Here it is, D. There's a spot right there, right in front. They must have heard us coming."

They were in downtown Royal Oak. Things were hopping. TJ and his brother Will owned a house right around the corner, so this was his turf and he knew the spots.

"Where we going, right here?"

"Yeah, D – Mr. B's. You'll like it. You can be as loud as you want and nobody will notice." True enough. Next to Dennis, the soft spoken TJ appeared catatonic.

"Don't worry," Dennis said. "They'll notice us before we sit down. Ladies and gentlemen, Mutt and Jeff are in the building."

Not far from the truth. Dennis was still a 6' 4" lumberjack of a college football lineman as wide as a Kentucky smokehouse, and TJ still looked the part of a taut curly-haired defensive back and ball carrier at 5' 9", undersized for even that. But he could run like the wind and he had fire in his belly.

Dennis remembered the second game of senior year against Bishop Gallagher, he had a spectacular run of 88 yards from scrimmage in the first quarter that resulted in a touchdown – but must of been the coaches didn't like his iconoclastic attitude so he ended up with only a handful of carries the whole game. Even though that 88-yarder set the table for a Cub High rout that day.

But mostly it didn't help his yard time that the starting tailback ahead of him a couple years later turned out to be the second leading rusher in the entire country on his college team at Cornell. Dennis nicknamed him Shank because that's how you felt when he hit you, like you got shanked in the head with a steel shillelagh. He was like a Jim Brown or an Earl Campbell type – he had the speed to run around you, but he just thought it was way more fun to run over you. Shank and another really good friend Dennis nicknamed Stenchie, who was the middle linebacker, they were the two toughest guys on the team and probably in the whole league.

But still, Coach should have found a way to play TJ more in some capacity, maybe as a wideout, because every time he touched the ball he made something happen.

They walked through the crowd to the only open spot in the whole place, the end of a long table in the middle.

A pitcher of amber liquid later, it was time to engage.

Not because he wanted to. Because he had to.

There was a hot brunette one table over. And he never met a pretty brunette he didn't like, or couldn't seduce given the opportunity, so it was time for a special drink order.

He sidled over after the waitress left and the rest was history, as they say. Turned out her name was Andrea Schwartz and of all things, even though they were in downtown Royal Oak, she was a Jewish American Princess from Oak Park, Michigan – his neighborhood.

Good thing TJ knew the spots.

In fact, she lived no more than five blocks over from the MulQueen bungalow, just across Nine Mile Road – within walking distance of the home pad. Can't get much more convenient love than that.

Turns out, she worked as a med tech at nearby Beaumont Hospital, so she had just hopped over after work. She was a very sweet beauty and they really hit it off and had a great time together. Later, they talked on the phone for hours. She was an absolutely beautiful woman, inside and out. They went to lunch and dinner and pretty soon it was time for the next step.

He pulled in her driveway to pick her up for another night on the town weeks later when she insisted he come inside. She said there was somebody he had to meet as she led him to the den in back.

He knew what was coming.

"No way, Andrea. Do we have to?"

"Yes way, Dennis MulQueen. I don't want him to find out through the grapevine I'm dating a gentile."

"Your Dad? No way."

He was actually nervous.

"He doesn't know I'm an Irish Catholic, does he?"

"He asked me your name. That's all I told him, that you are a writer and your name is Dennis McQueen. I'm sure he doesn't suspect a thing. "

"Okay, good. I'll tell him I'm Lithuanian Orthodox."

"Dennis."

They rounded the corner and there he was sitting on the couch. The All-American father, dressed in flannel shirt and gray slacks.

"Dad, I have somebody I want you to meet," she said.

They shook hands.

"Hi, I'm Jack Schwartz, Andrea's father. So tell me about yourself."

"I, ah, well, ahh." He cleared his throat nervously.

But no words came out. It wasn't that he was intimidated by Mr. Schwartz. He was flabbergasted by Mr. Schwartz.

When he sat back down on the couch after shaking Dennis' hand, he pulled on each pant leg midthigh, sliding his trousers up a couple inches on each leg as he crossed his right leg over his left – to reveal a rubber penis sticking out of the bottom of his right pant leg about three inches.

It was very realistic looking.

"You see."

"Yeah, I see."

They both burst out laughing at the same time, along with Andrea.

"Well, I see you have incredible genes, Andrea. As talented as I am, I don't know if even I can live up to these standards."

"Well, just let me know, darling," her father said as he winked at his daughter.

He looked back at Dennis.

"She will let me know if you measure up."

They engaged in a little more small talk, and then they were out the door.

They had a good dinner and a good time that night and I guess Dennis MulQueen measured up because it kept going from there with one incredible time after another.

She just couldn't resist.

His   charm,   of   course.

~ 24 ~

HOWE TO SPELL TOUGH

He was about to meet the Babe Ruth of Detroit.

So it was only apropos that when his father whipped that gorgeous snow-cone white Bonneville with the shiny chrome bumpers and sparkling silver trim into the driveway that day in late November 1962, he had a smile on his face to match one of The Babe's monolithic blasts.

Only this guy was bigger than The Babe.

In Detroit, this guy was God.

Only Joe Louis and Ty Cobb could compare.

And even they fell short. To his father at least. And a lot of other people this guy was a hero to.

"Okay, let's go. We're here, kid."

George MulQueen and his nine-year-old son exited the vehicle and sauntered up to the front door of 28780 Sunset Boulevard, Lathrup Village, Michigan, a modest red brick ranch house in this suburban neighborhood just west of Southfield road and north of 11 mile in suburban Detroit. The house looked pretty much like the other houses in the neighborhood, the red brick accented by a row of inlaid sandstone that framed in the picture window and heavy wooden front door and a similar chimney and tan roof the same pitch as everybody else's. The main difference was this

337

house was the last house on the block and was surrounded by a huge yard.

George MulQueen knocked on the front door.

A guy with dark wavy hair in a white golf shirt and dark slacks opened the door.

"Hi, George, how are you doing?"

"Good, Power. Just on our way over to Pete's and Hec was bugging me to see if we could get tikkies for the game coming up this weekend against Toronto. I told him I'd ask you, Power. I know it's not much notice but you know how he is about those Leafs."

"Yeah, we're playing those guys on Sunday, George. How many, just you and Hurricane?"

"Yes, just the two of us."

"Okay, George, I'll have it set up for you like last time, just go to Gate One again and ask for Harold, and he'll take care of you guys, okay?"

"Oh thanks, Power, really appreciate it. Sorry to bother you at home on an off-day, but you know that guy, he doesn't much care for those Toronto guys, the way they treated him. He wants to make sure you have enough fan support to make sure you, well, if you happen to knock out a couple Leafs for him, he wants you to know you will have his full appreciation."

"Yeah, I know how he loves those Leafs. Don't worry, George, if Baun or one of those buggers takes a run at me again they will wish they hadn't, that's for sure. I'll look for you guys at the game."

"Oh by the way, I have somebody here who wants to meet you."

He moved his overturned outstretched hand in the direction of the young kid standing next to him.

"Well, hello there. How are you doing today, young man? Are you a Red Wing's fan?"

"Yes, I am."

"Do you play hockey young, man?

"Yes, I do."

"And what team are you on?"

"I am on the Bruins."

"The Bruins. Oh my God. They are the enemy. Take him out of here, George."

The kid stiffened with silence as he inhaled a nervous short breath as George MulQueen and the man in the white shirt had a good laugh.

"I'm just kidding there, young man. You keep playing and having fun. I know one thing," he said as he pointed his beefy right index finger at George MulQueen, "if you are half as tough as this guy, you'll make out just fine, on and off the ice. Even if you do play for the Bruins."

"Thanks, Power. Again sorry to bother you at home, but I really appreciate everything, Hec and I look forward to seeing you at the game."

"Oh, you're welcome, George. I'd invite you guys in for a drink and a snack, but it's not an off-day actually. We're not playing today, but we do have a practice down at the old barn. I was just getting ready to go."

He extended his right arm to shake hands with George MulQueen and that's when the kid had one of those freeze-frame moments to be remembered forever.

The sinews in the guy's forearm stood out like nautical rope wrapped around a dock stanchion. His biceps were like carved marble on a Michelangelo piece. And he noticed his hands too. They were like a great ape's hands, totally disproportionate to any normal human body size. His fingers were fatter than a stone mason's.

"Thanks for stopping by, George. Tell Hurricane I said hi and I look forward to seeing you guys on Sunday."

"Thanks, Power. Can't wait to see what you do to Baun's face this time."

"As long as we win, George."

"Oh, you'll win. Me and Hurricane will be there."

The man and his son turned and walked back to the white 1960 Bonneville and took off around the corner on Roseland towards the house of a life-long friend of George MulQueen's who lived a couple blocks away.

George MulQueen turned to look at his son in the front seat next to him.

"Son, do you know who that was?"

"No, Dad," he said.

"Son, today is your lucky day."

He pointed behind him, toward the back window of the car.

"You just met the greatest athlete that ever lived. In any sport. For all time. Nobody has the skill he has. Or the heart he has. Nobody has what that guy has. He has already won us four Stanley Cups, Son. And he's not done yet. He is an even bigger champion off the ice."

~ ~ ~

Almost 18 years later, the evening of February 5, 1980, there was only one place George MulQueen and his son Dennis would be found.

In the living room, glued to the big-screen Zenith, waiting for the final introduction of the night.

The PA announcer didn't say his name.

He didn't have to.

All 21,002 fans, a record crowd for a hockey game at the time, were on their feet at the newly-minted Joe Louis Arena in downtown Detroit, Michigan.

"And from the Hartford Whalers, representing all of hockey, the greatest statesman for five decades, Number Nine."

There he was again. In front of the MulQueen's and this time the whole world, skating on the ice at the brand-spanking-new arena already nicknamed The Joe. The unforgettable Gordie Howe, appearing in his record 23rd All Star game.

Of course, Dennis MulQueen knew everything about this guy. He was practically raised with him. He had learned everything there was to learn about Gordie Howe over the years since that day when he was a little kid and his Dad took him to his house to meet him in person.

Gordie Howe and the Red Wings were as MulQueen as Molson Canadian.

Dennis MulQueen's affinity for the Red Wings started even before he met Gordie. When he was a young kid he would walk downstairs at the Oak Park house and gaze up at the MulQueen rafter of fame in the basement where with awe right next to his father's boxing gloves and a pair of Grandpa MulQueen's boxing gloves from his Golden Gloves days were hanging in the air right next to them a pair of old brown leather very famous hockey gloves.

Instead of just hanging in the MulQueen's basement Hall of Fame, these gloves really belonged in the NHL Hockey Hall of Fame.

These were the hockey gloves worn by George MulQueen's good friend Hec Kilrea, the hockey legend who would go down in NHL history as the guy who when he was wearing those very same gloves ended the longest game in NHL history in 1937 against Montreal, when Kilrea streaked in from the left wing in the third overtime to beat Montreal 1-0 in the first game of the playoffs that year.

Kilrea's goal not only provided the margin of victory in that game but provided the spark that lit the Wings' fire and propelled them to victory over the Canadiens in that series and provided the momentum that carried over into the finals where they beat the Rangers for their second consecutive Stanley Cup.

Kilrea was born in a small town named Blackburn near Ottawa and before he was a Wing he was a star for the Ottawa Senators, scoring an unbelievable 36 goals in little more than forty games played in the 1929-30 season. He won his first Cup with Ottawa in 1927 and he could do it all. Even fight, including some memorable ones, like the time he had a renowned bout with the legendary Toe Blake of those same Montreal Canadiens.

But his ticket to the Big Puck League was his speed. He was actually a champion speed skater before entering the NHL and he once even raced the legendary Howie Morenz, the first NHL superstar before Howe and Rocket Richard and Lemieux and Gretzky.

Morenz was considered the fastest skater ever.

Until he met Hec Kilrea.

Hec beat Morenz not once but twice in timed sprints around the ice.

Another huge NHL legend, Jack Adams, played with Kilrea on those Ottawa Sens teams and later when he became GM of Detroit, Adams brought Kilrea to the Red Wings where Kilrea proceeded to win two more Cups with the Red Wings, the first ever back-to-back NHL Cups in NHL history in 1936 and 1937. Adams nicknamed him Hurricane Hec, and Adams, who also brought Gordie Howe to the Wings, was also responsible for giving Howe his first nickname of "Power" before in his later years he was mostly known as "Mr. Hockey."

Kilrea was named one of the top 20 players of his era by one of the most respected hockey magazines of the time. And of course Howe would go down as the best ever, of any era.

Dennis MulQueen's dad and Hec met at Ford Motor Company, where George MulQueen was a safety engineer and where Hec also worked after he retired from the NHL after a stint in World War II that was just as stellar as his impressive NHL career.

Hec had moved to Detroit as a player and became an American citizen which allowed him to enlist in the US Army like many other hockey players did.

Hec was an infantryman and was on the front lines in Italy and France and won the Distinguished Cross and the Purple Heart for heroics under fire rescuing injured comrades and more. George MulQueen was also in that war, and served as a medic on a Navy ship where he mostly administered X-rays to injured troops before they had metal lined rooms and wore protective metal shields. That would not be good for his health, it would turn out.

It was at the Ford Rouge complex where their friendship blossomed and they remained close to the very end. He wanted his best buddy to have those gloves and he gave them to George MulQueen long before he died on September 8, 1969.

They always had great rapport and a great time together over the years, especially as Dennis and Chip tagged along together with their father on those weekend trips to Hec's cottage at the bend of the river in the town of Belle River, Ontario, Canada, where Hec Kilrea and George MulQueen would laugh and talk for hours about everything Red Wings under the sun and the great rivalries with the Leafs and the Habs, those great Montreal Canadiens. And of course, about their mutual friend Gordie Howe, a Saskatchewan native.

Dennis and Chip sat in rapt attention as Hec and their father traded old Gordie stories, possibly their favorite being that game in 1959 against the Toronto Maple Leafs when the Leafs' spark plug defenseman Bobby Baun blindsided Howe and took him down big-time and Howe just got up and skated off like nothing had happened.

343

Until late in the third period, after the Wings had the game in hand, when Howe and Baun went in the corner together after the puck and all of a sudden Gordie Howe was skating around the back of the net with Bobby Baun's face pinned to the glass by Howe's famous right elbow. He dropped Baun off onto the ice behind the net like a bloody sack of potatoes with his face in shreds.

That might have been Kilrea's favorite story because of his hatred for the Leafs in general. He was with the Leafs for a brief stint between the Sens and the Wings but they suspended him for drinking and fighting off the ice and he forever held it against the Maple Leafs' brass.

They also loved talking about the time in 1959 when the guy at that time considered the toughest fighter in the league challenged Howe to a fight. His name was Lou Fontinato and he played for the New York Rangers. Howe just killed him in front of a sold-out crowd and Hec recalled how after the game a friend of his named Gump Worsley, then the Ranger's goalie, said, "You could hear Howe's punches land on Fontinato *thump thump thump* like he was chopping wood." Fontinato's nose was off to the side and there was blood everywhere.

As usual George MulQueen was right about Howe's ability. The fastest NHL shot during the '60s was Bobby "The Golden Jet" Hull's slap shot which was clocked at 114 miles per hour, with a curved blade. By comparison, Gordie Howe's wrist shot – with a straight blade – was clocked at 109 miles per hour – and much more accurate – and a lot more deceptive too as he was ambidextrous. Maybe that's how you score 801 goals in the NHL.

And get to play in the Big Puck League until you are 52 years old – he was 51 that day at The Joe (his birthday was March 31) when he recorded an assist in the 3rd period of that All Star game on February 5, 1980.

It tells you a lot about the man that he was out there on the Joe Louis ice that day because he was only out there for one reason – he came out of retirement to play with sons Marty and Mark on the Houston Aeros of the World Hockey Association.

That first year Gordie came out of retirement in 1974 he scored 100 points, was league MVP, and his new team the Aeros won the league championship.

And included another legendary Gordie Howe moment:

That came late in the season, in a game against Edmonton, when a fight broke out and an Oilers defenseman named Roger Cote had Gordie's son Marty pinned to the ice. Howe skated over and told the guy to get off of his son. The guy told Howe to go eff himself. Gordie bent over and put his beefy fingers in Cote's nose and pulled him off of his son and held him up in the air like a rag doll or some kind of hunting trophy as the blood began to pour out of Cote's nose and down his jersey and onto the ice.

This was vintage Gordie Howe – at age 45. (He left Houston for Hartford which the next year, joined the NHL for the 1979-80 season (along with Gretzky's WHA team, which became the Oilers, and two other teams that joined the NHL in Quebec and Winnipeg).

It was a good thing the Joe was brand-new or it might have fallen down that night when Howe skated out on the ice. The building was definitely all done settling. After he was introduced, the Detroit fans gave their hero a five-minute standing ovation with chants of "Gordie, Gordie!" that continued even after he left the ice and sat down on the bench, an ovation that was only finally quelled by the PA guy interrupting to announce the National Anthem singers.

Howe said afterward the fans meant as much to him as he did to them. During the special ovation fans gave him that night, he said he deliberately skated over to Wings' trainer

Lefty Wilson to ask him to say something to prevent him from crying.

"Lefty was bilingual," Gordie Howe said. "He spoke English and profanity. I asked him to say something, and he did which I can't repeat and I was okay after that."

Throughout the rest of the evening it was the same, as every second Howe hit the ice the same gleeful pandemonium engulfed the arena with chants of "Gordie, Gordie, Gordie!"

In an ironic twist signifying an historic changing of the guard, while it was Howe's 23rd and final appearance in the All-Star Game, it was the up-and-coming superstar Wayne Gretzky's very first All-Star game.

But this was Gordie's night as Mr. Hockey upstaged the guy they would end up calling the Great One, and everybody else that night. Gordie's team won, and he stole the puck twice on one shift in the third period and made a needlepoint perfect pass from behind the net out front to a teammate who buried it, giving Gordie one more stellar point on the NHL ice in Detroit.

Every time he touched the puck, the "Gordie, Gordie, Gordie!" chants rattled the rafters with new vigor.

And to think it almost all never happened.

Howe's career was almost over, when he was just getting started, before Dennis MulQueen was even born.

In the first game of the 1951 playoffs, Gordie Howe was almost killed.

It was those darned Leafs again. He came across ice to check the Toronto Maple Leafs captain Teeder Kennedy, but Kennedy stopped and ducked and Gordie slipped and crashed head first into the boards at full speed and sustained a fractured skull, a broken orbital bone and a severe concussion.

346

Doctors at Harper Hospital operated on him to relieve the pressure on his brain and Detroit was on edge for several days. Doctors feared he might die, let alone never play hockey again.

That was the year the Wings won their first of the four Stanley Cups they captured with Gordie leading the way. Not only did he come back, but he won the League scoring championship the next four years in a row.

George MulQueen, after recalling Howe's near-death-on-the-ice moment, said he wanted his son to always remember one thing about the guy he introduced him to all those years ago that they were watching skate around the Joe Louis NHL ice at 51 years of age.

"That's how you spell tough, Son. Right there. H-O-W-E," he said.

~ 25 ~

DO YOU BELIEVE IN
MIRACLES?

If the huge cranes with huge metal hooks dangling from huge metal trestles reaching high in the afternoon sky and the giant earthmovers with tires twice as tall as a man and the piles of huge concrete piping you could drive a truck through didn't speak for themselves, the large wooden sign fastened to a chain-link fence walling off the site told him directly: "No Trespassing. The Detroit Water and Sewerage Department."

Unless you are a reckless newspaper man always in search of a good story.

He gingerly scaled the fence and walked on the site with the green-and-yellow flannel shirt he borrowed from his father blowing in the wind and with a white baseball cap on top deftly and sophisticatedly intended to mimic the white hard hats and dungaree look of the legitimate workers toiling the site. Just so as not to attract any attention.

His destination was the trailer off to the far side where he hoped to get close enough to talk to somebody who might really know what was going on here. The first thing he learned in journalism is you can hardly ever take a politician or government honcho's word at face value. You gotta get in the trenches to find out what the real deal is.

What he knew so far was a huge concrete pipe more than 50 feet underground that handled 15.6-million gallons of raw sewage per hour was caving in and in danger of imminent collapse, meaning the nearby Clinton River was going to become a giant sewer itself, or the giant sewage flow would back up into the 300,000 Oakland and Macomb County residences and businesses served by the broken line.

Dennis MulQueen smelled a rat and he was looking for some answers.

That's because as the sign on the fence indicated, the City of Detroit Water and Sewer Department was in charge of the operation. Therein lay the problem.

The City controlled the water and sewer systems for all of Metro Detroit and they had hired the same company to fix this break – and a previous break the year before – the same company the City hired to construct the entire defective sewer lines in the first place.

The biggest problem was when you said City of Detroit, you meant one thing – Detroit Mayor Coleman A. Young. The kingmaker extraordinaire, his control over the City put Mayor Daley of Chicago and Mayor Lindsay in New York to shame. It was his show. And you best not challenge him.

But Dennis MulQueen was eager to try. This situation made no sense to him.

He knocked on the trailer door and a middle-aged guy in a white hard hat answered the door and wanted to know who he was and what he wanted.

Dennis asked him details of the project, and what the likelihood was of a total catastrophic collapse which engineers and county and city officials were predicting.

Then he wanted to know how the same company that built the pipe was hired to repair two multi-million dollar breaks in the same line.

The guy he was talking to refused to be identified, and said the matter was simple: a "No Bid contract." Rules governing competitive bidding were thrown out the window because of the "emergency nature" of the situation.

Dennis thanked him, got a few more "official" statements on the situation, and climbed back over the fence and returned to the office to file his story.

The banner headline in the *Oakland Press* the next day read: "**Danger of Break Real, Kuhn Wants Probe of Sewer Bungling**." A big cutout quote from an engineer on site was blown up on the upper right of the page below a crane and piles of piping: "I think it's going to cave in. It's bad ... It could cave in tomorrow – Frank Bihl."

The journalism career at the *Oakland Press* was going great, he was getting lede story after lede story, and he thought it best to keep it going, so later that day he accepted the boss's invitation to work the cop beat on the weekend for extra cash. He was eager for any byline he could get even though he knew the 1980 Olympics were in progress.

When he walked in the downtown Pontiac Police Department that Friday, February 22, 1980, there they were in their red-white-and-blue uniforms plastered all over the TV screen above the main desk at the downtown Pontiac cop shop.

Erruzione and Craig and Pavelich and Broten – and numerous other kids, most between the ages of 18 and 21, because pro's were ineligible to play in the Olympics – had taken on what many still consider the greatest team ever assembled in any sport.

The US Olympic Hockey Team was playing the vaunted Red Army team that had won the previous four gold medals, a Soviet team with the best goalie in the world at the time, Vladislav Tretiak, with the best defense in the world lead by a guy named Viacheslav Fetisov, with elite scorers named Mikhailov, Kharlamov, Krutov, and Makarov, and the same long-time heralded coach in Viktor Tikhonov. They were by consensus considered the best team in history.

But this was a group of determined kids from the US who responded with zeal to the skating system and impassioned motivational speeches of Team USA Coach Herb Brooks, who personally spent a year preparing these youngsters he had hand-picked for the team.

The Soviets had crushed the USA team – with an average age of 21, the youngest Olympic team in US history – by a score of 10-3 in an exhibition game leading up to the games that counted on the Olympic schedule. This was the same Soviet team that the previous year routed a team of NHL All-Stars 6-0 to win the Challenge Cup.

Before the game, Brooks read his players a statement he had written out on a piece of paper, telling them that "You were born to be a player. You were meant to be here. This moment is yours."

Despite virtually everybody in the world feeling otherwise, Brooks truly believed his team could beat the Soviets. The young kids he personally recruited for the team believed him when he told them that, and bought into his system of relentless attack and fast skating and hard driving style that saw the guys fall behind early in the first period but with ferocious will power climb back in it.

Erruzione scored in the third period to break a 3-3 tie and put the Yanks up 4-3 with only minutes to play.

Brooks could be heard urging his players behind the bench to "keep playing your game, keep playing your game." Instead of sitting back in a defensive shell, the Americans kept pushing the pace and stayed on the attack and kept taking the play to the Russians which prevented the Soviets from unleashing the most potent puck possession offense in the world.

It was like a different version of the "shot heard round the world" as broadcaster Al Michaels counted down the final seconds of the game: "Eleven seconds, you've got ten seconds, the countdown going on right now! Morrow, up to Silk, five seconds left in the game. Do you believe in Miracles? Yes!"

The final score remained 4-3 for the Americans, a victory still considered by many to be the greatest upset in sports history.

The USA team then went on to beat Finland 4-2 for the Gold Medal.

Afterward, Brooks said, "The Russians were ready to cut their own throats. But we had to get to the point we were ready to pick up the knife and hand it to them. So the morning of the game I called the team together and told them, 'It's meant to be. This is your moment and it's going to happen.' It's kind of corny and I could see them thinking, 'Here goes Herb again.' But I believed it."

And so did they. A classic case of the Power of Positive Thinking overcoming impossible odds.

But Dennis MulQueen missed it that day – the Miracle On Ice – for nothing.

All the cops must have been hockey fans. There was hardly a ticket written, let alone an arrest – or anything else worth a story that day.

In the meantime, one week later, on February 29ᵗʰ, 1980, Gordie Howe became the first pro hockey player to ever score 800 goals.

Dennis missed that one, too, driving back from an out-of-town assignment.

But he would always have the memories.

Every time he thought of Gordie, he would see his Dad's face with that shake-and-bake hand-bob thing of his going and that belly-laugh-to-end-all-belly-laughs telling Hurricane Hec Kilrea that story about Gordie versus the Toronto Maple Leafs' Bobby Baun.

~ ~ ~

What happens when a priest leaves the priesthood for the entertainment world? He becomes a rock star.

That's certainly what it looked like.

The place was rocking to the tune of several thousand mostly drunk, mostly young revelers – packed like dots in a box into a huge sweaty hall on Telegraph Ave in suburban Detroit, Michigan.

So this is what can happen to you if you're not careful when you leave the priesthood for the entertainment world.

"What will we do with a drunken sailor?
What will we do with a drunken sailor?
What will we do with a drunken sailor?
Early in the morning!

"Way hay and up she rises,
Way hay and up she rises,
Way hay and up she rises,
Early in the morning!

Shave his belly with a rusty razor,
Shave his belly with a rusty razor,"
"Shave em with a rusty razor,
Early in the morning."

He spotted Dennis MulQueen saunter in with his girlfriend in hand and he waved from the stage – the former Fr. Pat McDunn, S.J., now Pat McDunn and the Gaels. The best teacher ever. Bar none. Now up on stage showing off his singing and carousing and smooching talent, with the best of them. All the while having the time of his life – and making tons of money doing it.

It didn't take much to see this one coming. The incompatibility with the Jesuit lifestyle was all too obvious. So McDunn left the order in the '70s and became a lay teacher at another great Metro Detroit institution, Brother Rice High School, run by the Christian Brothers of Ireland.

He married, had children, and became a tremendous success as a musician. And always a great teacher of men. Beautifully, it never went to his head.

"There he is, Dennis MulQueen, they gave him a day pass. He's out of Lyster College for the day so he could join us here. This one's for you, MulQueen. Good to see you, Dennis."

Then he broke into a rousing chorus of *The Merry Ploughboy*.

"I'm tired of this civilian life,
Since the day that I was born,
So I'm off to join the IRA,
And I'm off tomorrow morn'."

"And we're all off to Dublin in the green,
Where the helmets glisten in the sun,
Where the bay'nets clash,
and rifles crash,
to the echo of the Thompson gun.

"And when the war is over,
and dear old Ireland is free

355

I'll take her to the church to wed
and a rebel's wife she'll be
Well some men fight for silver
and some men fight for gold
But the IRA are fighting for the land
that the Saxon's stole.

How could it be less? It was St. Patrick's Day. Everybody laughed, everybody danced. And everybody had to have a healthy helping of corned beef and cabbage.

Couldn't be better. Until later on. In the car.

In the driveway. When they talked.

And broke up.

It was quite simple. They had a great time together – but there was no future.

She blurted it out of nowhere, that her Dad expected him to convert, and soon, if he was going to be with his daughter long term.

That threw him for a loop and he rebelled.

Wait a minute, he said. My next door neighbor Nate Garfinkel, he's a Holocaust survivor – and he celebrates both Christmas and Hanukkah.

I didn't demand that you become a Catholic, he told her. I would never do that.

He left out the part that he couldn't do that because he didn't believe in any of that either. The only time he ever went to church was to please his parents at major holidays.

How can it be more important anyway to join one organization over another when both purport to have the same God?

Well, that's the way it is, she said.

So that was that.

Ahh, where would we be without organized religion? And all those wars it has helped us fight?

Just business as usual.

Big business, right Ike?

~ ~ ~

Gordie Howe skated off the NHL ice for the final time on April 6, 1980, finishing his record 26th season, age 52. The greatest and longest run in professional sports history was officially over.

George MulQueen was correct. Nobody could ever compete at that level. Or ever would. At that age. In any pro sport. Any where, any time.

He tallied 41 points in his final year in the NHL, including 15 goals, making his final NHL totals 801 goals and 1,049 assists. That's 1,850 points in 1,757 games. Including his World Hockey Association days, the totals would be 2,358 points in 2,186 games.

His WHA team won the League championship the first three years Howe was on it, the last one coming when he was 48 years old. Gordie Howe, the Lafitte Rothschild of pro sports.

Those WHA numbers should count, too. Those teams had players like Gretzky and Howe and when they merged into the NHL as expansion teams they were immediately competitive. Gordie liked to point out the one year his WHA team played six exhibition season games against NHL teams, his team was 5-1. That's the League Gordie – at age 49 – had 100 points in.

Just as Gordie Howe's epic sports marathon was ending that April, another famous sports marathon involving another soon-to-be-iconic Canadian was just beginning.

Gordie would be the first to admit this marathon was going to be a physical – and mental – feat of endurance and strength and courage as great as any ever pulled off by any professional athlete.

This amazing feat was designed to last less than one year – and on one leg. But a marathon all right – an actual 26.2 mile run every single day for the estimated eight months it would take to run clear across North America, from one ocean to the other – an historic run all the way across Gordie's native Canada, from the North Atlantic to the North Pacific.

That's 26.2 miles per day for a total of more than 3,000 miles run from the starting line in Nova Scotia to the finishing line in British Columbia.

A run based on hope – hope for brighter days ahead for millions – hope not for just millions in Canada, but millions in North America, and before it was over, with all the publicity, hope for everybody the world over. Including for George MulQueen.

But hope most of all for the one-legged guy attempting the feat.

An amazing achievement for anybody to attempt – let alone a guy with one leg.

It all started back in 1976, when an 18-year-old college freshman was driving to his house in Port Coquitlam, British Columbia, when he was distracted by bridge construction and slammed into the back of a truck.

He was lucky, he thought – he only hurt his knee in the accident.

But the knee continued to hurt.

He was a basketball player on his college team, though, so he kept playing and ignored the pain.

In March of 1977, the pain intensified and he couldn't ignore it any longer. He was forced to seek medical intervention.

Shortly thereafter, doctors diagnosed osteosarcoma, a bone cancer that frequently develops in the knee area. He underwent an amputation and subsequent to that 16 months of chemotherapy.

Shortly afterward, he was recruited to play for a national wheelchair basketball team. He won three national championships and that's when he first heard of another amputee named Dick Traum, who was the first amputee to complete the New York City Marathon.

That's all that was needed to plant the seed.

The guy immediately set about making it happen, with the same determination he showed in just about anything he ever did. First he wrote the Canadian Cancer Society seeking funding and their support of an across-Canada run to raise money for cancer research.

In the letter he recounted his own experiences as a cancer patient when during "the 16 months of the physically and emotionally draining ordeal of chemotherapy I was rudely awakened by the feelings that surrounded and coursed through the cancer clinic. There were faces with the brave smiles, and the ones who had given up smiling.

"There were feelings of hopeful denial, and the feelings of despair ... I could not leave knowing these faces and feelings would still exist," he wrote, "even though I would be set free from mine. Somewhere the hurting must stop ... and I was determined to take myself to the limit for this cause."

He concluded with these words:

"We need your help. The people in cancer clinics all over the world need people who believe in miracles. I am not a dreamer, and I am not saying that this will initiate any kind of definitive answer or cure to cancer. But I believe in miracles. I have to."

He was in luck. The Cancer Society said they would support his run if he got medical clearance and lined up sponsors.

So he sent out another letter seeking a grant for a prosthetic leg.

"I remember promising myself that, should I live, I would rise up to meet this new challenge of fundraising for cancer research face-to-face and prove myself worthy of life, something too many people take for granted."

His second letter also worked and a special prosthetic leg for the run was specially engineered and built for him by prosthetic specialist Ben Speicher of Vancouver, British Columbia.

Then it was on to the next hurdle. He sent more letters seeking corporations to back him. Ford Motor Company was first in line, donating a special camper van for his cross country feat. Adidas agreed to sponsor him and contribute free shoes. And Imperial Oil agreed to sponsor free fuel to make the journey. Isador Sharp, a hotel magnate who had recently lost a son to melanoma, heard about this guy and offered free food and lodging at all of his Four Seasons hotels across Canada.

So with everything set, amid little fanfare, on April 12, 1980, this man by the name of Terry Fox dipped his new prosthetic right leg into the Atlantic Ocean near St. John's Newfoundland and thus began "The Marathon of Hope."

Fox filled two large bottles with ocean water. One was for a souvenir, and the other was to pour into the other big ocean, the Pacific, in a symbolic co-mingling of the waters upon completing his journey at Victoria, British Columbia.

His best buddy, Doug Alward, agreed to accompany him and drive the specially equipped Ford van.

Dennis MulQueen and his father were in Canada at their cottage that weekend and watched the spectacle kick off on television, sharing the excitement felt across Canada for Terry Fox and his courage and determination.

"I hope he gets his miracle, because that's what it takes for us guys" George MulQueen said that day from the black leather living room couch.

Terry Fox made Dennis think of Richard White.

Just then, out of nowhere his father looked at him and said, "Remember Richard White?"

That was the young Ferndale lad his mother took him to see as a child who lost his leg to osteosarcoma and later died from the disease. The same disease Terry Fox suffered from. Not that Dennis MulQueen needed any heightened interest, with his father now in the seventh year of his own marathon fight, but Dennis followed the Marathon of Hope on and off for most of the summer – he couldn't not follow it.

The coverage started out slowly but soon began to pick up to the point where it seemed like Terry Fox was on the CBC every night, not to mention regular radio spots and blanket coverage in the Windsor Star and the Canadian newspapers. And every time he saw or heard anything about Terry Fox, Dennis thought of Richard White – and his father.

In less than a month, on June 7, Fox hit his all-time high of 30 miles (48 km) in one day.

Despite the rigors of running an entire marathon each day Fox tenaciously kept at it and arrived in Montreal on June 22, with about a third of his journey already completed.

By now, the entire nation of Canada was paying attention, as were many south of the border and around the world as well.

On the last Saturday in June, Terry Fox made it to the Canadian capital of Ottawa, where the streets were lined with thousands of supporters and he met face-to-face with Prime Minister Pierre Trudeau.

And oh, how about those hockey players.

On July 11, a crowd of 10,000 cheering supporters met him in Toronto, where he was joined by National Hockey League star Darryl Sittler of the Maple Leafs, who presented Fox with his 1980 All-Star Game jersey.

A little farther down the road, he was met by Hockey Hall of Famer Bobby Orr, who presented him with a check for $25,000. The Great One, superstar Wayne Gretzky, also visited Fox along the way and gave him one of his sweaters.

No offense, Mr. Prime Minister, or Mr. Great One, but Terry Fox said meeting Bobby Orr was the highlight of his run.

~ 26 ~

MAKE AMERICA GREAT
AGAIN

This time the wall-to-wall pandemonium inside Joe Louis Arena had nothing to do with Gordie Howe or the Detroit Red Wings.

The "sit on my face" seat cushions told the story of this gathering.

When Dennis MulQueen walked inside the Joe and noticed the red-and-white plastic seat adornments scattered about, he figured it was going to be brutal – and it was.

"Sit on my face" was printed on the cushions above a caricature of a donkey with a head that looked like the sitting US President Jimmy Carter.

A tall, handsome, charismatic B-grade actor from California stood center stage at the podium and smiled as he regaled the cheering, colorful, sign-waving crowd with promises of a great life ahead.

"For those who have abandoned hope, we'll restore hope and we'll welcome you into a great national crusade to make America great again," said the up and coming GOP icon Ronald Reagan. The former California governor was at the Joe for the 1980 GOP convention to accept the Republican presidential nomination to run against President Carter.

Reagan and his fellow GOP brethren gathered at the Joe didn't spare Carter a lick. Republican after Republican took to the podium to expound on the official theme of the 1980 Republican party platform – "Make America Great Again" – by relentlessly bashing the beleaguered Jimmy Carter.

The official Grand Old Party platform, approved by delegates as the first order of business on Day One, lambasted Carter for the stalled economy that centered around the Arab oil embargo and a vulnerable foreign affairs performance highlighted by the ongoing Iran hostage crisis.

"In his first three years in the White House, Mr. Carter reduced defense spending by over $38 billion..." the platform stated.

"He cancelled production of the Minuteman missile and the B-1 bomber. He delayed all cruise missiles, the MX missile, the Trident submarine and the Trident II missile ...

"Mr. Carter postponed production and deployment of enhanced radiation (neutron) warheads ... He vetoed a nuclear aircraft carrier."

All this, the Republicans warned, while "The entire western world faces complex and multi-dimensional threats to its access to energy and raw material resources.

"The growth of Soviet military power poses a direct threat to the petroleum resources of the Persian Gulf now that its military forces deployed in Afghanistan are less than 300 miles from the Straits of Hormuz."

Since Carter took over in 1977, the Republicans went on to say, "The Soviets or their clients have taken over Afghanistan, Cambodia, Ethiopia, and South Yemen, and have solidified their grasp on a host of other nations in the developing world. The Soviet noose is now being drawn around southern Africa, the West's most abundant single source of critical raw materials."

Ironically, the 1980 GOP delegates included a special section on "Freedom in America" in their platform.

"The essence of freedom is the right of law-abiding individuals to life, liberty, and the pursuit of happiness without undue governmental intervention. Yet government in recent years, particularly at the federal level, has overwhelmed citizens with demands for personal information and has accumulated vast amounts of such data through the IRS, the Social Security Administration, the Bureau of the Census, and other agencies.

"We are alarmed by Washington's growing collection and dissemination of such data. There must be protection against its misuse or disclosure. The Republican Party commits itself to guaranteeing an individual's right of privacy."

The 1980 GOP platform's concluding statement read: "By reversing our economic decline, by reversing our international decline, we can and will resurrect our dreams.

"And so, in this 1980 Republican Platform, we call out to the American people: With God's help, let us now, together, make America great again; let us now, together, make a new beginning."

Aside from the political bashing, the biggest drama was over who was going to be the VP. There was a huge movement to make former President Gerald Ford of Michigan Vice President. Reagan wanted his friend Sen. Paul Laxalt of Nevada, but the GOP bigwigs said, please, no way, a guy that's from a state with legalized prostitution and legalized gambling is not a guy we want to be talking about during the campaign.

Reagan-Ford was considered a "dream ticket" but it would be the first time a former president returned as vice president.

Ford was interviewed by Walter Cronkite of CBS News during the convention and he sounded like he wanted to be more than your typical vice president.

Reagan was watching from his suite at the Westin Hotel in Detroit's downtown Renaissance Center and he heard everything Ford said. His aides reported he was not impressed. "Sounds like he wants to be co-president," Reagan was reported to have told one aide.

373

Game over.

For Ford.

The guy from Texas must have known something was up. The next to the last night of the convention, George H.W Bush was seen strolling down Monroe Street in Detroit's iconic Greektown neighborhood of shops and restaurants shaking hand after hand while introducing himself to total strangers. You would have thought he was running for President himself.

Reagan announced Bush as his VP choice later that night at almost midnight, from the Joe Louis convention floor.

The next day, in his acceptance speech, Reagan thanked Detroiters for their hospitality, and formally accepted the nomination while touting his selection of Bush as VP.

Then it was time to go after Carter again.

After focusing on the dismal economic times, exacerbated by the Arab Oil embargo and the long lines everywhere at gas stations and urban decay spreading and declining incomes and job levels mounting, he made the most out of it with another appeal to "make America great again" by electing him President.

"I pledge to you a government that will not only work well, but wisely, its ability to act tempered by prudence and its willingness to do good balanced by the knowledge that government is never more dangerous than when our desire to have it help us blinds us to its great power to harm us."

He asked for a new "compact" between government and the people.

These guys all have to have the same speech writers, Dennis MulQueen thought to himself as he listened to Reagan talk. Or it's just accepted business to plagiarize one another – throughout history, every four years, like a broken record, over and over and over.

Reagan wasn't done with all that.

"I ask you to trust that American spirit which knows no ethnic, religious, social, political, regional, or economic

374

boundaries; the spirit that burned with zeal in the hearts of millions of immigrants from every corner of the Earth who came here in search of freedom."

In his closing remarks, the great communicator said, "Can we doubt that only a Divine Providence placed this land, this island of freedom, here as a refuge for all those people in the world who yearn to breathe freely: Jews and Christians enduring persecution behind the Iron Curtain, the boat people of Southeast Asia, of Cuba and Haiti, the victims of drought and famine in Africa, the freedom fighters of Afghanistan and our own countrymen held in savage captivity.

"I'll confess that I've been a little afraid to suggest what I'm going to suggest – I'm more afraid not to – that we begin our crusade joined together in a moment of silent prayer.

"God bless America."

Human nature then took over – maybe it was the mention of the new crusade – but the delegates went nuts waving their flags and banners and jumping up and down and shouting "Reagan, Reagan, Reagan!" from the hallowed Joe Louis Arena floor.

The Gods must have heard. Or some special power that be that also really wanted Carter out. As if the Arab oil embargo and the American hostages still being held by the Iranians at the US Embassy were not enough to pre-determine the election outcome, there was Billy Gate.

The news broke at the convention that Carter's brother Billy was busted for being on the Libyan payroll. He accepted almost a quarter million dollar payment from Muammar al-Gaddafi for "lobbying."

Must have been when Billy would get drunk on all that Billy Beer, he thought he was a Secretary of State. Or maybe a President himself.

~ ~ ~

A couple of weeks later, in early August, Terry Fox had reached the Ontario town of Sudbury, as reports leaked out that almost four months of daily marathons were taking a heavy toll.

He suffered from shin splints, cysts on his stump, cramps and extreme pain and exhaustion from the summer heat. He was forced to seek medical help for the intense pain in his ankle, which he was relieved to learn was "only" tendinitis, treatable with steroids and pain meds.

But through it all, he never complained.

When asked in Sudbury about all the various issues he was facing, Fox would only say that nothing could compare to the almost 18 months of surgery and chemotherapy and other cancer treatments he had been through. Dennis MulQueen thought of his father again as he heard Fox interviewed on TV. How about my father's marathon now going on seven years, he asked himself?

Another journalist interviewing Fox in Sudbury asked if he was afraid he might not be able to finish.

He said he was taking it one step at a time, one mile at a time, but he was determined to stay on pace. He said matter of factly, the only thing he feared was not getting through the Rocky Mountains before the snow starts falling.

"You could be the richest man in the world but when I cross the finish line you couldn't buy what I am going to feel," Fox told the reporter for the *Ottawa Citizen* in Sudbury.

He might have kept it to himself, but inside he had to know what he was up against. That letter he wrote a long time ago spoke presciently of the reality of the cancer war he was now part of along with George MulQueen and millions of others.

"I'm not a dreamer ... But I do believe in miracles. I have to." he wrote to the cancer society people that day when he first proposed his "Marathon of Hope."

It wasn't going to get any easier, and he knew it.

Sure enough, his exhaustion continued to mount and on September 1, outside Thunder Bay, Ontario, he was forced to stop in the middle of the road from an intense coughing fit and pain in his chest.

He allowed himself a short break, and then got right back at it, out on the road running again as the near hysterical crowds on either side shouted him on.

Less than five miles later, however, he had to stop again, and this time he asked his friend and driver of the van, Doug Alward, to take him to the nearest hospital.

The next day, on September 2, 1980, Fox held a news conference outside the hospital and announced that the cancer had returned to his lungs. He said he was ending his run after 143 days and 2,570 miles covered.

He refused an offer from the hockey All-Star Sittler to complete the run in his stead. He said he hoped to recover and complete it himself.

"If there's any way I can get back out there and finish it, I will," Fox said.

He had already raised $1.7 million for cancer research, a sum that would soon be dwarfed by millions more in future contributions. The country of Canada continued to rally around their favorite son, and his cause, with a fervor never seen before.

~ 27 ~

LIFE IS A GOOD FIGHT

No wonder the MulQueens liked hockey. Like any good Irish gang, they liked to write, they liked to drink – and they liked to fight. It was in their blood.

The proof of course was in that Oak Park basement. The MulQueen rafter of fame down the steps and around the corner.

Hanging from the basement rafters alongside the Stanley-Cup-winning hockey gloves Hec Kilrea wore in Game 7 against Montreal still hung those two sets of very old boxing gloves, one set being from Grandpa MulQueen's days as a Golden Gloves boxer, the other George MulQueen Jr.'s from when he boxed in the Navy.

Not only was Chip MulQueen a terrific hockey player – he was a spark plug who always played with a fiery edge for the University of Detroit team – but Chip fought without gloves, or his would have to be part of the collection as well.

But make no mistake, Grandpa MulQueen was the undisputed king of the MulQueen fighting hill. George L. MulQueen Sr. was the MulQueen's Jack Dempsey, he was their John L. Sullivan. Or maybe he had a link to Muhammad Ali, whose grandfather was an Irishman from Ennis, Ireland, where the MulQueen family also originally came from.

For proof, look no further than the Detroit mayor's office.

This fight would be the MulQueen version of Joe Louis vs. Max Schmeling, or Ali-Frazier – only this fight only lasted one punch.

~ ~ ~

When George L. McQueen Sr. returned from WWI, where he was a pilot, he became politically active and became the long-serving president of the Ancient Order of Hibernians in Detroit.

Especially after the stock market crash in 1929 and the advent of the Great Depression, with jobs scarce and many families hurting, the AOH was a very important refuge for many in the struggling Detroit Irish community. And after Detroit Mayor Frank Murphy started the Irish political ascendency in Detroit politics back in the 1930s, the AOH gained even more clout as an important organization with influence over a critical block of voters.

As part of his AOH gig, Grandpa MulQueen regularly held weekend meetings at the house at 2828 Woodmere, in Southwest Detroit directly across from General George S. Patton Park, where jobs were discussed for neighborhood folks and organizing meetings set the political agenda for the Irish in the city. All this brought Dennis MulQueen's grandfather into regular contact with the top politicians in the Motor City, including a rising star in Detroit politics, a finance whiz named Albert Cobo.

Cobo, when he was city treasurer, an elected position at the time, attended a gathering at the Woodmere house one Saturday afternoon when George MulQueen Sr. demanded more city jobs for Irish workers.

"You goddamned Micks already have enough jobs in the city," Cobo said.

George MulQueen Sr. jumped up from the head of the dining room table, walked over to Cobo and knocked him out cold right then and there with a vicious over hand right, and there he laid bleeding from the nose on the MulQueen's brand new dining room rug, in front of a roomful of people including a couple aides who helped him to his feet and out the front door.

It would be a knockout punch forever famous in the MulQueen lore as Cobo, who was elected Detroit Treasurer in 1933 and went on to get elected Mayor of Detroit in 1949, would go down in history as the most racially divisive, polarizing, race-baiting politician in the long history of the Motor City.

"If you were there you would have done the same thing," George L McQueen Jr. said as he recalled Grandpa MulQueen's exploits to his son Dennis.

Well, brother Chip, I'm sure he would have knocked Cobo out as well. But Dennis MulQueen, maybe not.

Genes work in a funny way. Dennis MulQueen was taller and bigger and stronger and plenty fast enough, and he never backed down from anybody, and he certainly could take a punch. But he was never going to take his place in that line of accomplished Irish MulQueen fighters. Chip proved that growing up. He regularly beat the hell out of Dennis, who just didn't have the hand/foot speed to compete with a fighter of his older brother's talent. Chip's hands were so fast and his state meet high hurdle thighs so powerfully agile he would hit Dennis five times before he could even move. Dennis would have to run into his parent's bedroom and jump on the bed in the corner against the walls and do the rope-a-dope on his back with his legs to protect himself from getting killed.

Truth is, Dennis acted like he was walking the walk, because he was surrounded by it and he had to act the part, but inside he was really a pacifist. That would be an entirely euphemistic way of describing what happened that cold winter day at the Oak Park ice rink. Dennis had finished playing his Bantam hockey game, and he and his mother were standing behind the net at one end of the rink watching Chip's game when a local ruffian named Dale Camacho walked by them and spit on the ground in their direction narrowly missing his mother. Dennis stood there like

381

Ernie Harwell's "house beside the road" as his mother turned and glared at him.

Chip knew Camacho, they had already had a couple run-ins, and after he skated over to them after the game his mother informed him what his buddy Carmacho had just done.

"Did you beat the hell out of him, Denny?"

Now Dennis MulQueen stared silently at the ground with his head downcast like one of the Fatima nuns in church.

"Well? You better go find him and take care of this. Nobody is allowed to spit at our mother."

Inside the rink after unlacing his skates, Chip came running up to his little brother. "There he is. He's leaving now. Go take care of him."

Dennis MulQueen followed Carmacho out of the clubhouse and confronted him in the yard.

"Hey, Carmacho, why don't you spit at me and my mother again," he said. Carmacho turned around and bull rushed Dennis MulQueen and violently took him down on the ground, and now on top of him proceeded to methodically pound on Dennis MulQueen's head and every place else. He was trapped on the ground underneath a feared bully who outweighed him by about 50 pounds.

All of a sudden out of nowhere Chip MulQueen appeared from behind and grabbed Carmacho by the throat and ripped him off of his fallen brother and said, "Hey, fat boy, why don't you pick on somebody your own size?"

Chip MulQueen mercilessly beat the living hell out of Carmichael and only a passing adult who broke it up spared Carmichael an ambulance trip to the hospital. As it was, Carmichael's face was already a disaster, blood pouring out of his nose and his mouth, his fat lower lip split open in several places like an overcooked sausage.

So fast forward a couple decades, given that MulQueen affinity for fighting, what better way to celebrate a milestone birthday than with a good fight?

That's exactly what happened. Minus the good fight part.

On October 2, 1980, George L. MulQueen Jr.'s birthday, when they got the presents and the chocolate bumpy cake and the chocolate marshmallow ice cream out of the way, Chip, Dennis, and their father plopped down in front of the living room Zenith in anticipation of a classic bout.

It wasn't to be.

If you are a Muhammad Ali fan, which Dennis decidedly was – or a fight fan of any ilk – it wasn't much of a fight at all. This was like Chip versus Carmichael. Or George L. MulQueen Sr. against Cobo.

This was a travesty of brutal proportions.

Larry Holmes said it all without uttering a word when in one of the later rounds after repeatedly pummeling Muhammad Ali in the corner, he turned his gloves over and raised his hands in the air as he nodded his head and stared at the referee.

He punished Ali at will, repeatedly rocking the greatest's head back with lightning quick vicious left-hand jabs that kept coming like the *rat-a-tat-tat* of one of those Thompson guns Roger McCarville liked to sing about. Long past his prime, Ali was quite simply defenseless from start to finish.

Holmes earned a unanimous decision when the referee finally did step in and stopped the carnage in the 11th round. It never should have gone that far.

The public didn't know it, but months before this fight Ali had already begun showing signs of Parkinson's Disease. His fight doctor for many years, Dr. Ferdie Pacheco, quit several months in advance of the fight in protest of his guy continuing to get in the ring.

All the while, George L. MulQueen Jr. valiantly continued his fight, because – like Terry Fox said – there's no choice but to believe in miracles.

He continued to beat the odds, officially making it this October 2, 1980, to 58 years of age.

He was losing weight. Dennis could tell. Anybody could tell.

In fact, Dennis complimented him on it. "You look like you are in really good shape, Dad."

His father said nothing, continuing to look straight ahead at the TV screen. Moms Mabley peered at Dennis from the far corner of the room with a funny look on her face.

Otherwise, it was a good birthday – despite the brutal fight.

~ 28 ~

ADULTERY

John Lennon could have written his melodic and beautifully poetic song "Across The Universe" for exactly this moment. The huge white letters pasted high in the New York sky were indeed soon to slither on and off across that universe.

But not before the giant letters sculpted in the sky above like designer cotton candy clouds sent their message to all of New York City, and the world: "Happy birthday John and Sean, Love, Yoko." It was Thursday, October 9, 1980, and Yoko had hired an airplane skywriter to serenade the two men of her life with her sky-high birthday message.

John turned 40 this day, and it was Sean's fifth birthday. Her two Johns had the exact same birthday, and that was no coincidence as Sean was born by Caesarean section.

The occasion brought the fans out to the Dakota in droves. Yoko made an appearance on the roof with Sean and hollered down to the crowd that John was asleep, so they needn't bother waiting around all day. He had been recording all night again at the Record Factory, working on the Double Fantasy album set to come out soon.

Meanwhile, hundreds of miles away in Oak Park, Michigan, the sky was clear that day but Dennis MulQueen also knew what day it was the minute he got in his car in the morning and flipped on the dial.

"You say it's your birthday,
We're going to have a good time ..."

The local DJ's knew what day it was – this classic Beatles tune was the first song he heard that morning on his way in to the office, followed by a slew of other Lennon-authored tunes.

A day like this calls for a little celebrating, Dennis MulQueen said to himself at the end of a good day's work at the paper. When he strolled into the Mill Street Inn about 6 p.m., he immediately spotted Roger McCarville camped out at a booth along the far wall. No singing tonight, it was a weeknight.

He was sitting with Gary Bainbridge, a local insurance salesman, and another guy Dennis had seen in there before, a local cop.

"What are you doing out on a weeknight like this," Roger said. "Sit down and we'll have to discuss it."

It was easy to find Roger at the Mill Street on many nights. His company, Handicapped Transportation, had its offices in the same building across the hall from the bar, both the building and the bar owned by the same guy, Stan Stevens.

"Hey, it's John Lennon's birthday, gotta celebrate that, right?" Dennis said.

"It doesn't take much for you to celebrate then, does it? Forget that guy, Dennis. He is Irish and he has made a lot of great songs and made a lot of great contributions to the world but he is an atheist and an adulterer. I think he might have even neglected his first-born son. Other than that he's a great guy. How about celebrating something better. Like Tom Thum. He's bigger than Lennon, his birthday isn't just today, Tom Thum's birthday is celebrated the whole month of October."

"Oh yeah, Tom Thum? Who the heck is that, Roger?"

"You haven't heard of that guy? You must not be from Chicago. My relatives the Cronin's are from Chicago, Dennis. And it's also October in Chicago, you know. Nothing like it. All of October is Tom Thum Month in all of Chicago. That guy is my hero. Heck, he should be everybody's hero."

"Oh really? How come I haven't heard of him?"

"Because you're from Detroit, Dennis. You writers don't know nothin'," he said as he waved his right hand in the air at Dennis MulQueen. "You spend too much time in places like this, with you head in the sand. No, make that a bucket of Guinness. Speaking of which," Roger McCarville said as he banged his nearly empty pint glass on the table three times in rapid succession. "Hey, over there behind the bar," he said, "wake up, Stan. Let's please have another round of Guinness over here plus one."

He tilted his head back and drained the remaining dregs of black foam from his glass.

"Let me tell you why this guy's my hero, Dennis. This guy did it every day. Hands on. He sacrificed. He worked on practicing what he preached on a daily basis. He was true to himself every single day and what he believed in. His was not a fair weather calling. He was the rarest of the rare – a true believer, in himself, in humanity in general but most of all in the good Lord above. The hell with everything and everybody else."

"Oh yeah, what did he do?" Dennis said.

"He was a clown."

The whole table split up uproariously in unison, like a Rowan and Martin laugh track on max volume. Half the bar was now looking their way.

"Toughest job in the world," Roger McCarville said.

"Then I must be a hero, too, Roger," Dennis MulQueen said. "I'm a pretty good clown myself. And I work at it every day, too."

"No, this guy actually was a real professional clown, Dennis. He did clown shows all around town. I mean in addition to his day job. Really special shows for the kids, I'm talking troubled kids at juvenile homes, abandoned kids at orphanages, disabled kids in institutions, and he didn't just entertain them.

"He nurtured them and took them into his own house and gave them hope. He raised them, actually, dozens and dozens of them over the years as foster kids, and he used money from his day job to take care of them and feed and house them and send them back off into the big bad world out there where they were now prepared to withstand man's inhumanity to man and spread the message on their own."

A pretty blonde waitress arrived tableside with a fresh tray of Guinness's.

"Thank you, ma'am. Put it on my tab, please."

"Now what could be better than that," McCarville continued, as he hoisted a nice fresh dark glass full to the brim.

"Ahh, except for maybe this."

He took a swig of the creamy black nectar and set the glass down on the shiny lacquered wooden table with a clank of authority.

"But seriously, Dennis, how many guys you know like that? The hell with those Beatles, forget Elvis and Al Kaline, this guy is a real hero. Let's have a toast to Tom Thum."

All four of the guys raised their glasses simultaneously.

The ever-observant Roger McCarville licked the foam remnants from his lips as he pointed to a booth kitty-corner from their table.

"Okay, so I lied. That's my real hero," he said, nodding in that direction.

Dennis turned and looked.

"Oh jeez. She could be my hero, too," Dennis MulQueen said. "Everybody needs a hero like that."

"She is staring holes through you, Dennis."

"They all do, Roger."

"Forget that Lennon guy, now we know why you really came out tonight," Roger McCarville said.

The woman caught them looking at her; she had to figure they were talking about her too. She had long, dark tresses, olive-colored skin, very nice features, about mid-20s in appearance, maybe Italian, maybe Albanian, maybe a touch of Spanish Irish.

Dennis briefly locked eyes with her on a second gander.

About two minutes later she sauntered over to their table.

She was a very attractive woman, in very good shape. She reminded him of Stephanie Powers of "The Girl From Uncle" TV series. Everybody has an ideal and attractive brunettes were it for him. It must be the Oedipal thing.

His mother actually was a brunette. They were best friends, and she really was his ideal. Not only was she beautiful, but she was also classy, intelligent, funny, but moreover very strong in her beliefs and very tough. And successful. Her most stunning attribute was her character. She was a really extraordinary woman.

He didn't know about this woman, but at least she had the hair and the smile going for her, he said to himself as he broke out in a grin.

She introduced herself as Carol, an employee of the City of Pontiac in the engineering department. Several drinks later, after Roger and Gary and the cop had departed, they left together and ended up at a motel on Dixie Highway about 10 minutes away from the bar.

She was a woman on a mission. She attacked him. She ended up on top of him on the bed and he couldn't resist her, as his Number One weakness conquered his judgement once again. He was yet to learn how to say no to a beautiful woman.

Soon thereafter, before any Catholic guilt feelings had a chance to simmer to the surface, it was time to take her back to Mill Street to get her car.

Once they were back on the highway, she instructed him to turn right, the opposite direction from the Mill Street Inn.

"Are you taking us to a restaurant?"

"No, we're heading toward my house."

"What about your car? I thought we were going back to the Mill Street."

"No, I came to the bar with a girlfriend."

"Oh, okay."

She gave him more directions. Turn right here. Turn left the next street. Straight ahead six blocks. Turn right again. Okay, stop here.

"In the middle of the street?"

"Yes."

"Which house is yours.? Is that it right there, the white one? I'll pull in the driveway and maybe I will walk you to the door like the gentleman that I am."

"My house is back there. About three houses back there. This is fine right here."

"Huh? Wait a minute, why are you opening the door?"

"I'm getting out here so he won't see me."

"He won't see you? What? What are you talking about?"

"My husband. He's home now."

"Your husband? You've got to be kidding me. You didn't tell me —"

She cut him off instantly with an arm wave, and although she closed the door gently it felt to him like she had just slammed it in his face.

"*Shhhh.* I don't want him to hear you. It's quiet out here."

It was very quiet now. He was speechless. He gripped the steering wheel like it was a life ring keeping him from drowning in a sea of his own stupidity. That's how he felt. I can't get away with anything, he said to himself. I have to pay in spades – for everything.

Then she blurted out the reason he got sucked in.

"He's having an affair on me. I see you on the front page every day of the paper, I see your picture inside with your column, you're a star, I know you're going to be on the TV and the radio if you're not already. I just wanted it to be a level playing field. I'll tell you the truth, I just wanted to know what it feels like to be a woman again. And it feels pretty darn good, Dennis. I want to thank you for a wonderful time. I desperately needed this, Dennis, and I need it again. I mean I would like to stay in touch and see you again."

Why, so you can cheat on me the next time? He bit his tongue.

She fumbled in her purse for a moment then extended her right arm toward him with a white business card in her outstretched fingers.

"I haven't felt this good in a long, very long time. Thank you, Dennis. You are a very special man, I knew that instantly. Let's talk. Please call."

Yeah, real special. Her hand was still extended toward him with the business card in the air. He released his grip on the steering wheel and snatched it from her.

"Oh great. Now I'm an adulterer. Thanks, Carol," he said. "I just have one question. Why wouldn't you just divorce him, rather than play a game like this, a game I ended up playing with you?"

He didn't wait for her to answer.

"Good bye," he said.

He left her standing there in the road like a fence post as he crumpled the card up in a ball and threw it out the window in her direction as he slammed the gas pedal to the floorboard not caring who might hear those squealing tires on that cold hard pavement as he took off like a bat out of hell in the wee-hour pitch-black darkness of the Pontiac night.

~ ~ ~

When he exited the bathroom in his robe that morning his mother met him in the hallway lest she forget to hand him an envelope.

"I was asleep last night when you got home. I didn't even hear you. I was exhausted. I had to take your dad in again last night when you were gone."

"Oh jeez. Back in Sinai?"

"Yes. He's back in Sinai. He was getting dizzy and running a fever, he could barely walk, his gums were bleeding. We both knew."

He looked at her and said nothing.

"Your father is not in very good shape, Denny. He's on borrowed time, we all know that."

He shook his head back and forth.

"Terrible," he said.

She turned to walk away, then froze. "I will give you his room number."

"Thanks Mom. I'm going to run in and take care of a couple things for the weekend paper and then I will pop over to Sinai on the way home to see him."

"That would be great."

"By the way," she said, "that came in the mail yesterday. You better open it. It is from the Secretary of State.

"Okay. Thanks Mom."

He ripped the envelope open as soon as he got in the car.

A one-page letter inside informed him his license was suspended for failing to pay a ticket.

Instead of taking Coolidge north almost five miles to Woodward, he turned left on Nine Mile West and then north on Greenfield Road to the local Secretary of State's office.

There was nobody in line. He handed the lady behind the counter the envelope and his license and got his checkbook out. He signed and paid up and as he turned to leave she called out for him to wait.

She walked off and returned about half a minute later with a single piece of paper she handed him.

"Now, keep this in your glove box as it might take a month to six weeks or more to clear this suspension off of your record on the computer up in Lansing," she said. "In case you get stopped, just give them this piece of paper. It's an official document verifying that your suspension has been lifted. Our seal is on the document."

"Okay. Thank you very much, ma'am."

He was obviously late getting into the office, but it turned out to be a mostly uneventful day anyway. He spent the morning making calls to line up sources, and soon after an afternoon strategy session with his partner and the managing editor on an upcoming investigative project, it was time to head to the Mill Street for a little courage before heading over to Sinai to see his father.

He got to the club early, a little before five.

Pretty soon, after three Harvey Wallbangers, he looked at his watch and realized it was time to go. He said goodbye and as he was leaving he stumbled and almost tripped over a chair partially sticking out of the end booth near the front door just as Roger McCarville was walking in the door. Three Wallbangers inside of an hour will do that to you.

"Drive carefully there, okay, Dennis," Roger McCarville said.

"Okay, Roger, I will. Thank you."

"Sure you can't stay a while to cool down before driving home? I got a couple new jokes I wanna try out on you."

"I would love to, Roger, but I'm not driving home. My Dad is in the hospital again with real high counts and bleeding and a fever. I'm headed straight to the hospital. I gotta get down to see him before something happens."

"Oh my. What's kind of cancer is that your Dad has again, Dennis? Did you say leukemia?"

"Yes, chronic lymphocytic leukemia, CLL. He's had it going on seven years now, which is a long time for any kind of cancer, I guess. He's got a bad case of it. Some people live 20 years with it, I'm told. There are different grades of it, but it's not looking like that for him."

"Yeah, okay, Dennis. Be careful now. I'll say some prayers for you guys, okay?"

"Thanks, Roger. Sure could use 'em."

They said goodbye again and he was back behind the wheel of his new two-tone silver-blue and navy-blue Tornado cruising down Woodward when not five minutes into the drive he spotted a hitchhiker on the side of the road where Wide Track Drive accesses Woodward Avenue, a major four-lane boulevard running north and south from downtown Detroit to Pontiac.

Dennis never met a hitchhiker he didn't feel sorry for. Must have something to do with Birdsong Farms and his Green Lantern jacket. He really shouldn't have been driving and he knew it. Maybe this guy can help me navigate, he rationalized to himself as he pulled over.

He reached across the front seat and popped the passenger door open. A plain-looking ordinary Joe dressed in a red and blue checkered shirt and blue jeans jumped in.

"Thanks, man," he said.

"You're welcome. I'm headed down Woodward and then over to Oak Park. Will that cover you?"

"Yeah, man, that'll be great. I'm going that way. I'll let you know when it's time to hop out, okay?"

"Sounds good."

He flipped the radio on and concentrated on the road. John Lennon's voice immediately filled the car with "Instant Karma" about to get you. That would be an omen he failed to grasp.

There was no conversation with the hitchhiker to his right.

Suddenly, about 10 minutes and two songs later, the guy came alive and pointed frantically to the left and blurted out, "Hey man, turn left right here at this opening here. This is where I go, over there. I'll jump out about a couple blocks down, okay?"

It was the same feeling all over again, the same terror made famous in that rock and roll song about seeing the blue lights in the rearview mirror. They were barely in the middle of the intersection when the sirens rattled the car windows to go with the flashing lights. He pulled over and a youngish looking cop came up to the driver's side window.

"Hey, buddy, didn't you see that No Left Turn sign there? Give me your driver's license, registration, and proof of insurance."

"Sorry, officer, didn't see it."

"Have you ever been arrested before?"

"No, officer, I haven't."

"You been drinking tonight?"

"No, officer."

"Do you have any weapons in the car?"

"No sir, I don't."

He handed him the paperwork.

"Wait here and I'll be back in a few minutes."

"Okay, officer."

About five minutes later the police officer returned to the car with a distinctly different demeanor.

"Okay, buddy, get out of the car."

"Get out of the car, what for?"

"I said get out of the car and I mean now."

He opened the door and stood up.

"Okay, now close the door."

He closed the door.

"Now turn around."

"Officer, what the hell is going on?"

"Put your hands behind your back. You are under arrest. You are going to jail."

"Officer, what for?"

"Your license is suspended. You are driving on a suspended license. That's against the law. Now put your hands behind your back right now."

Dennis put his hands behind his back.

The cop retrieved his handcuffs from his belt.

Dennis had his hands about six inches apart behind his back. The handcuffs didn't quite reach. Then he remembered the piece of paper. The Harvey Wallbanger effect was probably responsible for the delayed recall.

"Officer, you can't arrest me. My license is not suspended."

Before he could even finish the sentence the cop shouted over him, "Look, I don't have time to listen to your bullshit. The law enforcement computer of the state of Michigan tells me your license is suspended and so your license is suspended, you understand? You are coming with me, pal. I said put your hands together."

"Officer, I have a document in my glove box stating that I have paid the ticket and my license is no longer suspended. I —"

The cop cut him off again.

"Put your hands together."

Dennis refused to put his hands together behind his back.

The cop grabbed his wrists and tried to force Dennis hands together behind his back.

Dennis was stronger than the cop and his hands didn't budge one inch closer together.

"Man, don't make me draw my weapon on you. This is your last chance, put your hands behind your back right now."

"Look, okay, my license is not suspended. You are going to find that out, if you insist on taking me in for no valid reason while I'm on my way to the hospital to see my father who is dying from cancer —"

"Nice try there. I don't need to hear any more of your bullshit, now are you going to cooperate or not?"

"Okay, I'll go with you," he said as he turned and started slowly walking toward the cop car.

Without handcuffs.

When he got to the cop car, he opened the back door himself and clambered inside without saying a word. Before he had a chance to straighten his legs the cop slammed the door behind him.

When they arrived at the station, there were several cops milling around in the booking room.

"You don't have handcuffs on him? How come?" said the older cop behind the desk with the big yellow sergeant bars on his uniform.

The officer that arrested Dennis MulQueen said nothing.

But in the bright lights of the police station you could almost see the steam of embarrassment rising from the back of the young arresting officer's neck.

His silent answer to the desk sergeant's question was explained by his next interactions with the arrested man he had just brought into the station sans handcuffs.

He grabbed Dennis MulQueen by the arms and spun him around towards the wall in front of the other cops in the room.

"Hands above your head against the wall and spread your legs," he sneered.

"What the fuck," Dennis said as he turned around to face the cop. At that exact moment the cop grabbed him and tried to forcefully turn Dennis around again and Dennis resisted the guy that was far less his equal physically and in an instant a violent scuffle broke out and a second cop in the room rushed over and jumped on Dennis' back. Dennis impulsively spun in a circle and the second cop was thrown up against the counter and the black fingerprint pad and the metal case that held it flew across the room and smashed into three pieces against the far wall and then Dennis felt a third cop tackle him from behind underneath and they all ended up on the floor in one happy pile punching and thrashing around violently on the floor as the shelf came crashing off the wall on top of them and they succeeded, the three cops together, in finally subduing him down on the floor after the third cop put him in a chokehold.

The guy behind the desk who was now in front of the desk said, "Cuff him and put leg restraints on him and take him to the county lockup. He has to be lodged over there now. Assault and battery of a police officer, that's a ten-year felony. And look at this shelf knocked off the wall all busted up and the fingerprint pad all busted up. Another felony.

Malicious destruction of police property. Two more felony counts right there. Two counts of malicious destruction of police property."

"Don't forget about resisting arrest," one of the cops chimed in.

"That's right,' the sergeant said. 'The county guys, they'll know what to do with him over there. I will call over there and warn them we've got a special delivery for them. I'll call the prosecutor's office first thing in the morning and we'll get everything taken care of after you guys file your reports. Let's go, guys. We gotta clean this mess up too. It looks like a Detroit riot in here."

Within the hour Dennis MulQueen was standing in the Oakland County Jail booking room with one cop on the right side of him and another behind him when out of the corner of his left eye he noticed a guy with tan slacks and brown shirt with the yellow star patches on the shoulders slowly advancing toward him from across the room.

Dennis was one foot from the counter, the wall behind him was 10 feet away.

The guy continued to walk straight at him. Dennis continued standing silently facing the glass wall and the lady behind the glass in front of him who was processing his paperwork before they threw him in the pokey.

Just as the deputy reached Dennis, he laid a vicious elbow into his left side.

"Oh, excuse me," he said with all the sincerity of a compulsive liar.

"Did you see that?" Dennis said to the lady behind the counter.

He turned and looked the deputy directly in the eyes. But otherwise he didn't move an iota.

"Nice try, officer," he said.

In short order after he was processed he was in the dog pen, about a 50' by 50' room with a tall ceiling that was like a small auditorium, filled with wall-to-wall prisoners, a room full of down-and-outers, mostly minorities, against the walls, on benches, sprawled out on the floor, everywhere, the few whites looking like they too just got out of rehab and also needed to take a shower and see a dentist.

His mother bailed him out in the morning and the minute he got home he went into the back bedroom to use the phone. He made one phone call and set up a meeting for later that day.

He drove to Pontiac, parked the car on Old Orchard Lake Road, and walked into the law offices of Elbert Hatchett for a one-on-one meeting.

He told Hatchett, a prominent attorney in Southeast Michigan at the time, about the illegal left turn he made, about the arrest, how the cop refused to look at the letter from the Secretary of State which he handed to Hatchett, and about getting roughed up at the police station. He added the part about the vicious elbow in his side at the Oakland County jail that felt like it broke a rib or two.

"False arrest and police brutality. I want to sue for both."

Hatchett leaned back in his maroon leather swivel chair with the indented bronze buttons and said, "I know you want to, Dennis, and I agree with you this is ridiculous, and your complaints are legitimate, but, Dennis, I'm sorry, you can't sue the police for this."

"What? You are joking, right?"

"No, Dennis, the police have government immunity. You can't sue them in this case even though your complaints are completely valid. I just looked at the document. I can see the bruises on your face and the marks on your neck. In fact, this is the same immunity a lot of the government employees have, Dennis. Sorry, that's just the way it is. You can't sue the police. They are immune. It's written into the law."

"Well, at least I got a few good shots in on them," he joked. "But seriously, what you are saying is they have no accountability and can do whatever they want, right, and get away with it?"

"That's the way it is, Dennis. I agree you were wronged, but again, it's just the way it is under the law."

"So what you are really saying is bad cops can brutalize people with no provocation and get away with it. What kind of government do we have in this country anyway? Is it really a democracy? What is that about a Constitution? And a Bill of Rights? Maybe the country needs to be renamed. And we need to get rid of a few statues, too. Like the one in the harbor with the torch that is supposed to stand for freedom. And justice. For all."

He wasn't done.

"But of course there's really no freedom or justice, is there Mr. Hatchett. And this really isn't a democracy, is it? As a black man, I'm sure you know that. Mr. Hatchett, we need change. Not the kind politicians talk about. I mean real change. If this country is going to make it."

~ 29 ~

LIFE IS A HERNIA

Better be careful. Don't want to get locked in here. This place would be tougher to break out of than Alcatraz. These aren't like those green doors in Oak Park. These are some big doors. Really big doors. About six inches thick. Gray, with a big black dial in the middle. Talk about a safe. What do they think this is, the Federal Reserve? Or a real bank, where the money has to be accounted for?

Actually, millions did move through those big doors. On a regular basis. This was the City of Pontiac safe, where all the records were kept. Now, about that being accounted for part.

He was only after an infinitesimally small part of that multi-million dollar pie. He was looking for receipts – specifically, expense reports involving an out-of-the-country trip by city officials. A tip came through that this was no ordinary trip. A Pontiac city councilman, a local promoter and the director of the Pontiac Silverdome, the home of the Detroit Pistons and the Detroit Lions, had travelled to Mexico City, Mexico, to supposedly arrange a fight at the Pontiac Silverdome between Pipino Cuevas, the Mexican champion, and Detroit's own superstar welterweight champion, Thomas Hearns.

Except the tipster claimed that wasn't what it was about at all. All three married guys took women with them who were not their wives. And they never met with any promoters on the trip, the anonymous tipster claimed.

The city editor of the paper, Tom the Bomb Walshinko, tapped Dennis MulQueen to get to the bottom of this one because he knew he would find whatever there was to be found, and verify everything methodically, especially if there was any stonewalling. He knew Dennis MulQueen would free dive to the bottom of the Mariana Trench for a great story. And surface with whatever there was to be had.

So here he was, up to his eyes in an ocean of paper, in the city of Pontiac safe, trying to do it the right way. Because he learned the right way, from the beginning, means knowing the answer to a question before you ask it. To preclude lies, and uncover truths yet unrecoverable.

He had the dates of the alleged trip, he just had to find the right box. Turned out not too tough, everything was in order. Five minutes in the vault, the evidence was right there, in his hands.

Like shooting canaries in a cage.

He looked at the documents.

The one expense report, dated 4-4-1980, in the name of Pontiac Silverdome Executive Director Charles McSwigan Jr., was from a restaurant named Pueblito Del Sol in Puerto Vallarta, Mexico.

The purpose was listed as "Discussion of Silverdome fight."

Those in attendance with Mr. McSwigan were listed as C. Valdazo and partner, promoter; Mr. Montoyo, also identified on the document as a promoter; Paul DiDio, a promoter; and Tom Padilla, City of Pontiac Commissioner.

Dennis MulQueen knew differently.

Valdazo and partner and Montoyo did not exist. These three were actually the three beautiful young women these married guys took with them on the trip which landed in Puerto Vallarta instead of Mexico City, where they were supposedly going to meet the promoter. Dennis interviewed one of the women, who was a waitress at the Pontiac Silverdome restaurant.

He never knew from the anonymous tip who specifically had blown the whistle. He would have guessed it to be one of the women. Maybe a promise not kept. A job promotion not forthcoming? That fury thing, right?. But the tip was nonetheless accurate, and Dennis had the goods. He hustled back to the office to share the good news.

Dennis and his partner quickly had it all laid out. Later on, when confronted, McSwigan, the head of the Silverdome, graciously admitted everything.

This became the lead story in the Thursday, November 20, 1980, *Oakland Press*. Another scalp on his belt, normally quite a thrill. This one felt different.

McSwigan was basically a decent guy. He had done a lot of good things for a lot of people over the years, but in this case, one mistake, one instance of very poor judgement and boom.

In an interview, he admitted he falsified the names to conceal the names of the three women, who were not their wives. Two months after the trip, McSwigan had second thoughts and repaid the city for expenses he said were personal. But the trip was still listed as "to meet a promoter in Mexico City to bring a Cuevas-Hearns fight to the Silverdome." They did fly to Mexico City for one day at the end of the trip, to supposedly meet promoter Rafael Mendoza – but he was in Texas that day promoting a fight for Cuevas going on there the exact same day.

By this time, the FBI had launched a full scale investigation into Silverdome activities.

As a result of the story, McSwigan was indicted by the Oakland County Prosecutor's office and was facing jail time and losing his job. Dennis MulQueen figured it also might be the end of his family life as he had known it – and he had a very nice wife and very nice kids too. He took no delight in any of this. It's not always what it's cracked up to be, being a big shot investigative journalist, Dennis MulQueen found out. Unless you are truly ruthless.

He was still working on that part.

Once the story hit, what was done was done and he headed to his favorite watering hole the next night to gauge the impact amongst the locals.

The next morning he jumped in the shower and froze a minute later like that classic deer in the headlights. He was washing himself and he felt a lump, on the right side of his groin, in the middle halfway between his waist line and the crease where his right leg met the trunk of his body.

What the hell is this, he wondered. He finished up in the bathroom and got dressed, but he pretty much thought about the lump on his groin on-and-off the rest of the weekend.

The following Monday he called Dr. Levy's office.

His office manager Liz answered the phone and told him he could come in later the same day.

When he got there Dr. Levy was out on an emergency call so he was examined by one of his associates.

"How long have you had this lump, Dennis?"

"I noticed when I was taking a shower on Friday. I don't know how long it's actually been there."

"Okay, today is Monday. Does it appear any different to you today?"

"It's hard to say, Doc. I don't think so."

"Well, you've got a hernia there, young man. Come back in a few weeks or a couple months after the holidays and if it's still bothering you, we can schedule a little surgical procedure for you with Dr. Sakwa. Otherwise, if it's not bothering you, you can leave it alone there as long as you want. It shouldn't be a problem; it's too small to strangulate. If it gets any bigger, and it is irritating you or causing a problem and you want to get it taken care of, just come on back in and we'll take care of it. By the way, I haven't seen your Dad in here for a little while, how's he doing?"

"Well, you know it's like Terry Fox says, Doc. Got to keep believing. He just got out of Sinai last week. He's losing a little weight, but thanks to you guys and Dr. Khilanani who you hooked him up with and Dr. Voravit, he's still here. He's tougher than Gordy Howe, my Dad."

"He sure is, isn't he?"

"Thanks, Doc. We'll be in touch."

~ ~ ~

He looked worse than thin. He was gray and his cheeks were hollowed out and he needed a shave.

When the 45th District Court doors swung open, Dennis looked up, and there he was. Just like that. His father, only a few days ago released from the hospital, slowly moving down the center aisle, with Oak Park Police Chief Glen Leonard tailing behind him.

He nodded at his son as he walked straight by him down the central aisle of Judge Marvin Frankel's courtroom to the front table on the right where he leaned over and said something to the prosecuting attorney seated there.

The government lawyer nodded, got up and led the two of them back behind the railing and behind the judges podium to a large wooden door, which he opened with a key and the three of them disappeared inside the judge's chambers as the door closed behind them.

407

About ten minutes later, the door swung open again.

George MulQueen Jr. paused in the aisle, looked at his son and winked.

"I think the prosecutor would like to speak with you now," he whispered. He turned and walked out of the courtroom with the police chief still on his heels.

The attorney in the gray sport coat sitting next to Dennis nodded his head forward and got up and walked to the front of the courtroom to speak to the prosecuting attorney who was once again seated at the same table.

Several minutes later Dennis' attorney returned to the back of the courtroom and sat down next to Dennis, holding a manila file folder in his left hand.

"All four felonies, gone," he said as he sliced the air with his right hand. "Two low misdemeanors to plead to. Adjudication withheld, one year clean and out. Is that okay with you?"

Being falsely arrested on top of the police brutality, he didn't think even petty misdemeanors were justified. But with his Dad involved, and given the MulQueen name in this town, with his father's service on the county board and his mother owning all the area newspapers, he figured he better take it.

"That'll be okay," he said.

"Okay. Here's the papers. I'll show you where to sign."

He couldn't sue them, but at least he wouldn't have a record.

~ ~ ~

It was time to pick up some more perspective. At the inspirational core.

When he got there, the winds of November were raging. And of course that meant the waves were crashing. If the blood wasn't pumping while taking in this scene, that would not be a good sign.

You just couldn't be around the big water over there and not think of Gordon Lightfoot and "The Wreck of the Edmund Fitzgerald."

It was November all right, but it wasn't Lake Superior – it was worse. This was Lake Erie. Even more feared, according to some mariners, than the dreaded Superior, where the *Fitzgerald* sank on November 10, 1975.

While Erie is almost 300 miles long, and more than 75 miles across in the middle, it is the shallowest of the freshwater oceans surrounding Michigan, particularly the western basin, where Colchester and the MulQueen cottage is located. The shallow depth can make the crests between waves closer together depending on the wind direction and location of the ship, which means a vessel can be struck rapidly in succession meaning less time for recovery and more stress on the hull, not to mention the shallow depths add to unpredictability, making for much quicker and unexpected storm formation.

Many times the big blows come out of nowhere and sometimes the weather services miss badly, predicting storm times and duration inaccurately or sometimes not at all. Moreover, the shallow depths, which average only 35 feet in the western basin, make passage all the more treacherous when westerlies move tremendous quantities of water down the lake 286 miles from the mouth of the Detroit River to Buffalo and nor'easters the opposite, each bringing hazardous reefs much closer to the surface in different parts of the lake.

This was the place the MulQueens sojourned to every year in November for Thanksgiving. This year, the 1980 Thanksgiving, would be no different.

In some respects.

Dennis arrived a couple days ahead of the big day, to those waves and winds and the one zillionth showing of the

Niagara and Lawrence paintings on the living room walls as he walked past them to the south picture window to ponder the white-capped scene stretching out in front of him as far as he could see.

It is amazing, he thought as he gazed out at the 10-foot swells crashing the beach, what that 27-year-old kid pulled off out here right in front of this place all those years ago. It dawned on Dennis he was currently the same age as Perry when he was out there on this very water risking his life for country back in 1813.

Oliver Hazard Perry. Now there's a name to never forget.

He didn't need to go to Gettysburg and stand on that field, or the fields of Verdun, or the beaches of Iwo Jima, for that matter, to know the feeling. The one you have to have, sooner or later, if you are going to make it. It was all right here in front of him. And more than that.

You have to have the courage, the determination, that was the lesson of this place, the message intended, from its inception, by his parents. Only then is it worth it – this life's journey – when it is worth fighting for.

He knew that much, as he was looking directly at Middle Sister Island, straight out just past the international line in US waters, when he suddenly caught himself involuntarily reaching down with his right hand to feel the lump on his groin again, through his tan khaki slacks.

Just then his mother strolled in from the kitchen and flipped the 19-inch RCA on in the corner and a familiar voice filled the room. It was Santa Claus – Mickey Rooney as Santa, in his third Christmas movie titled *Christmas in July*.

Didn't matter that it was November 25, 1980, not even close to July.

Seems that Santa and Mrs. Claus were trapped in a vicious storm by the evil Winterbolt and threatened with death. Mickey was singing a love song, "I see rainbows," to

Mrs. Claus, in the middle of it all as they appear about to perish. Oh jeez, he couldn't make it through this one. Time to go upstairs and read a couple more Doc Savage books.

"Where you going?"

"Oh, just upstairs to read a bit, Mom."

"You don't want to watch Mickey Rooney and Santa?"

"No, not really, Mom. I haven't been able to forget the first one."

"Oh, you mean *The Year Without a Santa Claus?*"

"How did you know?"

"Well, me too. That's how I knew you weren't coming home that year. When I saw that one it was two weeks before the Christmas of '74, remember? I just knew it was an omen. Thank God, we'll never have to watch that one again, right, Denny?"

"For sure, Mom. We're never going to see a script like that one again. I promise."

~ ~ ~

A couple days later, when the relatives showed up, he made a beeline for his uncle, his mother's adopted brother who was a physician in the Flint area.

"Doc, I want to ask you something personal. Could you come in here with me for a second, please?"

His uncle followed him into the small bathroom off of the kitchen.

He was an internist with a terrific reputation as a diagnostician and had helped out big time when Dennis had the collapsed lung.

Dennis dropped his drawers down halfway and pointed out the lump.

"That looks like a classic inguinal hernia, Denny. Go to your family guy and have him look at it and you can get it taken care of without too much trouble. Shouldn't take much to get it fixed, a very short and sweet procedure."

"Thanks, Doc. I actually already saw the family guy. He said the same thing. I just wanted to run it by you to make sure."

"How long have you had it?" he asked.

"Oh, I noticed it just about a week ago, I think it was."

"Okay, just curious. Call me next week up north if you have any other questions."

~ 30 ~

IMAGINE NO MORE

He didn't always need an alarm clock at 21471 Kipling Avenue. Like on the following Monday.

His father's dainty voice was far more effective than any electronic or wind-up device with bells or whistles or beeps or whirrs or all of the above could ever be.

No competition.

"Jesus Christ, get the hell out of the goddamned bed, will you for Christ's sake, it's almost the crack of noon, for God's sake. Don't you have a job to go to?"

"Sorry, Dad, feeling really bad lately, I can hardly get out of bed."

"You weren't too tired to get out of bed and go to the bars last week, were you? So how come you're too tired to go to work? I thought you went to the doctor last week. Didn't you just get a checkup? What did he say?"

"He told me I have a hernia."

"Jee-suzzz Chrr-iiiiiissstttt. Must be one hell of a hernia if you are too weak to get out of the damn bed and go to work."

He didn't have an assignment for that day. But if he went in, they might come up with something for him.

He got up and dressed and was out the door a short while later.

He didn't want to prove his father wrong, so if the hernia didn't prevent him from going to work that day, then it had no right to keep him from celebrating that night.

It didn't.

After all, it was Monday night football night.

This is how habits form.

After he got done filing a short little piece on an upcoming city council meeting, it was back to his favorite haunt, the Mill Street Inn. Like a repeat episode of "Twilight Zone," a different four Harvey Wallbangers later, he felt a lot less tired.

It was either the booze or the statuesque blonde he had met months ago, that night when he met Roger McCarville for the first time, who now ever-so-casually sidled up to his table. They made a little bit of small talk, but he wasn't in the mood. He quickly shooed her away. He had no interest in becoming a two-time adulterer.

He didn't need the distraction anyway because it was after nine, and his team graced the barroom's big TV screen: The Miami Dolphins.

They were playing on "Monday Night Football" against the New England Patriots in a great intra-conference rivalry game, and Dennis MulQueen was a Dolphins lunatic. He watched the game into the beginning of the third quarter when he decided that was enough Wallbangers and enough of the Mill Street. He said goodbye to Stan the owner and headed back down Woodward to catch the end of the game at home.

He grabbed one of his mother's Budweisers from the kitchen fridge for a night cap, a bag of Better Made chips from the kitchen cupboard and flipped the Zenith on in the living room. His father had just left for his midnight shift at Ford's.

He looked at his watch as he turned the dial to Chanel 7 to catch the end of the Dolphins' game. It was 11:36 p.m., December 8, 1980.

Howard Cosell and Frank Gifford and "Dandy Don" Meredith were in the middle of the second half of the broadcast when Cosell suddenly sputtered.

Then he said, "An unspeakable tragedy, confirmed to us by ABC News, in New York City. John Lennon, outside of his apartment building on the west side of New York City. Shot twice in the back, rushed to the Roosevelt Hospital, dead on arrival."

Oh my God. No Way.

Dennis MulQueen could not believe what he just heard.

It can't be true.

But it was.

John Lennon was dead.

Lennon and Yoko Ono were returning home from another session at the Record Plant recording studio, when they exited their limo onto the sidewalk in front of the Dakota apartment building at W. 72nd Street, when out of the shadows emerged a man named Mark David Chapman who shot and killed Lennon and who the police said then sat down and started reading a copy of *The Catcher in the Rye* by J.D. Salinger. The same Mark David Chapman who about 8 o'clock just a few hours ago came up to Lennon at almost the same spot and had him autograph an album for him.

Oh My God. It can't be true.

But it was.

John Lennon was dead.

The news filled Dennis with a profound sense of dread.

None of us are safe.

It's all over with the snap of two fingers. Just like that. No warning.

For any of us. For all of us.

Who's next in line, he wondered.

He got up out of his Dad's gold La-Z-Boy and walked about seven steps to the front closet where his Mother kept a series of medical encyclopedias.

Volume 8. He took it off the shelf and opened it. He fumbled through the pages.

His mother walked into the living room.

"What are you doing, Denny?"

"Oh just reading a little here, Mom."

"What are you reading?"

He didn't answer.

Okay. Here it is.

Under the diagnosis part, the passage read: "Hernias are generally pliable and can be gently pushed back through the tear in the muscle wall to prevent strangulation and lessen pain before surgery."

He felt the lump in his groin through his pants.

Oh Jeesus.

"What do you have one of my medical encyclopedias out for?"

"Mom, I think I have to go into the hospital for an operation."

"Oh, stop it. Are you worried about the hernia? Don't worry about that. Remember, the doctor told you that was nothing to worry about. And Dr. Bob told you that too."

"I know, Mom."

He couldn't get his favorite song out of his head. The same one he was singing in the shower about two weeks ago. The same one he heard when he turned the radio on in the car that night on the guy's birthday.

The one about how Instant Karma's gonna get us. About how we all better get ourselves together before we are dead.

He walked into the kitchen and picked up the phone. He dialed 411 and asked for the surgeon's phone number. He pushed the black bar in and let go of it until he heard another dial tone.

He dialed the number.

She followed him into the kitchen.

"Denny, who are you calling at this hour?"

"Do you believe it, Mom? John Lennon was just murdered. Nothing in the world is safe. We are all sitting ducks."

She said nothing. The recording chimed in.

"Hello, this is Dennis MulQueen calling. I am a patient of Dr. Levy's and his associate referred me to you. I have been diagnosed with an inguinal hernia and I would like to make an appointment to come in as soon as possible to get this taken care of, so please add me to the schedule at your earliest convenience. I can be reached at 313-546-6675. Thank You."

He hung up the phone.

"Denny, why did you call the doctor at this hour? Did it just start bothering you really bad right now?"

He didn't hear her. All he could think of was the guy who tried to give peace a chance. Say what you want, but he tried to make a difference.

Say what you want, but John Lennon had seen enough violence, he knew there was a better way. He was strong enough to get off the heroin, and he called Julian back, he made peace with Alf, he had mellowed – and now he was dead.

A guy that really tried to change things, to use his art to make a difference in the world. And damn, that music.

So many millions, all so sad now. Not bad for a guy with two really crappy parents and a strange aunt that raised him.

And hey, Alf tried to take you with him. You know that now. She made you choose and first you went with him and then she called for you and orchestrated it her way and you turned and walked back the other way.

Damn, you had a lot to overcome John Winston Ono Lennon.

And in the end, you were right about a lot of things.

Nothing more so than about being Irish.

If you have the luck of the Irish, you'd wish you were dead.

~ ~ ~

They called him back the next morning and he went in to see Dr. Sakwa on Wednesday, December 10th. The surgeon said the same thing as Dr. Levy's associate. The same thing as his uncle the medical doctor. To go home and enjoy the holidays and have a good time and come back in January if it was still bothersome and they would schedule surgery after the holidays. The third medical doctor to tell him the same thing.

"No, Doc, I want this taken care of right now."

"Bothering you that bad, is it? It's small, Dennis, and it's not strangulated. What's causing this sense of urgency?"

"I can't explain it, Doc. I'm not sure. I just want to get it taken care of now and put it behind me, Doc."

Dr. Sakwa pushed the little white button on the squawk box on his desk and said he needed a one-hour timeframe for right inguinal hernia repair.

The woman at the front desk replied that they had a cancellation and an opening for December 21.

"Is that the soonest, doctor?"

He said yes.

Dennis said to pencil him in.

"Now, I'm Jewish so it doesn't bother me, but with a name like MulQueen I can't imagine you are Jewish."

"I was almost Jewish there a while ago, Dr. Sakwa. She is an incredible woman. But we broke up."

418

Dr. Sakwa laughed.

"I just wanted to point out you realize this is right before the Christmas holiday. You know you're going to be a little sore, right? But that shouldn't be too much of a problem. JCPenney's has a nice catalogue."

"Yes, Doc, I know that. That will be fine."

Happy Day, Christmas. Why can't every day be Christmas, John Lennon? He still couldn't believe the guy that made peace his rallying cry left the world in such a violent way.

He was talking to himself now.

What's that about "Give Peace a Chance?"

What's that, Dad, about choosing when and how?

What about Lennon? What about you, Dad? What about me? What about all of us?

~ 31 ~

JOIN MY CLUB

His whole life he lived in fear of any kind of surgery. Even as a kid – even if it was relatively minor. Dr. Levy scheduled him for a tonsillectomy three times as a youngster to combat constant sore throats, but each time he came up with an excuse to not show up.

To be knocked out on a slab, hovered over by men and women in surgical scrubs wearing goggles with sharp knives in their hands, totally defenseless as they slice you open and cut out, rearrange, remove or splice body parts together – that was scary to him, and those who had gone through it he held in special awe, especially those who had survived the really big ones, like open heart surgery.

He preferred to live without this Red Badge of Courage for himself.

More so now that his moment of truth had arrived.

Sometimes it's just better not to read the fine print.

Would you rather be paralyzed for life or just dead? Or merely a brain-dead comatose creampuff attached to a breathing tube for perpetuity.

These, of course, were the worst-case-possible scenarios the hospital was forced by the legal department to reveal to him on the paperwork he had to sign in the pre-op conference room. Now he knew why he looked up to the surgical survivors.

Not that this was a heart transplant – this was simple basic hernia surgery, but still it was his first time under the knife and he had trouble quelling an irrational fear of being knocked out and never waking up again.

He decided he would rather be alive and paralyzed than in a coma or dead, so he chose a spinal (the worst complication here being paralysis) over general anesthesia, which according to the documents, patients once in a great while actually did not wake up from.

Even though the odds were minuscule, his fear of being knocked out and never waking up again made it an easy decision.

Until that moment of truth arrived.

Being his first-ever operation, and the unknowns that came with it, he was glad for the valium and whatever else they gave him because it was immediately apparent to him that being awake for all this was going to be more than he had bargained for.

Even though he couldn't feel a thing from the breastbone on down, he still felt helpless, tethered immobile and wide awake to a freezing operating-room table, not knowing exactly what was going on because he couldn't see anything. All he knew was he was getting carved up in some fashion.

Should have let them knock me out, he said with things barely underway in a sudden bout of rational thought.

Time for a little distraction.

"Let's play some ping-pong, guys. The heck with the hernia."

"What's that, Dennis?" Dr. Sakwa said.

"Oh nothing, guys, just jokin' around a little. I'm pretending I'm back at college instead of in this cold meat locker." He could make out a little strained laughter, too guttural and stilted to be genuine.

He certainly wished he was playing a little ping-pong about now. That's what this set up actually made him think of.

A blue-and-white spotted hospital gown folded in half, about a foot-and-a-half high, strung in the air across his belly, tied to two chrome-plated IV poles on either side of the operating table obscured his view of the action.

For reasons only known to God, this scenario somehow did remind him of a ping-pong net and the many hotly contested matches he had played against his dear friend Felipe at the old Newgy's Club in Miami where the top players in the country played. It was like the Flushing Meadows of ping-pong. He actually played three-time US national champion Bernie Biekut in that club in 1975, and even though Bernie was 55 at the time Dennis MulQueen was thrilled to get two points off of him. Dennis MulQueen fancied himself good at this game. He had won a couple tournaments in his day, including the Pittman Hall championship at Eastern Michigan U after he had retired from big-time college athletics, but maybe still felt he had a point to prove.

However, this guy wasn't a dorm player. In fact, Bernie Biekut was like the Gordie Howe of USA table tennis, if only in terms of longevity. He was a late bloomer (primarily because of WWII) and quite a character to talk to, but what a phenomenal player. He won the US Singles Championship three times (when he was 38, 44, and the last time when he was a record 47 years old). Only the year before Dennis played him, in 1974, when he was 54 years old, he was picked for the US National Team a record eighth time.

After Dennis and Felipe played themselves a few games, they would camp out in the stands and watch Bernie play some incredible matches usually against his favorite sparring partner, a guy named Dan Seemiller, one of the top US players at the time.

Dennis had to pay Bernie for the thrill of playing against him – a friendly $35 bet to see if he could get a measly three points against him. He was quite a character, and it was worth every penny just to get those two points against a world-class legend like that. It was no wonder they got along – Bernie was like his next-door neighbor Nate Garfinkel – he was a Polish Jew who also had to live through the Holocaust as a young man, one of the reasons his table tennis ride to the top took longer than anticipated. Maybe that's why he thought of Bernie on the slab – his momentary predicament paled in comparison to what Bernie and Nate endured.

Might have been some of the drugs they had him on, but Dennis MulQueen was still thinking about Bernie Biekut in that concentration camp as he wondered what was happening on the other side of his hospital ping-pong net.

Time for the net to go – at least part way.

He reached out with his right hand and lifted the blue-and-white cloth shield up about four inches in the middle so he could peruse the battle scene.

"What cha' doin' there, Dennis?"

"Just checkin' it out, guys, in case in the future I ever need to operate on myself."

When his eyes focused on what he didn't need to focus on in the first place, he dropped the makeshift drape like he had just touched a bare wire.

"What do you think, how we doing?" Dr. Sakwa said.

"I would definitely prefer bus driver school to med school after seeing that mess, guys."

He heard them laugh again; he tried to join in, but his diaphragm was so tight from the spinal it came out like he was trying to clear his throat.

"Just lie still there and relax, Dennis. It won't be too long."

He laid his head back down and was just starting to relax when a few minutes later he heard low-level chattering on the other side of the net. He couldn't tell who was saying what, then he recognized Dr. Sakwa's voice saying something about "his father."

Then the surgeon addressed him directly from behind the net.

"Tell me about your medical history, Dennis. Have you ever had any serious illnesses before?"

"No, Doc. Just a few concussions playing football and strep throats."

"Dennis, what is that your father has. His disease?"

"It's called chronic lymphocytic leukemia, or CLL, doctor."

"Okay. How long has he had it?"

"Oh, going on almost seven years now, I think, Doc."

"Okay. Just relax, we're almost done."

He heard some more mumbling on the other side of the cloth barrier.

Forget the ping-pong. He closed his eyes and thought of the waves crashing Westchester Beach and fell asleep.

~ ~ ~

When he awakened, she was hovering over his hospital gurney looking him in the eyes, hunched over like an invisible magnetic force was pulling on her from the top down.

She had dark circles under her eyes and when she leaned over the chrome railing to kiss him on the forehead he noticed her eyes were bloodshot.

"I hope I have all my parts, Mom. Did they forget some? Excuse me while I check.

425

"What's wrong, Mom, you look like you haven't slept in a week."

"Oh, I'm just tired, Denny. How are you feeling?"

"Oh, I'm doing great, Mom. No worries."

And no time for small talk. An orderly stepped up to his gurney and released the wheel brake with his foot and off they went in a cloud of dust out of recovery upstairs to a private room.

He made sure he requested a private room, a nod to his father, who had reminded him.

They had a few belly laughs already about the time Dr. Levy admitted his father to the same hospital a couple years ago and his roommate was a recovering colostomy patient who one day rolled over on his bag just as Dr. Levy walked in the room.

"George, light up one of those stogies of yours will you please," he said in low tones to his father. After that, it was a private room or else for George MulQueen.

Once they were situated in the room and the nurses took his vitals, his mother asked him a second time how he felt.

"Good, Ma."

"Okay then, I'm going to go now while you rest and I'll see you later after I get dinner ready for the kids."

"Okay, Mom, see you later."

She kissed him goodbye and left.

The timing was perfect as just as she was leaving another nurse arrived in his room with a nice shot of Demerol which she administered in his backside and he was in La La Land before his mother was in the car.

One of the surgical residents stopped in later in the afternoon and Dennis asked him how the surgery turned out and the doctor said fine. He removed the bandages and examined the surgical site and said everything looked good. He re-dressed the wound and left.

He took another cat nap and awakened a couple of hours later when dinner arrived. He nibbled a bit on a chicken cacciatore dish that tasted like cardboard soufflé, and picked up a copy of the *Detroit News* they delivered to the room, but he put it aside unread. At the moment, he wasn't much interested how the rest of the world was doing.

The phone rang about 6:30 p.m.

"How are you, Denny?"

"Oh I'm doing good, Mom."

"Just wanted to check on you. Have the doctors been in to see you? Have they told you anything?"

"No, Mom. Only thing they told me was I did real good with the surgery, they repaired my hernia and everything is good."

"Are you in a lot of pain, Denny?"

"No, Mom, they are giving me meds, not much pain."

"Okay, good. Then I'm going to stay home tonight. I wanted to come back down and see you again tonight, but Mickleberry isn't feeling good. He has a fever, so I'm going to stay home and watch him. Your Dad isn't home yet. So if you're doing good, we'll see you tomorrow, okay?"

"Okay, Mom. That will be great. You have a good night, thanks for being there for me today, Mom. Everything's just fine down here."

"Say your prayers, Son."

"Will do, Mom."

The following morning, he was in the bathroom when he heard Dr. Jacobs calling for him. He was an associate of Dr. Levy's and it was his day to make the rounds.

"Hi Doc. Just cleaning up a little. I'm coming out now. Do you have any news for me?"

"No, Dennis, take your time. Everything is fine. I'm just checking on you, I'll be back later."

He wanted to ask him some questions, but by the three seconds it took him to open the door, Dr. Jacobs was already gone.

His mother showed up a little while later in the early afternoon and she asked him if the doctors had been in.

He told her yes, they popped by in the morning.

"What did they say?"

"Not much, Mom. They said everything looks good."

The two of them chatted awhile and when the nurse came in to change his dressings and take his vitals, his mother got up to leave and said she would be back later in the evening with his father.

A couple of hours later, he was about five feet from his hospital bed after returning to his room from a mandatory post-surgical hallway stroll when he stopped in his tracks after hearing somebody enter the room behind him. He leaned on his IV pole for support as he turned around to see who it was.

"Hi, Dr. Sakwa."

"Hello, Dennis, how are you feeling? I guess you are okay, I see you are up and about."

"Yeah, Doc, but not by choice." He smiled as he looked at his surgeon.

He had no idea they would require him to walk the halls the very next day.

"So how did it go, Doc. As exciting as a hernia operation can be, eh, Doc?"

"Everything went well with your surgery, Dennis. But I want you to know while we were repairing your hernia, we observed something suspicious."

"What do you mean, Doc? What are you talking about?"

"Well, we found some suspicious tissue. We think it's actually uh, something, ah" – he hesitated, it sounded like he had a mouth full of marbles. "It looks like something, maybe something like what your father has, Dennis."

His mind instantly fought back, trying to play a trick on him.

"I remember my Dad had an appendectomy, and surgery on his hand, but I don't remember him having any hernias," he said.

"You didn't do hernia repair on my father, did you?"

"No, Dennis, I meant your father's malignancy. Something similar to that."

"What, Doc? Something similar to what?"

"Cancer, Dennis. Some type of cancer. "

The word came at him out of nowhere, and hit him like a blast from one of those War of 1812 cannons that had Perry cleaning guts and brains off of his uniform. He was still standing, but barely. It was like he was instantly transported to the middle of an Alfred Hitchcock movie with the eerie music in the background and the focus spiraling in and out as the monster jumps out of the closet in a dark room.

He was still standing, but his knees were literally trembling. They were about to buckle. He almost collapsed, his quad muscles quivered and shook and his vision was a blank black-and-white screen that faded in-and-out. He felt like he was blacking out, about to faint and fall out cold on the rock-hard hospital room tile floor. Luckily there was a chair about two feet away beside the bed that he was able to stutter step over to and turn around and fall back into. It was all he could do to not black out completely.

"Doc? You think I might have cancer? No way, Doc, no way, Doc."

"It could be, Dennis. Yes."

Now he knew fear wasn't about a grade point or a job. Now he knew fear wasn't being stared down by Dave

Purefiory or John Banaszak. Now he knew fear wasn't being tethered to a surgical slab.

Now he knew what real fear is. Fear that's a four-letter F-word born of a godawful six letter C-word that just exploded in his face like that Green Monster jumping out of the closet.

Fear that paralyzes your breathing. Fear that causes your knees to buckle and your vision to fade. Fear that is total powerlessness face-to-face with the sudden inescapable specter of death.

He had never experienced anything like it.

"So you think I might have cancer, Doc. Are you kidding me? What kind, Doc?"

"Dennis, we sent the samples to the pathology lab to be tested. Maybe something similar to what your father has, we can't be 100 percent sure. We have to wait and see how the tests come back."

"Now listen, Doc –"

His vision was back now, he was still sitting down, and he leaned forward in the chair and put one hand on the left arm as if to get up. With his elbow frozen in the air and still sitting, he looked Dr. Sakwa directly in the eyes.

"Doc, one thing very important, no matter what, listen. You cannot, do not, under any circumstances tell my parents about this, okay? Understand, no matter what the test results show, do not tell them one thing, okay? Not a word about this to anybody, okay? I will handle this myself. I don't want them knowing anything about this. They are going through enough hell right now, with my Dad's illness and a million other things."

Dr. Sakwa shifted his stance slightly from foot-to-foot and moved his head slightly down and then back up again an inch or two and inhaled robustly.

"I'll be back in tomorrow, and maybe we'll have the test results back and know the specifics then."

He turned and left.

A couple of hours later, the phone in his room rang again. It was his mother.

She asked how he was doing. He said fine. She asked if the doctors had been in and talked to him since she left about noon.

"No, Mom."

"Okay, well, Michael is still feeling bad and your father got called in for a double, so he can't come down tonight, so we will be down to see you tomorrow, okay, Denny?"

"That'll be fine, Mom. No problem."

The following morning the surgical resident who assisted on his surgery came back in again to examine him. Dennis asked him if he had any test results back yet.

He said no.

Dennis's mind was back to playing tricks on him again. He thought okay, good. No news is good news.

Maybe Dr. Sakwa was wrong. He focused on the "can't be sure" part of the conversation.

Everything must be okay. After all, it's been three days now since the surgery. They would have some test results by now, confirmation of some kind by now, if anything was certain.

He had no visitors all day. After dinner he turned the TV volume down and drifted off to sleep.

When he sat up in bed at 8:10 p.m. in room 2310 and opened his eyes he was met by the terribly worn visage of his father slouching silently in a chair at the foot of his hospital bed.

George MulQueen was staring blankly at the floor. He was wearing a green-and-yellow plaid shirt and green corduroy pants. Pat MulQueen was sitting in the chair next to him wearing a beautiful blue-and-white checkered pant suit. Dennis MulQueen didn't notice anything unusual about his mother other than she also looked tired, which she frequently did anyway these days if not for worrying about his Dad, then from her worry suppressors – the Carlton's and the double-olive martinis and too much late-night TV.

But his father, he had never seen him like this. His skin was a combination of sallow, gray, and chartreuse. He looked like he hadn't slept in a month and his cheeks were sunken in; there were dark circles under his eyes, it almost looked like he had black eyes. He was unshaven, with the gray stubble and the funeral-parlor pallor making him look like a very old man. He looked like a very old heart patient. But while he had no heart issues, Dr. Levy and Dr. Prem Khilanani had kept him alive for going on seven years now with high-grade leukemia that was supposed to kill him in a year-and-a-half, and this is the result, Dennis thought.

It was the first time he had seen his Dad since the week before his hernia surgery.

"Hi, Dad, how are you doing? How many doubles have you been working?"

"How are you doing, Son?"

"I'm fine. It feels a little sore there, but not too bad. I'm walking up and down the halls already, it's not too bad. Yesterday too, but even one day makes a big difference."

His father inhaled slowly and exhaled suddenly, like a balloon he was blowing up just got away from him.

"Anybody been in to see you?"

"No, not yet. Everybody's working anyway, Dad. I don't need visitors rushing down here for something like this. Not necessary."

"I mean the doctors. Have they been in to talk to you?"

"Yeah, Dad, they've been in. They took a look and said everything looks good and they left."

Before he could say anything else, his father grabbed the end of the bed and pulled himself upright, turned to the right and walked with a slow and unsteady gait out the door.

Dennis MulQueen leaned forward in his bed and watched his father leave as his mother abruptly stood up and silently followed him out the door.

Not more than five minutes later, they both returned.

His father looked older than five minutes ago, if that were possible. The effects of his seven-year struggle were even more vivid than five minutes ago, written all over his face in deep hanging flesh lines of indelible wear and tear. It didn't occur to Dennis that maybe it was much more than that now.

"You guys look tired. Now I'm doing great down here. You need to go home and rest. I can tell you guys have put in a lot of hours this week."

They both gazed at him with equally strained looks of sullen silence.

His father inhaled a deep breath again, his breathing seemed to flutter and sputter now in spurts, the air going in and out in fits and starts, his throat quivering a bit like you might see in the middle of a big yawn. Then he lowered his eyes to the floor again as he appeared to be looking off into deep space, then he raised his head and looked directly at his son again.

Their eyes locked on one another.

Now he noticed his father's eyes were red, cooked-lobster red. Redder than his mother's by several shades.

Then he said it.

"Well , Son, you'll just have to join my club."

"What, Dad? What are you talking about, Dad?"

There was a pause of about five seconds.

"No, Dad, sorry. I'm with Woody Allen on that one, if there's a club that'll take me as a member, I don't want to be in it. Thanks, but I'm not joining your club. I don't want to be in any club you're in."

His father said it again.

"You'll have to join my club, Son. You have no choice. You'll just have to be stronger than the drugs."

His father's words stuck in the middle of his son's chest like a sharp stick.

Join my club.

Dr. Sakwa said suspicious, we'll have to wait and see for sure. "Maybe" something like your father. Then he hadn't heard anything back. Three days, still no official test results. Then it dawned on him. All the docs, in and out, the same way. Nobody wanting to be the ultimate bearer of the worst kind of news.

He went back to Lennon that night. And that lump in the shower.

That night he was murdered. He felt it then. He just couldn't face it then. Now he had to face it. Now, he had no choice but to face the music.

Instant Karma. Pretty soon you're going to be dead.

The cat was out of the bag. Officially.

There was no mistaking those words now.

Join my club.

He had to be the one. He had to be the messenger. They went behind my back, Dennis MulQueen realized.

He tried to respond, but all that would come out was a subtle choking sound, like he was suffocating on his own tongue. That sharp stick was now lodged in his throat.

He gathered himself, momentarily. Now the words came out in whispered tones, defiant, garbled tones. The sounds of denial.

"No way am I ever joining your club, Dad. You know I never liked clubs anyway, Dad, never joined one and I'm not joining one now."

Their eyes locked on one another again. Looking at his father he saw that his words were empty vessels. He was blowing in the wind now, thank you Bob Dylan. Despite his protests, he knew he was in the club now, whether he wanted to join or not.

He looked deep into those red eyes at the end of the bed, and they shot red-hot geysers of regret at him deeper than the Red Sea.

The room was silent for what seemed like an eternity, but in reality was only one eternal minute. Then his father repeated himself again.

"Son, you'll have to join my club and you'll just have to be stronger than the drugs. And the Big C."

He bowed his balding head, moving it from side to side languorously as if in disbelief of what he was saying. Back and forth, slowly his head moved, like a giant slightly rusty pendulum in an antique grandfather clock stuck in the foyer of a haunted house.

He tried to continue.

Back and forth.

Still no words.

Then, he started to speak again

"You don't have –"

He froze in mid-sentence with a cough, then a slight gasp.

Back and forth again.

Then, "a choice."

He couldn't get another word out.

He could no longer stanch the veil of water that now cascaded down his face like the Falls of Niagara.

A mortally wounded father crying for his grievously wounded son.

The tears continued to flow down his father's mountain of pain into a pool on the floor. Never had his son seen sadness like this. He silently watched his father valiantly struggle as hard as he could, but it was hopeless. This was involuntary. He was heaving involuntarily now.

No more verbal communication.

Words – unnecessary.

Words – unspoken.

The tears spoke louder than any words ever could.

Nothing could hide the truth of those tears.

No more waiting for lab results. He already knew all he needed to know.

His father struggled to his feet, he took about three unsteady steps toward the door and stopped. He looked at the chart sitting in the wire basket against the wall, the room number listed on the chart, No. 2310.

"Should have known. I have been in this room before."

He moved slowly forward and out the door. His mother stood up and called out, "Be right there, George."

He didn't answer. Dennis could hear the sobs resume their pitiful sound as he passed from sight.

He looked at his mother, temporarily oblivious to the situation she was in.

They looked at each other, as if they both thought the same thing. Yeah, you've been in this room before, too, right Mom?

She walked up to the side of his bed, and grabbed his right forearm. He raised his hand, as if to recoil from her grasp, but stopped with only a short jerk disguised quickly by his left hand that he placed on top of her hand. He squeezed that hand as he inhaled deeply.

"It's so unfair, it's so unfair," she said as he felt her tears hitting the bed sheets with the same pitter-patter sounds of that day on the landing. Only now they fell like mortars from the sky.

He wished she would go. He wished his father would go.

He wanted to go.

He didn't want anybody.

He wanted to run away and hide, to never come back, to hide the reality of what in one split second changed the trajectory of his life – and that of his parents – forever.

He recalled his father's long ago warning. Now the moment was all the way here. Now all of the chickens have come home to roost.

"I busted my ass to get my act back together," he said to his mother. "I got outta that 'incestuous cess pool' as you called it, I came home again, and hell I even got a good job going now, Mom. And now this."

What she must be thinking never occurred to him. Her two favorite guys in the world – no offense brothers and sisters and family and friends – her two favorite men in the world in the same club now.

Oh, what his poor mother was now living.

Oh, what his poor father was now living.

Lives that through ten trillion years of eternity they would never deserve to have to live.

He would learn later why his father didn't come to see him for three days.

"It's okay, Mom, you better catch up with Dad. Everything's okay. Everything's going to be all right."

She kissed him and hugged him the longest time.

"I'll be home soon, Mom. We'll figure it all out. We'll come up with a plan. Don't worry. I'll talk to Dr. Levy. Everything will be okay. Please don't worry."

"No, I'm not worried, Denny. I already called the monastery for you, Son. Everything will be all right. You'll have to do what your father said and beat this thing."

"Thanks, Mom. How long have you known about all this?"

"Since about 10 in the morning the day of your surgery. Dr. Sakwa came directly from the operating room and told me they found cancer in you. He was very upset. A type of Non-Hodgkins lymphoma, he said, something similar to what your father has."

"Oh my God, you were all alone, and you found out right after the surgery. Why didn't you tell me, Mom?"

"I, well, I had to tell your father first."

"When did you tell, Dad? "

"I drove straight from the hospital to home and told him when he got back from work."

"How come you didn't tell me then, Mom?"

"We didn't want to say anything, Denny, because we were praying the surgeon was wrong, and we wanted confirmation from the pathologist. We didn't get the report until this morning."

"Okay. Thanks, Mom. You better go get Dad and go home and rest. Tell Dad to rest. Everything's okay. Now be careful going home now, okay?"

"Yes, Son, it is after visiting hours now. I guess we better get going."

She slowly stood and grabbed her purse and prepared to leave.

"Love you, Mom. Tell Dad I love him too. Don't worry, Mom, everything will be okay. I promise."

"Okay, Son. Love you too. God be with you."

Then the room was quiet.

Dead quiet.

The sounds of silence.

Dennis MulQueen and the four walls – and the suffocating sounds of silence slowly closing in.

The silence of eternity now speaking to his soul through the empty four walls.

"With very few exceptions, we all choose when and how we are going to die," he'd said in the car that day when they narrowly avoided death on the highway.

Partying, womanizing, boozing, smoking, terrible sleep, terrible nutrition.

Terribly out of control stress.

And the chickens come home to roost.

They didn't know exactly what kind it was, just some kind of Non-Hodgkins lymphoma, a cousin of the lymphocytic leukemia his father had. But the specifics didn't matter.

Nothing mattered now.

Just him and the green dragon now, alone in the room, in the dark of the night.

With the four walls closing in.

The monster stalked him everywhere that night in Room 2310, everywhere it popped up in his mind's eye, over and over, whether in the bed or in the bathroom, whether he rolled over or stood up, walked around or sat silently.

No matter what when or where, everywhere the monster stalked him now disguised as a black-and-gold-hued box, resting on top of a brass and stainless steel gurney, with black and gold wheels, there it was resting on top, a black-and-gold coffin.

Everywhere he turned in Room 2310 that night, every waking moment there it was, a black box, a black-and-gold coffin, all night long stalking him like a starving dog.

Everywhere he looked, there it was, the black box, at the front of a flower-filled room, at a funeral parlor, the funeral parlor of his destiny.

There, inside this black-and-gold box, there he laid, cold and dead, pasty makeup and closed eyes, a vapid and expressionless face.

439

There, in his mind's eye, the scene played itself out over and over, like a slow-motion movie he was forced to watch, over and over, the same flower-filled room, the same black-and-gold coffin, at the front of the room, as a steady stream of people, one after another, passed by in succession.

First came by his mother and father, then Chip and his other brother and sisters filed past, followed by Grandma MulQueen and his Aunt Peggy and Uncle Jack, then Mary Lou and Jim and Barbara and Bob, Aunts Florence and Virginia then TJ and Hondeau and Aurelius and Bokker Lee and all his friends and acquaintances.

Then came the tears.

Tears of self-pity and abandonment.

Tears of pain and loneliness.

Tears of bitter disappointment for all that could have been.

Tears of wanting, and wishing, that for God's sake it could somehow be different, that if God could be willing, if God could be forgiving, if there is a God, please please if I could just have one more chance to do it all over again, the right way, some way, to make it all better again, a chance to live the right way, to make better choices. Maybe the world could be a different place.

The tears fell continuously, the tears of his mother in the line, the tears of his father in the line, the tears of all the others in the line, the tears of a lifetime that were drowning him in the dark of the night.

The tears that fell steadily, on and off throughout the night, until suddenly dawn began approaching and he stood up and got out of his hospital bed and walked the few short steps to the window facing east.

Totally exhausted, he slowly raised the wood-framed window and gingerly climbed onto the window frame and sat sill, his feet dangling many stories high. He peered silently outward at the vast darkness, his hands holding onto the back of the sill. *Déjà vu*, Valdosta, Georgia. On the top floor of that parking garage, on the way back from Florida, contemplating the end. All the years of struggle. For what?

Should I stay or should I go?

He gazed steadfastly into the dark nothingness outside the window for several minutes contemplating the end once more and suddenly he noticed the stars in the distance slowly fading as Old Man Night slowly shook the twinkling lights out one by one, furtively unfurling a vast rose-gray carpet of forgotten beauty across dawn's far eastern edge.

He continued to gaze in wonder until quickly it was all the way there – God's golden orange bubble of life slowly appearing fully risen now above the horizon, hoisting gold and orange and red streaks of resplendent glory hearkening the beauty of a new day amid the sounds of silence in room 2310.

"No way," he said out loud.

"Let's prove it," he said out loud again, as he lifted his legs and turned around and hopped off the ledge back into the room and walked to a wastebasket beside the head of the bed. He reached inside and retrieved a bottle cap from a bottle of Coca-Cola the nurse had brought him earlier in the day. He returned to the window and looked through the pink-and-granite morning lights to a brown brick building across the courtyard. It looked like maybe it was a large power plant for the hospital, a tall smoke-stacked structure of height equal to his fourth-story room.

Approximately 30 to 40 yards separated him from this building.

Dear God, he prayed, if you are out there, you know I despise the hypocritical Catholic Church hierarchy that can't even protect the children, you know I haven't gone to church or believed in you or any kind of your religion forever, but please, dear God, if you exist at all and if you can hear me now please give me a sign. Dear Jesus, please make this bottle cap make it as a sign of hope I can make it. Please, please, dear God, hear my prayer. I don't want to die now, please, for my mother, my father, my brothers and sisters, Hondeau and TJ and Aurelius and Bokker and all the others. And for me."

He raised his right arm almost perpendicular and whipped it sideways like Dan Quisenberry on the mound and snapped his wrist and the tiny metal sphere spun and careened through the air towards the building off in the distance.

"Please dear Sacred Heart of Jesus, let the bottle cap make it. Tell me I can make it. Please give me hope."

The corrugated tin cap sliced the air in a slightly upward arc to the left towards the building only to turn downward about halfway there. "No, no," he said as it veered straight for the brick wall. Then suddenly, when it was almost at the wall, it suddenly angled back to the right and up about three feet now, like a rising Nolan Ryan fastball. Now it soared like a miniature motorized frisbee on its own course, and just like that, like a skipping magical stone jumping off an invisible ripple of air, it jumped to the very top edge of the building and up, up, and over it went, he couldn't see it in the gray shadows any more but he heard it skip once, twice and then a rapid confluence of ringing tinny noises echoed in his ears as it bounced helter-skelter across the roof and the noise came to a sudden, silent, eternal stop.

A surge of adrenaline lifted him off the ground and he felt weightless. He was feverishly levitating now on a moment of hope as ridiculous as it was phenomenal. It was a phenomenal trajectory, virtually physically impossible, to toss or spin or flick or whatever it was he did to that tiny piece of tin to have it traverse such an impossible distance, to do the totally impossible.

Ah, do you believe in miracles? Yes I do, Al Michaels, he told himself as he silently looked out the window at the scene of the feat he had just accomplished that was more improbable than those guys beating the Soviets that day.

He closed the window and laid back down on the bed. He inhaled slow deep breaths and sighed over and over again as he exhaled, as if by those concentrated deep breaths and that bottle cap he could now exorcise from his very being every bad thought, every doubt, every fear of death.

He felt the certain peace of resignation to his plight settle over him like a warm blanket.

He closed his eyes and tried to return to the funeral parlor and the black-and-gold box.

He couldn't.

He wouldn't and he couldn't ever go back there again.

He would never go back there again.

He had seen death, he had confronted death. His own death. Now it was time to look in the eye of the dragon.

And spit.

And start living again.

He would never go back to that black-and-gold box again.

Every day from now on, life to be lived, life worth fighting for. Life to be savored. No worry, Mom and Dad. We're going to make it. All of us.

Yes, no jump here. Now or ever.

But first, a little promise for the Green Monster.

Bring it on baby. I want you to know something. You're gonna wanna get the hell out of here soon, real soon. I promise you I will make you wish you never came around, I promise I will make you so miserable I promise you will want out and you will get out.

Join My Club

Please read JOIN MY CLUB: The Ultimate Survivor Story,
Volume II: Do You Believe in Miracles? to find
out what happens to this father and son duo as they fight to
the wire against formidable odds to stay alive.

Both volumes are available at:
www.AbsolutelyAmazingeBooks.com or your
favorite online bookseller.

Thank you for reading.
Please review this book. Reviews
help others find Absolutely Amazing eBooks and
inspire us to keep providing these marvelous tales.
If you would like to be put on our email list
to receive updates on new releases,
contests, and promotions, please go to
AbsolutelyAmazingEbooks.com and sign up.

About the Author

D Basil MulQueen is an old-time investigative journalist and musician who recently moved to Key West, Florida, to follow in Hemingway's footsteps. the Detroit Medical Center's Harper Hospital – His recently released *Join My Club* duology will be followed by his fourth book due for release in early 2022. He has one cat and several pet iguanas who love to hang out with him at his Grinnell Street writer's retreat. During the summer he can be found chilling out at his Lake Erie beach house in Canada or his 1824 historical home in downtown Farmington, Michigan. His three favorite things in life, besides chasing love and inspiration at Sloppy Joe's when he's not cruising around town on his Townie, are writing and reading, reading and writing, and writing and reading – in addition to still pounding out Rock and Roll Never Forgets on his timeless white Pearl drum kit.

Acknowledgements

Special thanks to those who helped make *Join My Club* possible, starting with Kimberly Marie Comer MulQueen, without whose undying support it never would have happened, and all the friends and other dear family members whose encouragement and support helped see it through to print, including Chuckinson, Burzey, Sondein, T.J., Hondeau, Mouse and The Professor. Special thanks also to Elizabeth Atkins, whose early-on encouragement and editing suggestions helped push *Join My Club* forward. Special thanks also to Janzy and Peep for their friendship and support, and Peep's main man RG Seger, who encouraged and inspired in the very beginning and never ceases to inspire, and to Hope Black Bull Ravenallure, a/k/a Olivia Munn, who was inspired by the author's writing and gave encouragement to this book, and to Dutch Leonard, who also urged publication of the book, and last but way beyond least, to the memory of Roger McCarville, who exacted a final promise the book would be published.